ACUTE MEDICAL EMERGENCIES

USEFUL WEBSITE ADDRESSES

Advanced Life Support Group	http://www.alsg.org
Best Evidence in Emergency Medicine	http://www.bestbets.org
Evidence based on-call	http://cebm.jr2.ox.ac.uk/eboc/eboc.html
Royal College of Physicians	http://www.rcplondon.ac.uk/

ACUTE MEDICAL EMERGENCIES

The Practical Approach

Advanced Life Support Group

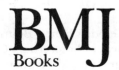

© BMJ Books 2001
BMJ Books is an imprint of the BMJ Publishing Group

First published in 2001
by BMJ Books, BMA House, Tavistock Square,
London WC1H 9JR

www.bmjbooks.com

British Library Cataloguing in Publication Data

A catalogue record for this book is available from the British Library

ISBN 0-7279-1464-2

Cover design by Goodall James, Bournemouth, Dorset
Typeset by Phoenix Photosetting, Chatham, Kent
Printed and bound by J W Arrowsmith Ltd, Bristol

CONTENTS

WORKING GROUP

P Driscoll	Emergency Medicine, Manchester
R Kishen	Anaesthesia/ICU, London
K Mackway-Jones	Emergency Medicine, Manchester
G McMahon	Emergency Medicine, Manchester
F Morris	Emergency Medicine, Sheffield
TD Wardle	General Medicine, Chester
B Waters	Anaesthesia/ICU, North Wales
J Whitaker	Care of the Elderly, Harrogate
S Wieteska	ALSG, Manchester

CONTRIBUTORS

M Bhushan	Dermatology, Manchester
P Davies	Emergency Medicine, Bristol
P Driscoll	Emergency Medicine, Manchester
CEM Griffiths	Dermatology, Manchester
C Gwinnutt	Anaesthesia, Manchester
J Hanson	Emergency Medicine, Preston
R Kishen	Anaesthesia/ICU, London
K Mackway-Jones	Emergency Medicine, Manchester
A McGowan	Emergency Medicine, Leeds
G McMahon	Emergency Medicine, Manchester
F Morris	Emergency Medicine, Sheffield
C Moulton	Emergency Medicine, Bolton
K Reynard	Emergency Medicine, Manchester
P Sammy	General Practice, Manchester
P Terry	Emergency Medicine, Manchester
D Wallis	Emergency Medicine, London
TD Wardle	General Medicine, Chester
B Waters	Anaesthesia/ICU, North Wales
J Whitaker	Care of the Elderly, Harrogate

PREFACE

This book has been written to enable health care workers to understand the principles of managing an acute medical emergency safely and effectively. To achieve this aim it provides a structured approach to medical emergencies, describing relevant pathophysiology that will also help to explain physical signs and the rationale behind treatment. The first edition of this manual (written by Terry Wardle) has undergone significant modification directed by the working group and also, in particular, candidates from the first MedicALS courses. The requirements of these contributing doctors has meant that the contents and associated information may initially appear skewed – but this is evidence based.

Most text books are out of date by the time they are published – this manual is different in that it is both pragmatic and dynamic. Medicine is a rapidly evolving discipline and in order to ensure that this manual remains dynamic and up to date, reference web sites are available to ensure that the reader has constant access to relevant information. This will facilitate continual professional development that is the responsibility of the individual.

The book provides a structured approach that is applicable to all aspects of acute medicine, ensures the early recognition of signs of critical illness and will empower the individual to take immediate and appropriate action.

The text alone cannot provide all the necessary knowledge and skills to manage an acute medical emergency, therefore readers are encouraged to attend the MedicALS course to further their theoretical and practical knowledge.

This book will continue to change to include new evidence based practices and protocols to ensure a solid and safe foundation of knowledge and skills in this era of clinical governance.

Continued professional development is mandatory for all medical practitioners. This manual and the associated course will ensure both new knowledge acquisition and revision – and stimulate further learning.

ACKNOWLEDGMENTS

We would like to thank members of faculty and candidates who have completed the MedicALS course for their constructive comments that have shaped both the text and the course.

We would also like to thank Helen Carruthers, MMAA for her work on many of the figures within the text.

Finally, our thanks to the members of staff both at the BMJ and within ALSG for their on-going support and invaluable assistance in the production of this text.

INTRODUCTION

PART

I

INTRODUCTION

CHAPTER

1

Introduction

INTRODUCTION

After reading this chapter you will understand:

- the current problems in the assessment of acute medical emergencies
- the need for a structured approach to the medical patient.

THE PROBLEM

A medical emergency can arise in any patient, under a variety of circumstances, for example:

- a previously fit individual
- acute on chronic illness
- post surgical
- precipitating or modifying the response to trauma.

The acute problem can be directly or indirectly related to the presenting condition, an associated complication, any treatment instituted, and the result of inappropriate action.

> **Key point**
> Inappropriate action costs lives

Furthermore, with the increase in the elderly population there is a corresponding increase in the number and complexity of medical problems. The management of such patients is compromised by the drive to cut costs, but maintain cost effective care; ensure efficient bed usage; reduce junior doctors' hours; and increase medical specialisation.

There is an annual increase of emergency admissions in excess of 5% and they account for over 40% of all acute National Health Service beds. In the UK the mean hospital bed complement is 641, but only 186 are allocated for medical patients with an average 95% of these housing medical emergencies.

The common acute conditions can be broadly classified according to the body system affected (Table 1.1).

Table 1.1. Classification of medical emergencies

Type	%
Cardiac	29
Respiratory	26
Neurological	21
Gastrointestinal	13

This information may be broken down further to reveal the common reasons for admission:

- myocardial infarction
- stroke
- cardiac failure
- acute exacerbation of asthma
- acute exacerbation of chronic obstructive pulmonary disease
- deliberate self harm.

Despite the fact that these are common conditions, frequent management errors and inappropriate action result in preventable morbidity and mortality.

A recent risk management study examined the care of medical emergencies. One or more avoidable serious adverse clinical incidents were reported. Common mistakes are listed in the box.

Common mistakes

- Failure to recognise and treat serious infection
- Error in investigating – acute headache
                              acute breathlessness
                              epilepsy
- Misinterpretation of investigations
- Inadequate assessment of abdominal symptoms

This was only a small study but of the 29 patients who died, 20 would have had a good chance of long term survival with appropriate management. In addition, of the 11 patients who survived, three were left with serious neurological defects, three underwent avoidable intestinal resection and four patients suffered unnecessary prolonged hospital admission.

Diagnostic errors were made in 80% of patients because of inadequate interpretation of the clinical picture and initial investigations. These errors are given in the box.

Errors in patient assessment

- Available clinical evidence incorrectly interpreted
- Failure to identify and focus on very sick patients
- Investigations misread or ignored
- Radiological evidence missed
- Standard procedures not followed
- Inadequate assessment or treatment
- Discharge from hospital without proper assessment

The overall problems were identified as follows:

- medical emergencies were not assessed by sufficiently experienced staff
- a second opinion was not obtained
- assessment was inadequately performed before discharge
- X-rays were not discussed with radiologists
- protocols were not used for standard conditions.

Furthermore, the assessment of medical patients for intensive care was either incomplete, inappropriate or too late to prevent increased morbidity and mortality.

Therefore, there are problems in the **fundamental** areas of medical patient care, i.e. clinical examination, requesting appropriate investigations and their correct interpretation, and communication. However, probably most important of all, knowing when and who to ask for help. One answer to this important problem is to provide a structured approach to patient assessment that will facilitate problem identification and prioritise management.

All that is required to manage medical emergencies is focused knowledge and basic skills. These will ensure prompt accurate assessment and improve patient outcome. Avoidable deaths are due to inappropriate management, indecision or delays in treatment. Another important issue is the time patients wait for appropriate medical care. The average time for initial review after admission is 30 minutes with a further 130 minutes passing before definitive management occurs.

In the United Kingdom, numerous studies have shown that specialist care is better than that provided by a generalist; for example, prompt review by a respiratory physician has been shown to reduce both morbidity and mortality from asthma. The mortality from gastrointestinal haemorrhage falls from 40% to approximately 5% if the management is provided by a specialist in gastroenterology. Further supportive evidence has been provided by studies in the United States where mortality from myocardial infarction or unstable angina was greater in patients managed by generalists.

However, there are insufficient numbers of "specialists" to manage all of these conditions and some will require review by a general physician.

Thus, physicians need to know how to manage medical emergencies. This course will teach a structured approach for assessment that will enable you to deliver safe, effective, and appropriate care.

Traditional medical teaching dictates that a history should always be taken from the patient before the clinical examination. This will subsequently allow a diagnosis or differential diagnosis to be postulated and dictate the investigations required. Unfortunately this approach is not always possible; for example, trying to obtain a history from a patient who presents with breathlessness may not only exacerbate the condition but also delay crucial therapy.

This course has been developed by observing how experienced physicians manage medical emergencies. The results have shown quite an interesting cultural shift. Most of us, as we approach the patient, quickly scan for any obvious physical signs, for example breathlessness, and then focus our attention on the symptoms until the diagnosis is identified. Only when the patient's symptoms have been improved can a history be taken and the remainder of the examination performed. This process has been refined and formalised to produce a structured approach to patient assessment. This will ensure that the most immediately life threatening problems are identified early and treated promptly. All other problems will be identified subsequently as part of the overall classical approach to the medical patient, i.e. taking a history and examining the patient.

However, if the patient deteriorates at any stage a reassessment should start at the beginning. Thus, this structured approach considers the conditions that are most likely to kill the patient. If these are excluded the physician will then have time to approach the patient in a traditional fashion.

The key principles of MedicALS are shown in the box.

Key principles of MedicALS

- Do no further harm
- Focused knowledge and basic skills are essential
- A structured approach will identify problems and prioritise management
- Prompt accurate assessment improves patient outcome

SUMMARY

The number and complexity of acute medical emergencies are increasing. However, the majority of mistakes result from a failure to assess acutely ill patients, interpret relevant investigations, and provide appropriate management. This manual and the associated course will equip you with both knowledge and skills to overcome these difficulties and provide safe, effective, and appropriate care.

CHAPTER

2

Recognition of the medical emergency

OBJECTIVES

After reading this chapter you will be able to:

- understand the clinical features of potential respiratory, cardiac, and neurological failure
- describe these clinical features and use them to form the basis of the primary assessment.

Irrespective of underlying pathology, the acute medical patient will die from failure of either the respiratory, circulatory or central neurological systems, or a combination of these. It is therefore of paramount importance that the physician can recognise **potential failure** of these three systems as early recognition and management will reduce morbidity and mortality. The ultimate failure, a cardiorespiratory arrest, is too large a topic to be added to this course.

This chapter will provide an overview of the clinical assessment of patients with potential respiratory, circulatory, and neurological failure. The chapters in Part II will then use this format to develop an in-depth assessment that will eventually produce a structured approach to the patient with a medical emergency.

RECOGNITION OF POTENTIAL RESPIRATORY FAILURE

This can be quickly assessed by examining the rate, effort, symmetry, and effectiveness of breathing.

Respiratory rate

The normal adult respiratory rate is 14–20 breaths per minute. Tachypnoea (greater than 30 breaths per minute at rest) indicates that increased ventilation is needed because of hypoxia associated with either disease affecting the airway, lung or circulation, or metabolic acidosis. Similarly, a respiratory rate ≤10 breaths per minute is an indication for ventilatory support.

Effort of respiration

If the patient can count to 10 in one breath there is usually no significant underlying respiratory problem. Other features which suggest increased respiratory effort are

7

intercostal and subcostal recession, accessory muscle use, and a hoarse inspiratory noise while breathing (stridor; this is a sign of laryngeal/tracheal obstruction). In severe obstruction, stridor may also occur on expiration but the inspiratory component is usually more pronounced. In contrast, lower airway narrowing results in either wheezing and/or a prolonged expiratory phase.

Symmetry of breathing

Asymmetrical chest expansion suggests an abnormality on the side with reduced movement.

Effectiveness of breathing

Chest expansion will indicate the volume of air being inspired and expired. Similar findings will be obtained from auscultation.

> **Key point**
> A silent chest is an extremely worrying sign

Pulse oximetry can be used to measure the arterial oxygen saturation (SaO_2). These instruments are inaccurate when the SaO_2 is below 70%, there is poor peripheral perfusion, and in the presence of carboxyhaemoglobin.

Effects of respiratory inadequacy on other organs

Heart rate
Hypoxaemia produces a tachycardia; however, anxiety and fever will also contribute to this physical sign, making it non-specific. Severe or prolonged hypoxia eventually will lead to a bradycardia – a preterminal sign.

Skin colour
Hypoxaemia, via catecholamine release, produces vasoconstriction and hence skin pallor. Cyanosis is a sign of severe hypoxaemia. Central cyanosis in acute respiratory disease is indicative of imminent respiratory arrest. In the anaemic patient, cyanosis may be difficult to detect despite profound hypoxaemia.

Mental status
The hypoxaemic patient will appear agitated and eventually will become drowsy. Similar features will also occur with hypercapnoea and the patient will also exhibit vasodilatation and a flapping tremor (asterixis). If the hypoxaemia is not treated cerebral function will be affected.

RECOGNITION OF POTENTIAL CIRCULATORY FAILURE

Heart rate

This increases in the shocked patient due to catecholamine release, e.g. secondary to a decreased circulatory volume. There are many reasons why a normal adult may experience a tachycardia (pulse rate >100). Other signs should be sought to confirm the clinical suspicion of circulatory failure.

Effectiveness of circulation

Pulse
Although blood pressure is maintained until shock is very severe (loss of at least one third of the circulating volume) a rapid assessment of perfusion can be gained by examining peripheral and central pulses. The radial pulse will disappear if the systolic blood pressure is below 80 mm Hg. Thus the combination of absent peripheral pulses and weak central pulses is a sinister sign indicating advanced shock and profound hypotension.

Perfusion
Capillary refill following pressure on a digit for five seconds should normally occur within two seconds. A longer time indicates poor skin perfusion. However, this sign is not valid if the patient is hypothermic.

Blood pressure
Hypotension in circulatory failure is an indicator of increased mortality. Always ensure that an appropriate cuff size is used to take the blood pressure.

Effects of circulatory inadequacy on other organs

Respiratory system
A rapid respiratory rate with an increased tidal volume, but no signs of increased respiratory effort, is predominantly caused by a metabolic acidosis associated with circulatory failure.

Skin
Mottled, cold, pale skin peripherally indicates poor perfusion.

Mental status
Agitation, confusion, drowsiness, and unconsciousness are the progressive stages of dysfunction associated with circulatory failure. These features are attributed to poor cerebral perfusion.

Urinary output
A urine output of less than 0.5 ml/kg/hour indicates inadequate renal perfusion during shock.

RECOGNITION OF POTENTIAL CENTRAL NEUROLOGICAL FAILURE

Both respiratory and circulatory failure will have central neurological effects. The opposite situation also occurs; for example, patients who have status epilepticus will have respiratory and circulatory consequences.

Conscious level

A rapid assessment of the patient's conscious level can be made by assigning the patient to one of the categories shown in the box.

> **AVPU grading of consciousness**
>
> A **a**lert
> V response to **v**oice
> P response to **p**ain
> U **u**nresponsive

A painful stimulus should be applied by pressure over the superior orbital ridge. An adult who either only responds to pain or is unconscious has a significant degree of coma equivalent to 8 or less on the Glasgow Coma Scale.

Posture

Abnormal posturing such as decorticate (flexed arms, extended legs) or decerebrate (extended arms, extended legs) is a sinister sign of brain dysfunction. A painful stimulus may be necessary to elicit these signs.

Pupils

Many drugs and cerebral lesions have effects on pupil size and reactions. The most important pupillary signs to seek are dilation, unreactivity, and inequality. These indicate possible serious brain disorders.

Respiratory effects of central neurological failure on other systems

There are several recognisable breathing patterns associated with raised intracranial pressure. However, they are often changeable and may vary from hyperventilation to periodic breathing and apnoea. The presence of any abnormal respiratory pattern in a patient with coma suggests brain stem dysfunction.

Circulatory effects of central neurological failure

Systemic hypertension with sinus bradycardia indicates compression of the medulla oblongata caused by herniation of the cerebellar tonsils through the foramen magnum. This is a late and preterminal sign.

TIME OUT 2.1

List the clinical features that can be used to diagnose potential failure of:

a. respiration
b. circulation
c. central neurological function.

Note how many features assess more than one system. Rearrange your list of clinical features into a logical order to produce a system for rapid assessment.

SUMMARY

In the acutely ill medical patient a rapid examination will detect potential respiratory, circulatory, and neurological failure. The clinical features are:

- respiratory – rate, effort, and effectiveness of respiration
- circulatory – heart rate and effectiveness
- neurological – conscious level, posture, and pupils.

These features will form the framework of the primary assessment. The components will be discussed in detail in Part II.

STRUCTURED APPROACH

CHAPTER

3

A structured approach to medical emergencies

OBJECTIVES

After reading this chapter you will be able to describe the:

- correct sequence of priorities to be followed when assessing an acutely ill medical patient
- primary and secondary assessments
- key components of a patient's history
- techniques used in the initial resuscitation, investigation, and definitive care of a medical emergency.

INTRODUCTION

The management of a patient with a medical emergency requires a rapid assessment with appropriate treatment. This can be achieved using a structured approach.

> **Structured approach**
>
> - Primary assessment and resuscitation
> - Secondary assessment and emergency treatment
> - Reassessment
> - Definitive care

The aim of the primary assessment is **to identify and treat any life threatening conditions**. This differs from the traditional clinical teaching where a history is taken from the patient and followed by clinical examination. Such an approach can potentially delay the diagnosis of a lethal condition. Most acutely ill medical patients (approximately 75%) do not have an immediately life threatening problem. However, a rapid primary assessment is still required.

The primary assessment should be repeated following any deterioration in the patient's condition so that appropriate resuscitative measures can be commenced immediately.

Once any immediate life threatening conditions have been either treated or excluded, the clinician can proceed to take a comprehensive history and complete a thorough examination; this is known as the secondary assessment. Following any emergency treatment the patient should be reassessed. Definitive care can then be planned including transportation to the appropriate ward and further investigation.

> Always use universal precautions before assessing an acutely ill patient

---

PRIMARY ASSESSMENT AND RESUSCITATION

> The aim of the primary assessment is to **IDENTIFY** and **TREAT** all **immediately life threatening** conditions

Key components of the primary assessment (ABCDE) are:

A – Airway and administer oxygen
B – Breathing
C – Circulation
D – Disability
E – Exposure

A – Airway and administer oxygen

Aims = assess potency; if necessary clear and secure the airway
= administer oxygen
= appreciate the potential for cervical spine injury

Assessment
Assess airway patency by talking to the patient. An appropriate response to "Are you okay?" indicates that the airway is clear, breathing is occurring, and there is adequate cerebral perfusion. If no answer is forthcoming then open the airway with a chin lift or jaw thrust and reassess the patency by:

- looking – for chest movement
- listening – for the sounds of breathing
- feeling – for expired air.

A rapid check for other causes of upper airway obstruction should include inspection for foreign bodies, including dentures, and macroglossia.

Resuscitation
If a chin lift or jaw thrust is needed, then an airway adjunct may be required to maintain patency. A nasopharyngeal airway is useful in the conscious patient. In contrast, a Guedel "oropharyngeal" airway may be a necessary temporary adjunct in the unconscious patient before endotracheal intubation.

Once definitive control of the airway has been achieved supplemental oxygen should be given to all patients who are breathless, shocked or bleeding. If the patient is not intubated oxygen should be delivered using a non-rebreathing mask and reservoir. This enables the fractional inspired oxygen (FiO_2) concentration to reach a level of approximately 0.85. Even patients who have chronic obstructive pulmonary disease (COPD) should receive high flow oxygen; this can subsequently be reduced according to its clinical effect and arterial blood gas results.

Cervical spine problems are very rare in medical patients – except in those with rheumatoid disease, ankylosing spondylitis and Down's syndrome. The clinical features of these conditions are usually easily identifiable. However, be wary of the elderly patient found collapsed at the bottom of the stairs after an apparent "stroke". If you suspect cervical spine injury ask for immediate help to provide in-line immobilisation.

> Hypoxia kills and therefore should be treated *first*!
> Hypercarbia is not a killer providing the patient is receiving supplemental oxygen

Monitor
End tidal carbon dioxide should be measured after endotracheal intubation to check correct tube placement.

B – Breathing

Aim = detect and treat life threatening bronchospasm, pulmonary oedema, and a tension pneumothorax

Assessment
A patent airway does not ensure adequate ventilation. The latter requires an intact respiratory centre along with adequate pulmonary function augmented by the coordinated movement of the diaphragm and chest wall.

Chest inspection

- Colour/marks/rash
- Rate
- Effort
- Symmetry

Examine for the presence of cyanosis, respiratory rate and effort, and symmetry of movement. Palpate the trachea feeling for any tracheal tug or deviation. The position of the trachea and apex beat will also indicate any mediastinal shift. Percuss the anterior chest wall in the upper, middle, and lower zones, assessing the difference in percussion note between the left and right hemithoraces. Repeat this procedure on the posterior chest wall and also in the axilla to detect areas of hyper-resonance (air), dullness (interstitial fluid) or stony dullness (pleural fluid). Listen to the chest to establish whether breath sounds are absent, present or masked by added sounds. Further information will be provided by a pulse oximeter.

> Some physical signs will be elicited that suggest a "non breathing (non-B)" cause for respiratory difficulty. Thus corroborative evidence must be sought to confirm a clinical diagnosis of, for example, left ventricular failure

Resuscitation

Life threatening bronchospasm should be treated initially with nebulised salbutamol (β_2-agonist) and ipratropium bromide (muscarinic antagonist).

As a tension pneumothorax can embarrass both respiratory and cardiac function, it requires urgent decompression with a needle thoracentesis followed by intravenous access and chest drain insertion.

Further clues as to the underlying cause may be gained from examination of the patient's circulation.

Monitor

Arterial oxygen saturation (SaO$_2$) should be monitored continuously.

C – Circulation

Aim = detect and treat shock

There are many causes of shock that require specific treatment, for example, anaphylaxis and adrenaline.

Assessment

Rapid assessment of the patient's haemodynamic status is necessary by monitoring both cardiovascular indices and the patient's level of consciousness. Examine a central pulse, ideally the carotid, for rate, rhythm, and character. It is important, however, to compare both carotid pulses, but **not simultaneously**, as a reduction or absence in one pulse may reflect focal atheroma or a dissecting aneurysm. Measure the blood pressure and assess peripheral perfusion using the capillary refill time. Do not forget that reduction in blood volume can impair consciousness due to reduced cerebral perfusion.

Resuscitation

Intravenous access is needed in all acutely ill patients. If there is a suspicion of hypovolaemic shock then two large-bore cannulae should be inserted. The antecubital fossa is usually the easiest and most convenient site (for the doctor). At the same time, take blood for baseline haematological and biochemical values including a serum glucose and, in appropriate cases, a cross match. Arterial blood gases should also be taken.

> **Key point**
> Fluid, antibiotics, adrenaline, and inotropes are crucial in the management of shock

Treat hypovolaemia, especially from gastrointestinal tract bleeding, with vigorous fluid replacement with two litres of warm crystalloid immediately. Further fluid will be titrated according to the patient's clinical signs. If after two litres of fluid the patient remains hypotensive and haemorrhage is suspected, then blood is needed urgently. Specific treatment will be dependent on the clinical situation. Early surgical referral is advised. A similar pale, cold, and clammy picture will be found in cardiogenic shock. The presence of pulmonary oedema is a useful differentiating factor. Inotropes such as dobutamine will be required.

In contrast, the hypotensive, warm, vasodilated pyrexial patient is "septic" until proven otherwise. Actively seek the non-blanching purpuric rash of meningococcal septicaemia. This condition requires immediate treatment with intravenous benzyl penicillin 2.4 g and ceftriaxone 1 g. Subsequent investigations should include blood cultures and C-reactive protein as a marker of infection/inflammation.

The tachypnoeic, dehydrated, hypotensive patient may have diabetic ketoacidosis, possibly with underlying sepsis. The treatment is intravenous insulin 6 units/hour and antibiotics in addition to oxygen and fluids.

Any rhythm disturbance causing haemodynamic instability needs to be identified at this stage and treated according to UK and European resuscitation guidelines.

Occasionally, shock may have more than one cause. If there is no evidence of either ventricular failure or a dysrhythmia all patients should receive a fluid challenge. Subsequent management will depend upon the patient's response and blood test results.

Monitor

Continuous monitoring of pulse, blood pressure, and ECG will provide valuable baseline information in addition to the patient's response to treatment. Always check the patient's core temperature. The clinical situation will dictate whether a urinary catheter is needed.

D – Disability (neurological examination)

Aim = carry out a rapid neurological assessment and begin treating any immediately life threatening neurological condition such as a prolonged fit, hypoglycaemia, opioid overdose, and infection.

Assessment

The rapid evaluation of the nervous system comprises measuring pupillary size and reaction to light along with evaluation of conscious level using either the AVPU system or the Glasgow Coma Score (GCS) (Table 3.1). Signs of meningeal infection should be sought. The GCS has the added benefit of identifying unilateral weakness.

AVPU system

A = Alert
V = Responding to verbal stimulus
P = Responding to pain
U = Unresponsive

Table 3.1. The Glasgow Coma Score

Response	Score
Eye opening response	
Spontaneous	4
To speech	3
To painful stimuli	2
Nil	1
Motor response	
Obeys commands	6
Localises pain	5
Withdraws from pain	4
Abnormal flexion	3
Abnormal extension	2
Nil	1
Verbal response	
Orientated	5
Confused	4
Inappropriate words	3
Incomprehensible sounds	2
Nil	1

In the presence of any neurological dysfunction, assessment of the serum glucose is necessary. If the result is not immediately available then a bedside glucose estimation should be done with a glucometer or a BM stix.

Resuscitation

In the unconscious patient it is vital to clear and secure the airway, and give supplemental oxygen until further clinical information and the results of investigations are available.

"Tonic, clonic" seizures usually resolve spontaneously and no action is required except to ensure that the patient has a patent airway, is receiving supplemental oxygen, and that their vital signs are monitored regularly. It is also important to place the patient in the recovery position to prevent aspiration and injury on any adjacent objects. If the fit is prolonged then intravenous benzodiazepines are the treatment of choice, e.g. 2 mg of diazemuls (to a maximum of 20 mg). If two doses fail to control the fit then start intravenous phenytoin at 15 mg/kg over 30 minutes with ECG monitoring. This drug does not impair the conscious level and will facilitate early neurological assessment (unlike benzodiazepines). If this combination fails to control the fit then liaise with an anaesthetist as the patient should be sedated, paralysed, and ventilated.

Coma associated with either hypoglycaemia (common) or hyperglycaemia (rare) will have been appropriately treated (i.e. A, B, C). However, with hypoglycaemia the addition of intravenous dextrose (i.e. 10% infusion) and/or intravenous glucagon (1 mg) is immediately necessary. In contrast, intravenous insulin will be tailored according to the type of hyperglycaemic coma (Chapter 19). The unconscious patient showing signs of opioid excess should be treated with naloxone. The unconscious or confused patient will need a CT scan. However, this must not delay antibiotic and/or antiviral treatment for suspected meningitis/encephalitis.

Monitor

Glasgow Coma Score, pupillary response, and serum glucose.

E – Exposure

Aim = gain adequate exposure of the patient

Assess

- Rash – non-blanching purpura?
        – erythroderma?

Resuscitation

- Intravenous antibiotics

Monitor

- Temperature

It is impossible to perform a comprehensive examination unless the patient is fully undressed. However, care must be taken to prevent hypothermia, especially in elderly patients. Therefore, adequately cover patients between examinations and ensure all intravenous fluids are warmed.

MONITORING

The effectiveness of resuscitation is measured by an improvement in the patient's clinical status as described earlier. It is therefore important that repeat observations are measured and recorded frequently. The following should be considered as a minimum level of monitoring by the end of the primary assessment.

Minimal patient monitoring

- Pulse oximetry
- Respiratory rate
- Blood pressure, ideally monitored automatically
- Continuous ECG monitoring augmented by a 12 lead ECG
- Chest X-ray
- Arterial blood gases
- Core temperature estimation
- Central venous pressure when appropriate
- Urinary output
- Glasgow Coma Score and pupillary response when appropriate

It is important to realise that during the primary assessment the patient is reviewed regularly, especially after treatment has been started. This will ensure that the patient has responded appropriately and not deteriorated.

Key point
The most important assessment is the reassessment

The majority of medical patients will not require formal primary assessment and resuscitation. In clinical practice the usual patient–doctor introduction will provide a rapid assessment of the A, B, Cs. A patient who is sitting up and talking has a patent airway and sufficient cardiorespiratory function to provide oxygenation and cerebral perfusion. Thus one can skip, virtually immediately, to the traditional style of taking a history followed by a physical examination. This is referred to as the secondary assessment.

Key point
If the patient deteriorates repeat the primary assessment starting at A

TIME OUT 3.1

After reading the case history, answer the following question:

A 54 year old man is admitted to hospital because of an acute onset of confusion.

Briefly describe your primary assessment of this patient.

SUMMARY

- The aim of the primary assessment is to identify and treat immediately life threatening conditions.
- In most medical patients this can be done rapidly from the end of the bed.

- Do not proceed to the secondary assessment until the patient's vital signs have been stabilised.

SECONDARY ASSESSMENT

> The aim of the secondary assessment is to identify and treat all conditions not detected in the primary assessment, seek corroborative evidence for provisional diagnosis and prioritise the patient's condition.

The secondary assessment starts once the vital functions have been stabilised and immediately life threatening conditions have been treated.

History

Nearly all medical diagnosis is made after a good history has been obtained from the patient. Occasionally, for a variety of reasons this may not be possible. Therefore facts should be sought from relatives, the patient's medical notes, the general practitioner, friends or the police and ambulance service. A well "phrased" history is required, and also serves as a useful mnemonic to remember the key features.

A well "phrased" history

P Problem
H History of presenting problem
R Relevant medical history
A Allergies
S Systems review
E Essential family and social history
D Drugs

The history of the presenting problems is of paramount importance. A comprehensive systems review will ensure that significant, relevant information is not excluded. In addition it will ensure that the secondary assessment focuses on the relevant system/s.

Examination

Aims = find new features – often related to clues in the history
     = comprehensively reassess conditions identified in the primary assessment
     = seek corroborative evidence for the diagnosis considered in the primary assessment

The examination should be directed by the history and primary assessment findings. It is a methodical, structured approach comprising a general overview and the detection of specific features.

General
A clinical overview of the patient's overall appearance "from the end of the bed" can give clues to underlying pathology.

> **Clinical overview**
>
> - Posture
> - Pigmentation
> - Pallor
> - Pattern of respiration
> - Pronunciation
> - Pulsations

Specific features

Hands Inspect the hands for stigmata of infective endocarditis, chronic liver disease, thyrotoxicosis, carbon dioxide retention, polyarthropathy, and multisystem disease. Palpate the radial pulse for rate, rhythm, character and symmetry, comparing it to the contralateral radial pulse and the femoral pulse.

Face Examine for facial asymmetry, cyanosis, and the presence of any pigmentation as well as stigmata of hyperlipidaemia, titubation, and cutaneous features of internal pathology. Inspect the mouth, tongue, and pharynx for the presence of ulcers as well as blisters, vesicles, and erythema which may suggest ingestion of toxic compounds. Pigmentation of the buccal mucosa should be specifically sought as this may indicate Addison's disease.

Neck Assess the height, wave form, and characteristics of the internal jugular venous pulse. Following this palpate both internal carotid arteries in turn to compare and determine the pulse character. Check the position of the trachea and the presence of any lymphadenopathy.

Chest Assess the shape of the chest and breathing pattern. Inspect for the rate, effort and symmetry of respiration, and the presence of surgical scars. Palpate the precordium to determine the site and character of the apex beat, the presence of a left and/or right ventricular heave, and the presence of thrills. Listen for the first, second, and any additional heart sounds. Percuss the anterior and posterior chest walls bilaterally in upper, middle, and lower zones comparing the note from the left and right hemithoraces. Auscultate these areas to determine the presence, type, and quality of breath sounds as well as any added sounds.

Abdomen Systematically examine the abdomen according to the nine anatomical divisions. Specific features that should be sought include hepatosplenomegaly, peritonism/itis, abdominal masses, ascites as well as renal angle tenderness. Examination of the external genitalia and rectum is necessary but not always in the acute setting.

Locomotor Inspect all joints and examine for the presence of tenderness, deformity, restricted movement, synovial thickening, and inflammation. The patient's history, however, will indicate the joints that are affected. Although inflammatory polyarthropathies may present acutely, acute monoarthropathies are potentially more sinister.

Neurological A comprehensive neurological examination is rarely required in the acutely ill patient. A screening examination of the nervous system can be accomplished as follows.

1. Assess the conscious state using the Glasgow Coma Scale.
2. A Mini Mental State Examination (See box below).

23

Abbreviated mental-status examination

1 Age
2 Time (to nearest hour)
3 Address for recall at end of test – this should be repeated by the patient to ensure it has been heard correctly: 42 West Street
4 Year
5 Name of institution
6 Recognition of 2 people (doctor, nurse, etc)
7 Date of birth (day and month sufficient)
8 Year of World War I
9 Name of present Monarch
10 Count backwards 20–1

Each correct answer scores one mark. Healthy people score 8–10

Source: Qureshi KN, Hodkinson HM. Evaluation of a ten-question mental test in the institutionalized elderly. *Age and Ageing* 1974; 3: 152–7.

3. Examine the external ocular movements for diplopia, nystagmus or fatiguability. Elicit the pupillary response to light and accommodation (PERLA, i.e. pupils equally react to light and accommodation). Examine the fundi. The absence of dolls eye movement (oculocephalic reflex) indicates a brain stem problem. Assess the corneal reflex, muscles of mastication and facial movement followed by palatal movement, gag reflex, and tongue protrusion.
4. Test the tone of all four limbs, augmented by the power of muscle groups, and reflexes including the Plantar (Babinski) response and coordination.
5. Sensory testing, although subjective, is useful in the acute medical setting especially when a cord lesion is suspected.
6. Further CNS examination will be dictated by the patient's history and the examination findings, especially from the screening neurological assessment.

Skin   The skin and the buccal mucosa must be thoroughly inspected. Lesions may be localised to the skin and mucous membranes, and possibly a manifestation of internal pathology.

REASSESSMENT

The patient's condition should be monitored to detect any changes and assess the effect of treatment. If there is any evidence of a deterioration reevaluate by returning to A in the primary assessment.

Many patients presenting with an apparent medical problem may require surgical intervention. It is, therefore, of paramount importance to obtain an early surgical opinion when appropriate, e.g. when treating patients with gastrointestinal haemorrhage.

Key point
Remember to examine the back of the patient either during the primary or secondary assessment

---

DOCUMENTATION

Always document the findings of the primary and secondary assessments. This record, along with subsequent entries into the patient's notes, should be dated, timed and signed. The patient's records must also contain a management plan, a list of investigations requested, and the related results, as well as details of any treatment and its effect. This will not only provide an *aide-mémoire* but will also enable the patient's condition to be monitored and provide colleagues with an accurate account of a patient's hospital admission.

DEFINITIVE CARE

Management plan

This needs to list further investigations and treatment required for the particular patient. This is a dynamic plan that may change according to the clinical condition.

Investigations

These will be dictated by the findings from the initial assessment and liaison with colleagues. Tests are not without risks; therefore tests should only be done if they directly influence patient care.

Transport

All patients will be transferred sometime during their hospital stay. Irrespective of the transfer distance, appropriate numbers and grades of staff are required along with relevant equipment.

TIME OUT 3.2

Your primary assessment of the confused 54 year old man has revealed the following.

A	Assessment	patent
	Resuscitation	$FiO_2 = 0.85$
	Monitor	not required, as yet
B	Assessment	rate 30/minute
		no accessory muscle use
		symmetrical expansion
		no focal features
	Resuscitation	not required, as yet
	Monitor	pulse oximetry ($SaO_2 = 99\%$)
C	Assessment	pulse – radial 140/min
		atrial fibrillation
		blood pressure 90/60
		jugular venous pulse visible when flat
		remainder of examination was normal

	Resuscitation	cardioversion ($\times$ 3) failed to convert patient to sinus rhythm following sedation therefore intravenous digoxin commenced
	Monitor	pulse
		blood pressure
		blood glucose, haemoglobin, urea and electrolytes
D	Assessment	PERLA
		Glasgow Coma Score 14/15: E = 4; V = 4; M = 6

a. What would be your next action?
b. What is the problem with this patient?
c. What is your management plan?

A WORD (OR TWO) OF WARNING

The structured approach is a safe comprehensive method of assessing any acutely ill patient. It should be regarded as the "default method" in that it will prevent any further harm and cater for all medical problems. However, as most patients do not have an immediately life threatening problem, a rapid primary assessment is needed. Many patients do not require high flow oxygen, intravenous access ($\times$ 2), and a fluid challenge. Clinical judgement is still needed combined with a modicum of common sense. If in doubt revert to A.

SUMMARY

The acutely ill patient must be evaluated quickly and accurately. Thus, you must develop a structured method for assessment and treatment. In most acutely ill medical patients the primary assessment is rapid and resuscitation is rarely required. Diagnosis is based on a well "phrased" medical history obtained from the patient. However if this is not possible then further information must be sought from medical records, relatives, general practitioners or colleagues from the emergency services.

Assessment and treatment are divided into two key assessment phases:

- **Primary assessment and Resuscitation**
  To identify and treat immediately life threatening problems.

Assessment of:
A – Airway
B – Breathing
C – Circulation
D – Disability
E – Exposure

Resuscitation by:

1. clearing and securing the airway and oxygenation
2. ventilation
3. intravenous access and shock therapy – fluids, antibiotics, inotropes, dysrhythmia management
4. exclude/correct hypoglycaema; anti-epileptic drugs, specific antedotes
5. monitoring respiration rate, pulse, blood pressure, oxygen saturation, urinary output, pupillary response, AVPU, and blood gas (monitored previously)

- **Secondary assessment and emergency treatment**

To gain corroborative evidence for primary diagnosis; to identify and treat new conditions.

Comprehensive physical examination including:

1. general overview
2. hands and radial pulse
3. facial appearance
4. neck – jugular venous pulse, carotid pulse, trachea
5. chest – precordium and both lungs
6. abdomen and genitalia
7. locomotor system
8. nervous system
9. skin.

- **Definitive care**

1. management plan
2. investigations
3. transport

CHAPTER

4

Airway assessment

OBJECTIVES

After reading this chapter you will be able to:

- recognise the signs of airway obstruction
- understand how to use simple airway adjuncts
- describe advanced airway control and ventilation.

INTRODUCTION

- Airway problems are common in acute medical emergencies.
- The immediately life threatening problem is airway obstruction.

In the unconscious patient it is essential to rapidly assess and control the airway; these simple manoeuvres can be life saving. Therefore, in both basic and advanced life support, management of the airway is the first priority – the A of "ABC".

An obstructed airway can result in or be caused by a loss of consciousness. The obstruction can occur at many levels:

- pharynx   by tongue displacement
  swelling of the epiglottis or soft tissues
- larynx   oedema
  spasm of the vocal cords (laryngospasm)
  foreign body
  trauma
- subglottic   secretions or foreign body
  swelling
- bronchial   bronchospasm
  pulmonary oedema
  aspiration
  pneumothorax

In the unconscious patient, the most common level of obstruction is the pharynx. This has always been thought to be due to a reduction in muscle tone allowing the tongue to fall backwards (Figure 4.1). However, this is not the whole explanation as obstruction

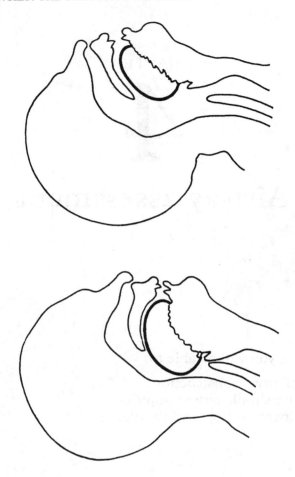

Figure 4.1 Obstruction of the airway by the tongue

may still occur when the patient is placed prone. An additional contribution comes from abnormal muscle activity in the pharynx, larynx, and neck. This situation can be rectified and an airway provided by using manoeuvres described in this chapter.

Primary assessment and resuscitation

Look at the chest for depth, rate, and symmetry of movement. In complete airway obstruction paradoxical movement of the chest and abdomen (see-sawing) will occur as a result of the increased respiratory effort. In addition, there may be use of accessory muscles; intercostal and supraclavicular recession may be visible and a tracheal tug may be palpable. Look in the mouth for blood, gastric contents, frothy sputum (pulmonary oedema), and foreign bodies.

Listen for breath sounds. Partial obstruction may be accompanied by the following.

- Inspiratory noises (stridor) commonly indicate upper airway obstruction.
- Expiratory noises, particularly wheezing, usually occur in obstruction of the lower airways as they collapse during expiration.
- "Crowing" accompanies laryngeal spasm.
- "Gurgling" indicates the presence of liquid or semisolid material.
- "Snoring" indicates that the pharynx is still partially occluded by the tongue.

Feel for:

- expired air against the side of your cheek
- chest movement, comparing one side with the other
- the position of the trachea, and for any subcutaneous emphysema.

If indicated, a finger sweep will ensure that the obstruction is not due to a foreign body. Remove broken or very loose dentures, but well fitting ones should be left in place as they help to maintain the contour of the mouth and make using a bag–mask system easier (see later).

The possibility of an injury to the cervical spine must always be considered. However, medical patients are more likely to die from hypoxia than be rendered quadriplegic as a consequence of carefully conducted airway opening manoeuvres.

AIRWAY ADJUNCTS

These are often helpful to improve or maintain airway patency, either during resuscitation or in a spontaneously breathing patient. Both oropharyngeal and nasopharyngeal airways are designed to overcome backward tongue displacement in the unconscious patient. In both cases, however, the head tilt or jaw thrust techniques usually need to be maintained.

Oropharyngeal (Guedel) airways

These are curved plastic tubes, flanged at the oral end and flattened in cross-section so that they can fit between the tongue and the hard palate. They are available in a variety of sizes which are suitable for all patients, from newborn babies to large adults. An estimate of the size required can be obtained by comparing the airway with the distance from the centre of the incisors to the angle of the jaw.

The oropharyngeal airway is inserted either upside down and rotated through 180° or under direct vision with the aid of a tongue depressor or laryngescope (see Chapter 27 for further details).

Incorrect insertion can push the tongue further back into the pharynx and produce airway obstruction. It can also cause trauma and bleeding, and force unrecognised foreign bodies further into the larynx. Furthermore, in patients who are not deeply unconscious, an oral airway may irritate the pharynx and larynx and cause vomiting and laryngospasm, respectively.

Nasopharyngeal airways

This type of airway is made from malleable plastic, that is, bevelled at one end and, flanged at the other. It is round in cross-section to aid insertion through the nose. Nasopharyngeal airways are sized according to their internal diameter, which increases with increasing length. The patient's little finger gives an approximate guide to the correct size of nasopharyngeal airway.

Nasopharyngeal airways are often better tolerated than oropharyngeal airways. They may be life-saving in a patient whose mouth cannot be opened, for example with trismus or in the presence of maxillary injuries. They should, however, be used with extreme caution in patients with a suspected base of skull fracture (very rare in the acutely ill medical patient).

Even with careful insertion, bleeding can occur from tissue in the nasopharynx. If the airway is too long, both vomiting and laryngospasm can be induced in patients who are not deeply unconscious.

A further problem with both of these types of airway is that air may be directed into the oesophagus during assisted ventilation. This results in inefficient ventilation of the lungs and gastric dilatation. The latter splints the diaphragm making ventilation difficult and also predisposes to regurgitation of gastric contents. This commonly occurs if high inflation pressures are used to try and ventilate a patient. In these circumstances carefully check that ventilation is adequate and gastric distension is minimised.

VENTILATORY SUPPORT

If adequate spontaneous ventilation follows these airway opening manoeuvres place the patient in an appropriate recovery position – providing there are no contraindications. This will reduce the risk of further obstruction.

Exhaled air resuscitation

If spontaneous ventilation is inadequate or absent, artificial ventilation must be commenced. If no equipment is available, expired air ventilation will provide 16% oxygen. This can be made more pleasant, and the risks of cross-infection reduced, by the use of simple adjuncts to avoid direct person-to-person contact; an example of this is the Laerdal pocket mask. This device has a unidirectional valve to allow the rescuer's expired air to pass to the patient while the patient's expired air is directed away from the rescuer. The masks are transparent to allow detection of vomit or blood. The more modern version has an additional attachment for supplemental oxygen.

Oxygen

Oxygen should be given to all patients during resuscitation, with the aim of increasing the inspired concentration to greater than 95%. However, this concentration will depend upon the system used and the flow available. In spontaneously breathing patients, a Venturi mask will deliver a fixed concentration (24–60%) depending upon the mask chosen. A standard concentration mask will deliver up to 60% provided the flow of oxygen is high enough (12–15 l/min). Some patients are more tolerant of nasal cannulae, but these only raise the inspired concentration to approximately 44%. The most effective system is a mask with a non-rebreathing reservoir in which the inspired concentration can be raised to 85% with an oxygen flow of 12–15 l/min. This is the most desirable method in spontaneously breathing patients.

ADVANCED AIRWAY CONTROL AND VENTILATION

Airway control

In the deeply unconscious patient, airway control is best achieved by tracheal intubation. However, the technique requires a greater degree of skill and more equipment than the methods already described.

Tracheal intubation may be indicated for a variety of reasons but the most obvious is that all other methods of providing an airway have failed. In addition it allows:

- suction and clearance of inhaled debris from the lower respiratory tract
- protection against further contamination by regurgitated stomach contents or blood
- ventilation to be achieved without leaks, even when airway resistance is high (e.g. in pulmonary oedema and bronchospasm)
- an alternative route for drugs.

Tracheal intubation

This is the preferred method for airway control during cardiopulmonary resuscitation, for the reasons already outlined. Considerable training and practice are required to acquire and maintain the skill of intubation. Repeated attempts by the inexperienced are likely to be unsuccessful and traumatic, compromise oxygenation and delay resuscitation. Orotracheal intubation is common, nasotracheal is rare.

The technique of orotracheal intubation is described in Chapter 27. Nevertheless this is not intended as a substitute for practice using a manikin or, better still, an anaesthetised patient under the direction of a skilled anaesthetist.

Tracheal intubation is frequently more difficult to perform during resuscitation. The patient may be in an awkward position on the floor, equipment may be unfamiliar, assistance limited, cardiopulmonary resuscitation (CPR) obstructive, and vomit copious. In these circumstances, it is all too easy to persist with the "almost there" attitude. This must be strongly resisted. If intubation is not successfully accomplished in approximately 30–40 s (about the time one can breath-hold during the attempt), it should be abandoned. Ventilation with 12–15 l/min (95%) oxygen using a bag–valve–mask should be recommenced before, and in between, any further attempts at intubation.

In certain circumstances, such as acute epiglottitis, laryngoscopy and attempted intubation are contraindicated because they could lead to a deterioration in the patient's condition. These specialist skills may be required including the use of anaesthetic drugs or fibreoptic laryngoscopy.

> **Key point**
> It is not appropriate to learn or practise endotracheal intubation during resuscitation

ALTERNATIVES TO TRACHEAL INTUBATION

Currently endotracheal intubation is the optimum method of managing the airway in an unconscious patient. For most people, acquiring this skill is time consuming, continuous training is unavailable, and skill retention is poor. The laryngeal mask airway is a recognised acceptable alternative.

The laryngeal mask airway (LMA)

This comprises a "mask" with an inflatable cuff around its edge that sits over the laryngeal opening. Attached to the mask is a tube that protrudes from the mouth and through which the patient breathes or is ventilated (Figure 4.2). Originally designed for spontaneously breathing anaesthetised patients, however ventilation is possible providing that inflation pressures are not excessive. The main advantage of the LMA is that it is inserted blindly, and the technique may be mastered more easily than laryngoscopy and tracheal intubation. However, if the seal around the larynx is poor or if the mask is malpositioned, ventilation will be reduced and gastric inflation may occur. Furthermore, there is no guarantee against aspiration. Whenever possible insertion of a LMA must be preceded by a period of preoxygenation. Any attempt at insertion must be limited to 30–40 s, after which ventilation with 12–15 l/min oxygen using a bag–valve–mask should be recommenced before further attempts.

The latest development is the use of the LMA as a conduit to allow the insertion of a tracheal tube to secure the airway in cases of difficult tracheal intubation. The technique of insertion is described in Chapter 27.

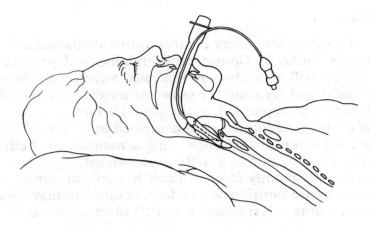

Figure 4.2 Laryngeal mask *in situ*

Cricoid pressure

This is a manoeuvre used by anaesthetists to prevent regurgitation and aspiration of gastric contents during induction of anaesthesia – often in acutely ill patients or those with a full stomach.

The cricoid cartilage forms a complete ring immediately below the thyroid cartilage. Pressure is applied on the cricoid by an assistant forcing the ring backwards, occluding the oesophagus against the body of the 6th cervical vertebra (Figure 4.3). Thus preventing the flow of any gastric contents beyond this point. This manoeuvre is maintained until:

- the tracheal tube is inserted into the larynx
- the cuff is inflated
- the person intubating indicates that pressure can be released.

If the patient vomits cricoid pressure must be released immediately because of the slight risk of oesophageal rupture. If pressure is incorrectly applied, intubation may be made more difficult.

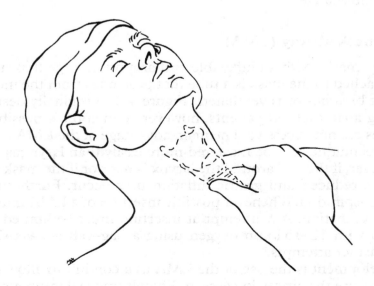

Figure 4.3 Technique for cricoid pressure

Ventilation

The ultimate aim is to achieve an inspired oxygen concentration of greater than 95%. The most common device used is the self-inflating bag with a one-way valve that can be connected to either a facemask or a tracheal tube (Figure 4.4).

Squeezing the bag delivers its contents to the patient via the one-way valve. On release the bag reinflates, refilling via the inlet valve at the opposite end. At the same time, the one-way valve diverts expired gas from the patient to the atmosphere. Using the bag-valve alone (attached to mask or tracheal tube), the patient is ventilated with 21% oxygen, as the bag refills with ambient air. However, this can (and should) be increased during resuscitation to around 50% by connecting an oxygen supply at 12–15 l/min directly to the bag adjacent to the air intake. If a reservoir bag is also attached, with an oxygen flow of 12–15 l/min, an inspired oxygen concentration of 95% can be achieved.

Although the self-inflating bag–valve–mask will allow ventilation with higher concentrations of oxygen, it is associated with several problems.

- It requires considerable skill for one person to maintain a gas-tight seal between the mask and the patient's face, whilst at the same time lifting the jaw with one hand and squeezing the bag with the other.

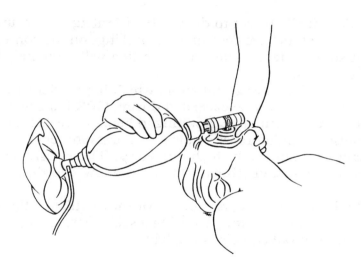

Figure 4.4   Self-inflating bag–mask and reservoir

- Any air leak will result in hypoventilation, no matter how energetically the bag is compressed.
- Excessive compression of the bag when attached to a facemask results in gas passing into the stomach. This further reduces effective ventilation and increases the risk of regurgitation and aspiration.
- The valve mechanism may "stick" if it becomes blocked with secretions, vomit or heavy moisture contamination.

As a result of some of these problems, it is now recommended that a two-person technique should be used during ventilation of a patient with a bag–valve–mask. One person holds the facemask in place using both hands and an assistant squeezes the bag. In this way a better seal is achieved, the jaw thrust manoeuvre is easier to maintain and the patient can be ventilated more easily.

Clearly these problems can be overcome by tracheal intubation, which eliminates leaks and ensures that oxygen is delivered directly and only into the lungs (always assuming the tube is in the trachea!).

The ultimate method of ventilating patients during resuscitation is with a mechanical ventilator. When using these devices the most important feature to remember is that **they are good servants, but poor masters**. They will only do what they are set to do, and will not automatically compensate for changes in the patient's condition during resuscitation. Therefore, it is imperative that they are set correctly and checked regularly when used.

A variety of small portable ventilators are used during resuscitation (e.g. pneuPAC) and are generally gas powered. If an oxygen cylinder is used as both the supply of respiratory gas for the patient and the power for the ventilator, its contents will be used more rapidly. This is of particular importance if patients are being transported over long distances because adequate oxygen supplies must be taken.

Gas powered portable ventilators are classified as time cycled and often have a fixed inspiratory:expiratory ratio. They provide a constant flow of gas to the patient during inspiration and expiration occurs passively to the atmosphere. The volume delivered depends on the inspiratory time (i.e. longer times, larger breaths) with the pressure in the airway rising during inspiration. As a safety feature, these devices can often be "pressure limited" by a relief valve opening to protect the lungs against excessive pressures (barotrauma).

A ventilator should initially be set to deliver 10–15 ml/kg tidal volume at a rate of 12 breaths/min. Some ventilators have coordinated markings on the controls for rapid initial setting for different sized patients. The correct setting will ultimately be determined by analysis of arterial blood gases.

Care should be taken when using ventilators which have relief valves fixed to open at relatively low pressures. This may be exceeded during CPR if a chest compression coincides with a breath from the ventilator, resulting in inadequate ventilation. Furthermore, by the same mechanism, ventilators with adjustable pressure relief valves, if set too high, may subject patients to excessively high pressures. These risks can be reduced by decreasing the rate of ventilation (breaths/min) to allow coordination of breaths and compressions.

If there is any doubt about the performance of the ventilator, the safest option is to temporarily disconnect it and continue by using a self-inflating bag–valve assembly with oxygen and reservoir, until skilled help is available.

Suction (endotracheal)

Once the trachea has been intubated, suction is performed to remove secretions, vomit or blood. To avoid making the patient hypoxic and bradycardic this must be done carefully in the following way.

- Ventilate the patient with 100% oxygen.
- Wear gloves.
- Introduce a sterile catheter through the airway into the trachea **without** suction applied.
- The diameter of the catheter should be less than half that of the tracheal tube or surgical airway.
- Suction and withdraw the catheter using a rotating motion over 10–15 s.
- Irrespective of the amount of blood/mucus removed do not reintroduce the catheter without a further period of oxygenation.
- Loosen tenacious secretions by instilling 10 ml of sterile saline followed by five vigorous manual ventilations. Suction as described earlier.

Key point
Suction must not be applied directly to the tracheal tube or surgical airway, as this will result in life threatening hypoxia and dysrhythmias

TIME OUT 4.1

Take a break and list the clinical features of airway obstruction.

SUMMARY

Airway control and ventilation are essential prerequisites for successful resuscitation. Airway obstruction should be recognised and managed immediately. Endotracheal intubation remains the best method of securing and controlling the airway, but requires additional equipment, skill and practice. The ultimate aim is to ventilate the patient with greater than 95% oxygen. Occasionally, when all other methods of ventilation have failed, a surgical airway may be required as a life saving procedure.

CHAPTER

5

Breathing assessment

OBJECTIVES

After reading this chapter you will be able to:

- understand the physiology of oxygen delivery
- describe a structured approach to breathing assessment
- identify immediately life threatening causes of breathlessness
- describe the immediate management of these patients.

INTRODUCTION

The acutely breathless patient is a common medical emergency that is distressing for both the patient and the clinician. Often the effort required for breathing makes it virtually impossible for the patient to provide any form of medical history and questioning may only make the situation worse. Information should be sought from any available source. The clinician's skills will help to determine the underlying cause and dictate appropriate management.

Key point
Breathlessness can result from a problem in breathing (B), circulation (C), and disability (D)

Immediately life threatening causes of breathlessness

Airway
- Obstruction

Breathing
- Acute severe asthma
- Acute exacerbation of chronic obstructive pulmonary disease (COPD)
- Pulmonary oedema
- Tension pneumothorax

Disruption of oxygen delivery is a fundamental process in these conditions. Therefore it is important to understand the mechanisms that maintain their integrity in health.

PRIMARY ASSESSMENT AND RESUSCITATION

Relevant physiology

Oxygen delivery

The normal respiratory rate is 14–20 breaths per minute. With each breath 500 ml of air (6–10 litres per minute) are inhaled and exhaled. This air mixes with alveolar gas and, by diffusion, oxygen enters the pulmonary circulation to combine mainly with haemoglobin in the red cells. The erythrocyte bound oxygen is transported via the systemic circulation to the tissues where it is taken up and used by the cells.

Consequently the delivery of oxygen (DO_2) to the tissues depends on:

- concentration of oxygen reaching the alveoli
- pulmonary perfusion
- adequacy of pulmonary gas exchange
- capacity of blood to carry oxygen
- blood flow to the tissues.

Concentration of oxygen reaching the alveoli

The two most important factors determining the amount of oxygen reaching the alveoli are:

- the fraction of inspired oxygen (FiO_2)
- ventilation.

Providing supplementary oxygen to a person increases the number of oxygen molecules getting to the alveoli. Consequently common medical practice in dealing with ill patients is to use various types of oxygen masks so that the **fraction of inspired oxygen** is increased.

However, the effectiveness of this procedure depends on the lungs' ability to draw the inspired gas into the alveoli. The mechanism for transporting inspired air to, and expired gas from, the alveoli is called **ventilation** (V). As ventilation is essential for life it is subject to several regulatory processes which are summarised in the box.

Key components in regulating ventilation	
Brain stem	medullary respiratory centre
Receptors	pulmonary stretch chemoreceptors for CO_2, O_2, H^+
Vagus and phrenic nerves	increased ventilation
Respiratory muscles	chest wall and diaphragm
Mechanics	air passages
	compliant lungs and chest wall

The normal ventilatory volumes and rates are summarised in Figures 5.1 and 5.2.

The **normal resting respiratory rate** is 15 (range 14–20) breaths per minute. The amount of air inspired per breath is called the **tidal volume** and is equivalent to

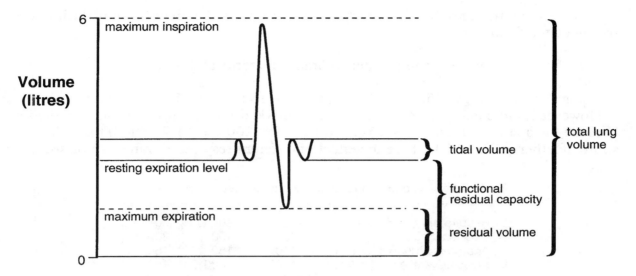

Figure 5.1 Normal ventilatory volumes as measured by spirometry

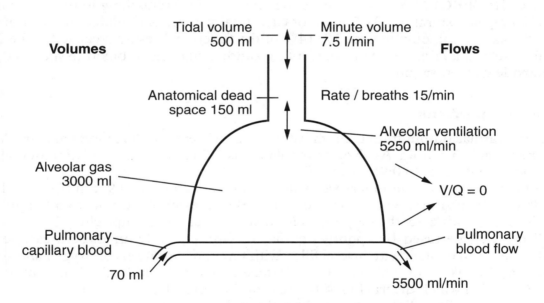

Figure 5.2 Normal volumes and flows

7–8 ml/kg body weight (or 500 ml for the 70 kg patient). Therefore the amount of air inspired each minute, the **minute volume**, can be calculated by multiplying the **respiratory rate** by the **tidal volume** (15×500 ml) to produce a value of 7·5 l/min.

The tidal volume (500 ml) is distributed throughout the respiratory system but only 350 ml (70%) mixes with alveolar air. The remainder (150 ml) occupies the airways that are not involved in gas transfer. This volume is referred to as the **anatomical dead space**. In addition, there are certain areas within the lungs which are also not involved with gas transfer because they are ventilated but not perfused. The volume produced by the combination of these areas and the anatomical dead space is called the **total or physiological dead space**. In healthy individuals these two dead spaces are virtually identical because ventilation and perfusion are well matched.

It follows that the amount of air reaching the alveoli, i.e. the **alveolar ventilation**, can be calculated from:

$$respiratory\ rate \times (tidal\ volume - anatomical\ dead\ space)$$

Using data from Figure 5.2, this corresponds to $15 \times (500 - 150) = 5250$ ml/min. However rapid shallow respiration causes a marked reduction in alveolar ventilation because the anatomical dead space is fixed i.e. $30 \times (200 - 150) = 1500$. This is demonstrated further in Table 5.1 where the effect of different respiratory rates can be seen.

Table 5.1   The effect of respiratory rate on alveolar ventilation

Respiratory rate (/min)	10	20	30
Tidal volume (ml)	600	400	200
Anatomical dead space (ml)	150	150	150
Alveolar ventilation (ml/min)	4500	5000	1500

Finally it is important to be aware of a crucial volume known as the **functional residual capacity** (FRC) (2·5–3·0 l). This is the amount of air remaining in the lungs at the end of a normal expiration. As 350 ml of each tidal volume is available for gas transfer, fresh alveolar air will only replace 12–14% of the functional residual capacity. The FRC therefore acts as a large reservoir, preventing sudden changes in blood oxygen and carbon dioxide concentration.

Pulmonary perfusion

At rest the cardiac output from the right ventricle is delivered to the pulmonary circulation at approximately 5·5 l/min. As alveolar ventilation is 5·25 l/min, the ventilation:pulmonary perfusion ratio is equal to 0·95 (5·25/5·5).

The pressures in the pulmonary vascular bed are low (around 20/9 mm Hg) and therefore affected by posture. As a result there are differences in blood flow to different lung regions, contributing to the physiological dead space. In the upright position, basal alveoli are well perfused but poorly ventilated. Consequently, in these areas, venous blood comes into contact with alveoli filled with low concentrations of oxygen and so less oxygen can be taken up. This effect is minimised in healthy individuals by pulmonary vasoconstriction which diverts blood to areas of the lungs that have better ventilation.

There are also direct links between the right and left side of the heart. These normally allow 2% of the right ventricle's output to bypass the lungs completely and are collectively known as the **physiological shunt**. As the blood in this shunt has had no contact with the alveoli, its oxygen and carbon dioxide concentrations will remain the same as those found in the right ventricle.

Pulmonary gas exchange

Oxygen continuously diffuses out of the alveolar gas into the pulmonary capillaries with carbon dioxide going in the opposite direction. The rate of diffusion is governed by the following factors:

- partial pressure gradient of the gas
- solubility of the gas
- alveolar surface area
- alveolar capillary wall thickness.

The lungs are ideally suited for diffusion as they have both a large alveolar surface area (approximately 50 m^2) and a thin alveolar capillary wall. It is also easy to understand why gas exchange would be compromised by a reduction in the former (e.g. pneumothorax) or an increase in the latter (e.g. interstitial pulmonary oedema).

Gases move passively down gradients from areas of high to low partial pressure. The partial pressure of oxygen in the alveoli (PAO_2) is approximately (13·4 kPa), 100 mm Hg whereas that in the pulmonary artery is (5·3 kPa) 40 mm Hg. In contrast the gradient for carbon dioxide is only small, with the alveolar partial pressure being (5·3 kPa) 40 mm Hg compared with (6·0 kPa) 46 mm Hg in the pulmonary artery. However, carbon dioxide passes through biological membranes 20 times more easily than oxygen. The net effect is that, in health, the time taken for exchange of oxygen and carbon dioxide is virtually identical.

Although alveolar ventilation, diffusion and pulmonary perfusion will all affect the alveolar PO_2 (PAO_2) and hence the arterial PO_2 (PaO_2), the most important factor in determining the PaO_2 is the ratio of ventilation to perfusion.

Ventilation:perfusion ratio
To understand this concept it is helpful to divide each lung into three functional areas: apical, middle, and basal (Figure 5.3).

Remember that the overall ratio of ventilation to perfusion is nearly one (0·95).

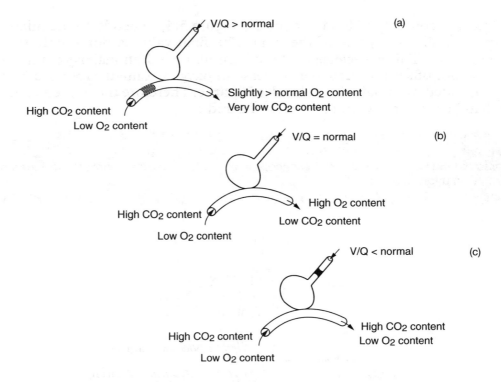

Figure 5.3 Three different ventilation (V) perfusion (Q) ratios (a) normal ventilation with reduced perfusion; (b) normal ventilation with normal perfusion; (c) reduced ventilation with normal perfusion

The apical segment is well ventilated, but unfortunately poorly perfused. Therefore, not enough blood is available to accept all the alveolar oxygen, however, the red cells that are available are fully laden (saturated) with oxygen. Thus, the unused oxygen is simply dissolved in the plasma.

43

> **Tip**
> In the apical segment there is more ventilation than perfusion, i.e., the V:Q ratio > 1

The middle segment has ventilation and perfusion perfectly matched. Alveolar oxygen diffuses into, and is correctly balanced by, the pulmonary capillary blood ensuring that the red cells are fully saturated. The remaining small amount of oxygen is dissolved in plasma.

> **Tip**
> In the middle segment ventilation and perfusion are matched, i.e., the V:Q ratio = 1

The basal segment alveoli are well perfused, but poorly ventilated. All the available oxygen is bound to red cells but they are not fully saturated, i.e. there is spare oxygen carrying capacity. This is similar to the physiological shunt as described earlier.

> **Tip**
> In the basal segment ventilation is reduced when compared to perfusion, i.e., the V:Q ratio < 1

The oxygen content of blood at point X (Figure 5.4) depends on the mixture of blood coming from all three parts of the lung. The final value is not simply the mid point between a and c. This is because the **small** amount of additional oxygen dissolved in the plasma cannot offset the **massive** decrease in oxygen content produced by the incompletely saturated haemoglobin molecules in part c. Therefore the oxygen content is much lower than half way between the values of a and c.

> **Key point**
> An area of lung with a high V:Q ratio cannot offset the fall in oxygen content produced by an area of lung with a low V:Q ratio

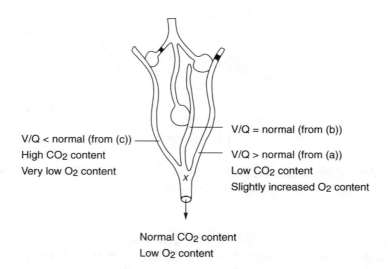

V/Q < normal (from (c))
High CO_2 content
Very low O_2 content

V/Q = normal (from (b))

V/Q > normal (from (a))
Low CO_2 content
Slightly increased O_2 content

Normal CO_2 content
Low O_2 content

Figure 5.4 Mixed blood returning from three sites at point *X*

Oxygen content of arterial blood

The oxygen content of haemoglobin (Hb) going to tissues depends on the:

- saturation of haemoglobin with oxygen
- haemoglobin concentration
- oxygen carrying capacity
- oxygen dissolved in plasma.

Haemoglobin is a protein comprising four subunits, each of which contains a haem molecule attached to a polypeptide chain. The haem molecule contains iron which reversibly binds oxygen; hence it is oxygenated but **not** oxidised. Each haemoglobin molecule can carry up to four oxygen molecules. Blood has a haemoglobin concentration of approximately 15 g/100 ml, and normally each gram of haemoglobin can carry 1·34 ml of oxygen if it is fully saturated. Therefore the **oxygen carrying capacity** of blood is:

$$\text{Hb} \times 1\cdot34 \times 1$$
$$15 \times 1\cdot34 \times 1 = 20\cdot1 \text{ ml } O_2/100 \text{ ml of blood}$$
(A value of one indicates that Hb is fully saturated.)

This is approximately 60 times greater than the amount of oxygen dissolved in plasma.

> **Key point**
> Nearly all of the oxygen carried in the blood is taken up by haemoglobin with only a small amount dissolved in the plasma

The relationship between the PaO_2 and oxygen uptake by haemoglobin is not linear, because the addition of each O_2 molecule facilitates the uptake of the next O_2 molecule. This produces a sigmoid shaped oxygen dissociation curve (Figure 5.5). Furthermore, because haemoglobin is 97·5% saturated at a PaO_2 of 100 mm Hg (13·4 kPa) (i.e. that found in the normal healthy state), increasing the PaO_2 further has little effect on oxygen transport.

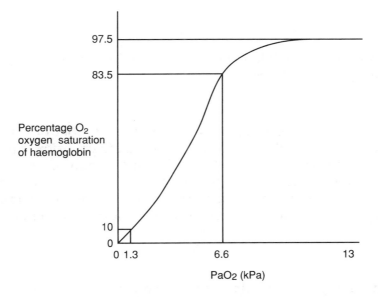

Figure 5.5   Percentage of oxygen saturation of haemoglobin

The affinity of haemoglobin for oxygen at a particular PO_2 (commonly known as the O_2–Hb association) is also affected by other factors. A decreased affinity means that oxygen is more readily released. Thus the oxygen dissociation curve is shifted to the right. This is caused by:

- ↑ hydrogen ion concentration (fall in pH)
- ↑ $PaCO_2$
- ↑ concentration of red cell 2,3-diphosphoglycerate (2,3-DPG)
- ↑ temperature.

(The opposite of these factors increases the affinity and these will be discussed later.)

The normal haemoglobin concentration (as measured by the haematocrit) is usually just above the point at which the oxygen transportation is optimal. Consequently a slight fall in haemoglobin concentration will actually increase oxygen transportation by decreasing blood viscosity.

In addition to the oxygen combined with haemoglobin, there is also a smaller amount dissolved in plasma. This amount is directly proportional to the PaO_2 and is approximately 0·003 ml/100 ml blood/mm Hg of PaO_2.

It follows from the description above that the total content of oxygen in blood is equal to the oxygen associated with haemoglobin and that dissolved in plasma.

$$\text{Oxygen blood concentration} = (\text{Hb} \times 1{\cdot}34 \times \text{saturation}) + (0{\cdot}003 \times PaO_2)$$

For example, in arterial blood with a haemoglobin content of 15 g and a PaO_2 of 100 mm Hg the oxygen content would be:

$$(15 \times 1{\cdot}34 \times 97{\cdot}5\%) + (0{\cdot}003 \times 100) = 19{\cdot}8 \text{ ml/100 ml}$$

Alternatively, in venous blood with a haemoglobin content of 15 g and a PaO_2 of 40 mm Hg the oxygen content would be:

$$(15 \times 1{\cdot}34 \times 75\%) + (0{\cdot}003 \times 40) = 15{\cdot}2 \text{ ml/100 ml}$$

Airway

This has been described in detail in Chapter 4. The following summary contains the relevant facts relating to the breathless patient.

Assessment

Most breathless patients will have a patent airway. The number of words said with each breath is a useful indicator of illness severity and the effects of treatment. If the patient can count to 10 in one breath, then the underlying condition is unlikely to warrant immediate intervention. Occasionally, however, the patient will be severely distressed with stridor, possibly coughing and making enormous but ineffectual respiratory efforts. Stridor is a sinister sign and should be regarded as indicating impending airway obstruction.

Resuscitation

High flow oxygen ($FiO_2 = 0{\cdot}85$) may relieve some of the patient's distress. If airway obstruction is suspected, immediate review by an anaesthetist is required. If, however, further history is forthcoming that a foreign body has been inhaled then a Heimlich or modified Heimlich manoeuvre should be attempted. In contrast, if the patient has a respiratory arrest then examine the larynx with a laryngoscope and remove any identifiable foreign body. If this is impossible proceed to needle cricothyroidotomy and jet insufflation followed by formal cricothyroidotomy.

Breathing

Assessment
This is summarised in the box.

Summary of breathing assessment

- **Look**   colour, sweating
  posture
  respiratory rate, effort
  symmetry
- **Feel**   tracheal position
  tracheal tug
  chest expansion
- **Percuss**
- **Listen**

The immediately life threatening conditions were identified in the primary assessment of breathing earlier.

Specific clinical features
By the time "B" is assessed all breathless patients should have received high flow oxygen (FiO_2 = 0·85 at 15 l/min). Do not be concerned about patients who retain CO_2. Providing that FiO_2 equals 0·85, a rise in $PaCO_2$ will not increase mortality – but untreated hypoxaema will! After the primary assessment has been completed then the FiO_2 can be titrated according to the arterial blood gas results or the pulse oximeter reading.

A hyperinflated chest is indicative of asthma or chronic airflow limitation (COPD). In an acute exacerbation of these conditions the trachea moves downwards during inspiration. This is referred to as tracheal tug and implies airway obstruction or increased respiratory effort. In addition, the internal jugular pressure may be elevated and accessory muscle use will be prominent, as will intercostal recession over the lower part of the chest during inspiration. Patients often adopt a seated or standing posture to facilitate respiration.

Although bronchospasm is common to both asthma and COPD, in acute asthma the inspiratory phase is snatched and expiration is prolonged. With chronic airflow limitation, however, the clinical picture ranges widely from a patient with preserved respiratory drive with pursed-lip breathing to one who is cyanosed, lethargic, and mildly dyspnoeic. Wheezes may be heard on inspiration, but especially on expiration.

Acute pulmonary oedema can mimic or coexist with either of these conditions. The commonest cause of pulmonary oedema is left ventricular failure associated with ischaemic heart disease. Although these are many other causes, these will be seen only occasionally in most hospitals.

An idea of the "chance" of meeting such a condition is displayed on an arbitrary scale in the box.

Causes of acute pulmonary oedema and "chance" of meeting the condition*

Cause	Chance
Ischaemic heart disease	Daily
Myocardial infarction	
Cardiac dysrhythmias	
Fluid overload	Weekly
Severe hypertension	
Aortic stenosis/regurgitation	Monthly
Mitral stenosis/regurgitation	
Cardiomyopathy	
Non-cardiac	
Left ventricular aneurysm	Annually
Infective endocarditis	
Cardiac tamponade	
Left atrial myxoma	Only in examinations

---

* Patients with some of the more common causes of pulmonary oedema may also feature in examinations.

However, features that would support a diagnosis of pulmonary oedema include absence of both neck vein distension and chest hyperexpansion. In addition, the percussion note is often dull, particularly at the lung bases, and there are usually fine inspiratory crackles on auscultation. Occasionally, signs of a pleural effusion may also be evident.

A deviated trachea (a very late sign) should alert the clinician to the possibility of a tension pneumothorax. Other signs, in particular raised neck veins, a hyperresonant percussion note and absent breath sounds, should be sought on the opposite side to the tracheal deviation.

Resuscitation
Irrespective of the underlying cause of the bronchospasm, treat the patients with nebulised bronchodilators whilst clues to the underlying diagnosis are sought. The clinical features described above will have helped distinguish bronchospasm due to asthma, COPD or pulmonary oedema.

Immediate management of a tension pneumothorax is needle thoracentesis followed by intravenous access and then chest drain insertion.

TIME OUT 5.1

a   Define (i) tidal volume
               (ii) minute volume

b(i)   How does the respiratory rate affect alveolar ventilation?

b(ii) Sketch a graph showing the relationship between PaO_2 and % SaO_2.

c   List the immediately life threatening conditions that affect "B".

SUMMARY

Breathing is rapidly assessed using the look, feel, percuss, and listen sequence to identify life threatening:

- bronchospasm
- pulmonary oedema
- tension pneumothorax.

CHAPTER

6

Circulation assessment

OBJECTIVES

After reading this chapter you will be able to:

- understand the physiology of tissue perfusion
- describe a structured approach to circulatory assessment
- identify the immediately life threatening causes of shock
- identify the anatomy for peripheral and central venous cannulation.

INTRODUCTION

The immediately life threatening ones are shown in the box. Clinical features are used to assess circulation that can be affected by a variety of conditions.

Immediately life threatening conditions

Airway
- Obstruction

Breathing
- Acute severe asthma
- Acute exacerbation of chronic obstructive pulmonary disease (COPD)
- Pulmonary pneumothorax
- Tension oedema

Circulation
- Shock

Therefore it is important to understand the mechanisms that maintain tissue perfusion in health before considering the effects of disrupting the circulation.

Relevant physiology

Blood flow to the tissues

The amount of blood reaching a particular organ depends on several factors:

- venous system
- cardiac output
- arterial system
- organ autoregulation.

Venous system

This is capable of acting as a reservoir for over 70% of the circulating blood volume and is therefore often referred to as a **capacitance system**. The amount of blood stored at any one time depends on the size of the vessel lumen. This is controlled by sympathetic innervation and local factors (see later) which can alter the tone of the vessel walls. If the veins dilate, more blood remains in the venous system and less returns to the heart. Should there be a requirement to increase venous return, sympathetic stimulation reduces the diameter of the veins and hence the capacity of the venous system. A change from minimal to maximal tone can increase the venous return by approximately one litre in an adult.

Cardiac output

This is defined as the volume of blood ejected by each ventricle per minute. Clearly, over a period of time, the output of the two ventricles must be the same (or else all the circulating volume would eventually end up in either the systemic or pulmonary circulation). Thus, the cardiac output equates to the volume of blood ejected with each beat (stroke volume in ml) multiplied by the heart rate (beats per minute) and is expressed in litres per minute.

$$\text{Cardiac output} = \text{stroke volume} \times \text{heart rate} = 4\text{--}6 \text{ l/min (normal adult)}$$

To allow a comparison between patients of different sizes, the cardiac index (CI) is used. This is the cardiac output divided by the surface area of the person and hence is measured in litres per square metre.

$$\text{Cardiac index} = \text{cardiac output/body surface area} = 2 \cdot 8\text{--}4 \cdot 2 \text{ l/min/m}^2 \text{ (normal adult)}$$

The cardiac output can be affected by:

- preload
- myocardial contractility
- afterload
- heart rate.

Preload This is the volume of blood in the ventricle at the end of diastole. The left ventricular end diastolic volume (LVEDV) is about 140 ml and the stroke volume (SV) is 90 ml. Therefore the end systolic volume is approximately 50 ml and the left ventricular ejection fraction (SV/EDV) ranges from 50 to 70%.

During diastole, the cardiac muscle fibres are progressively stretched as the ventricular volume increases in proportion to the venous return. Remember that **the more the myocardial fibres are stretched during diastole, the more forcibly they contract during systole; hence more blood will be expelled** (Starling's Law). Therefore, the greater the preload, the greater the stroke volume. However, this phenomenon has an upper limit (due to the internal molecular structure of muscle cells) so that if the muscle is stretched beyond this point then a smaller contraction is produced.

Thus, the end diastolic fibre length is proportional to the end diastolic volume or force distending the ventricle. A clinical estimate of this volume, or force, is the end diastolic pressure (EDP). As the ventricular end diastolic pressure (LVEDP) increases so does the stroke volume. If the end diastolic pressure exceeds a critical level then the force of contraction declines and eventually ventricular failure ensues (Figure 6.1).

Current haemodynamic monitoring is based upon measurements from a pulmonary artery flotation catheter (PAFC). A commonly used recording is the pulmonary artery occlusion pressure (PAOP) because it is considered a useful estimate of the left ventricular end diastolic pressure.

Myocardial contractility This is the rate at which the myocardial fibres contract for a given degree of stretch. Substances affecting myocardial contractility are termed **inotropes**, and they can be positive or negative in their actions. A positive inotrope produces a greater contraction for a given length (or EDP clinically) (Figure 6.1). Adrenaline, noradrenaline and dopamine are naturally produced substances which have this effect. Dobutamine is a synthetic catecholamine with positive inotropic activity. Therefore, depending on where you work, you may find some (or all) of these agents are used to treat cardiogenic and septic shock.

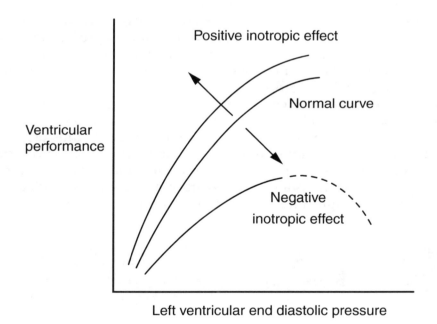

Figure 6.1 *Ventricular performance*

Negative inotropes reduce contractility for a given muscle length (Figure 6.1). These substances are often drugs, for example, antiarrhythmics and anaesthetic agents. Many of the physiological states produced by shock will also depress contractility, for example, hypoxia, acidosis, and sepsis. Myocardial damage also has a negative inotropic effect.

Afterload As the left and right ventricular muscle contracts, pressures within the chambers increase until they exceed those in the aorta and pulmonary artery, respectively. The

53

aortic and pulmonary valves open and the blood is ejected. The resistance faced by the ventricular myocardium during ejection is termed the afterload. In the left ventricle this is mainly due to the resistance offered by the aortic valve and the compliance (stiffness) of the arterial blood vessels. Usually this latter component is the most important and is estimated by measuring the **systemic vascular resistance** (SVR).

Using Ohm's law where resistance equals pressure divided by flow, the systemic vascular resistance is defined as the mean arterial and venous pressure difference divided by the cardiac output.

$$\text{(mean arterial pressure} - \text{central venous pressure)} \times 80/\text{cardiac output} = 770 - 1500 \text{ dyn/s/cm}^5 \text{ (normal adult)}$$

(The value of 80 comes from converting mm Hg to SI units.)

> **Key point**
> Reducing the afterload for a given preload will allow the myocardial fibres to shorten more quickly and by a greater amount. It therefore increases the stroke volume and cardiac output

Heart rate   An increase in heart rate is mediated via β_1 adrenoreceptors. These can be stimulated by the sympathetic nervous system (SNS), the release of catecholamines from the adrenal medulla and drugs (e.g. Isoprenaline). This is termed a **positive chronotropic effect**. Conversely, the parasympathetic nervous system (PSNS) supplies the sino-atrial node and atrioventricular node via the vagus nerve. Stimulation of the PSNS decreases heart rate, i.e. it has a **negative chronotropic effect**. This effect can also be produced by drugs that inhibit the sympathetic nervous system such as β blockers. In contrast, an increased heart rate may follow inhibition of the parasympathetic nervous system muscarinic (M) receptors.

An increase in heart rate can lead to an increase in cardiac output (see equation earlier). However, ventricular filling occurs during diastole and this phase of the cardiac cycle is predominantly shortened as the heart rate increases. A sinus tachycardia, above 160 beats/minute in the young adult, drastically reduces the time for ventricular filling. This leads to a progressively smaller stroke volume and a fall in cardiac output. The critical heart rate when this occurs is also dependent on the age of the patient and the condition of the heart; for example, rates over 120 beats/minute may cause inadequate filling in the elderly.

> **Key point**
> Increasing the heart rate will only lead to rise in the cardiac output if the rate is below a critical level

The main factors affecting the cardiac output of the left ventricle are summarised in the box.

> **Main factors affecting cardiac output**
>
> - Preload, or left ventricular end diastolic volume
> - Myocardial contractility
> - Afterload, or systemic vascular resistance
> - Heart rate

The arterial system

The walls of the aorta and other large arteries contain relatively large amounts of elastic tissue that stretches during systole and recoils during diastole. In contrast, the walls of arterioles contain relatively more smooth muscle. This is innervated by the sympathetic nervous system that maintains vasomotor tone to a large extent. Stimulation of α adrenoreceptors causes vasoconstriction. Therefore, a total loss of arterial tone would increase the capacity of the circulatory system so much that the total blood volume would be insufficient to fill it. As a consequence, the blood pressure would fall and the flow through organs would depend upon their resistance. Some organs would receive more than normal amounts of oxygenated blood (e.g. skin) at the expense of others which would receive less (e.g. brain). To prevent this, the arterial system is under constant control by sympathetic innervation and local factors to ensure that blood goes where it is needed most. This is exemplified in the shocked patient where differential vasoconstriction maintains supply to the vital organs (e.g. heart) at the expense of others (e.g. skin). Hence the skin is cold and pale.

Blood volume

- Adult male = 70 ml per kilogram ideal body weight
- Adult female = 60 ml per kilogram ideal body weight

Systemic arterial blood pressure

This is the pressure exerted on the walls of the arterial blood vessels. Systolic pressure is the maximal pressure generated in the large arteries during each cardiac cycle. In contrast the diastolic pressure is the minimum. The difference between them is the pulse pressure. The **mean arterial pressure** is the average pressure during the cardiac cycle and is approximately equal to the diastolic pressure plus one third of the pulse pressure. As the mean arterial pressure is the product of the cardiac output and the systemic vascular resistance, it is affected by all the factors already discussed.

Autoregulation

Organs have a limited ability to regulate their own blood supply so that perfusion is maintained as blood pressure varies. This process is known as autoregulation and is brought about by the presence of smooth muscle in the arteriolar walls. By altering the calibre of the vessels, flow to the organs is maintained. Furthermore, other local factors, such as products of anaerobic metabolism, acidosis and a rise in temperature, all cause the local vascular tree to dilate. Such effects enable active tissues to receive increased quantities of nutrients and oxygenated blood.

PRIMARY ASSESSMENT AND RESUSCITATION

A summary of the circulatory assessment is shown in the box.

> **Summary of circulatory assessment**
>
> - **Look**: pallor, sweating, venous pressure
> - **Feel**: pulse – rate, rhythm, and character
>   capillary refill time
>   blood pressure
>   apex beat
> - **Listen**: heart sounds, extra sounds

The aim of this brief assessment is to identify the patient who is shocked. This is a clinical syndrome resulting from inadequate delivery, or use, of essential substrates (e.g. oxygen) by vital organs. The causes of shock are described in detail in Chapter 11 and summarised in the next box.

> **Causes of shock**
>
> | | | |
> |---|---|---|
> | Preload reduction | – hypovolaemia | – haemorrhage |
> | | | – diarrhoea |
> | | – impaired return | – pregnancy |
> | | | – severe asthma |
> | Pump failure | – endocardial | – acute valve lesion |
> | | – myocardial | – infarction |
> | | | – inflammation |
> | | – epicardial | – tamponade |
> | Post (after) load reduction | – vasodilation | – sepsis |
> | | | – anaphylaxis |

Specific clinical features

All patients with respiratory distress will have a tachycardia as described in the previous chapter. With severe airways obstruction, however, pulsus paradoxus may be present. Normally there is a reduction in systolic blood pressure of up to 10 mm Hg on inspiration. This is attributed to a fall in intrathoracic pressure (i.e. it becomes more negative on inspiration) which enlarges the pulmonary vascular bed and reduces return of blood to the left ventricle. There is partial compensation by a simultaneous increase in right ventricular output. In severe asthma and COPD there is a more substantial fall in intrathoracic pressure on inspiration. This greatly increases the capacity of the pulmonary vascular bed that in turn reduces output from the left ventricle, resulting in pulsus paradoxus. This is an exaggeration of the **normal** systolic fall on inspiration and not a paradoxical change in the pulse as the name would imply. The abnormality is the extent by which the arterial pressure falls. If severe, the pulse may disappear on inspiration and this can easily be palpated at the radial artery. In contrast, if the fall in systolic pressure is not so marked, it can be detected using the sphygmomanometer. This physical sign indicates critical circulatory embarrassment and can also occur in patients with cardiac tamponade.

Another pulse abnormality is pulsus alternans where evenly spaced beats (in time) are alternately large and small in volume. As this can indicate left ventricular failure the clinician should check for corroborative signs such as a displaced apex beat, a third heart sound and a pansystolic murmur of mitral regurgitation. A third heart sound in patients over 40 years usually indicates elevated ventricular end diastolic pressure. With increasing age, the myocardium and associated valvular structures become less compliant, i.e. stiffer. Thus, an increase in end diastolic pressure is needed to ensure adequate ventricular filling during which sudden tension in these structures generates vibrations which correspond to the third heart sound.

Shock associated with a dysrhythmia is due to either pulmonary oedema or hypotension or a combination of these conditions. Under these circumstances tachy-dysrhythmias, irrespective of the QRS complex width, will require cardioversion (see Chapter 31). Unfortunately, atrial fibrillation may either fail to cardiovert (especially when chronic) or only transiently return to sinus rhythm. The remaining options include:

- chemical cardioversion. Of the many potential drugs available, intravenous amiodarone is well tolerated. Flecainide is an excellent alternative, but has been shown to increase mortality in patients with ischaemic heart disease.
- control the ventricular response with intravenous digoxin.

In contrast, a patient with a bradydysrhythmia may require temporary support with either atropine and an inotrope (e.g. isoprenaline) or external pacing whilst preparations are made for transvenous pacing (see Chapter 9 on Shock for further details).

Hypovolaemia, commonly due to blood loss, can present with tachypnoea and a variety of other physical signs including tachycardia, hypotension and reduced urine output.

The remaining two immediately life threatening causes of breathlessness are pulmonary embolus and cardiac tamponade. The size and position of the embolus will determine the haemodynamic effects. Non-fatal emboli blocking the major branches of the pulmonary artery (PA) provoke a rise in PA pressure due to hypoxia and vasoconstriction. In addition, tachypnoea follows stimulation of alveolar and capillary receptors. An acute increase in pulmonary vascular resistance and hence right ventricular afterload causes a sudden rise in end diastolic pressure and dilatation of the right ventricle. This produces a raised jugular venous pressure, a fall in systemic arterial pressure and a compensatory tachycardia.

The signs of cardiac tamponade include pulsus paradoxus, raised internal jugular venous pressure that increases on inspiration (the opposite of normal; Kussmaul's sign), and an impalpable apex beat. As fluid accumulates, the elevated pressure in the pericardial sac is raised further during inspiration (this may be related to the downward displacement of the diaphragm). A corresponding increase is seen in the right atrial and central venous pressures. In contrast, pressures on the left side of the heart may be lower than that in the pericardium. As a consequence, filling of the left ventricle is compromised, stroke volume is reduced and the interventricular septum bulges into the left ventricular cavity. Thus, the stroke volume of the right ventricle is maintained at the expense of the left ventricle which collapses on inspiration. With further increases in pericardial pressure there is diastolic collapse of the right atrium and ventricle. The venous pressure is always raised and is due to abnormal right heart filling. Kussmaul's sign can also be seen in right ventricular disease and pulmonary hypertension.

Treatment

All patients should receive high flow oxygen and have their oxygen saturation, pulse, blood pressure, and cardiac rhythm monitored. Intravenous access is needed and at least one large venflon (12–14 gauge) is required in the antecubital fossa.

Hypovolaemia

In acute hypovolaemia a fluid challenge can then be given whilst the cause, usually haemorrhage, is sought (see Chapter 9). In contrast, chronic fluid depletion often presents as dehydration with features of acute renal impairment. Oxygen and careful fluid replacement are required, especially in patients with preexisting cardiac conditions. Diuretics and angiotensin converting enzyme (ACE) inhibitors are a common cause of this problem in patients with a history of left ventricular failure. These drugs should be stopped and fluid replacement titrated against the patient's clinical condition and central venous pressure.

Acute severe left ventricular failure

The blood pressure is probably the most important feature in determining treatment. The combination of acute pulmonary oedema and hypotension demands inotropic support. Any patient who has a systolic pressure of **less** than 90 mm Hg should **not** be given diuretics, nitrates or opiates as their immediate action is to cause venodilatation. This, in turn, will reduce the cardiac preload and potentially exacerbate hypotension.

Dysrhythmia – tachycardia

The presence of a tachydysrhythmia in the shocked or compromised patient necessitates electrical cardioversion (see Chapter 28). If this fails then drug treatment according to UK and European resuscitation committee guidelines is advocated (Figure 6.2). Remember that a sinus tachycardia can be the response of a failing ventricle. However, if the patient has another baseline rhythm such as atrial fibrillation, the increased sympathetic drive would result in atrial fibrillation with a rapid ventricular response. It can be difficult to decide whether a dysrhythmia is the cause of heart failure or vice versa. Previous ECGs are invaluable in this circumstance. If no such information is available the treatment is dictated by the clinician's judgement. The following key points can help in this dilemma.

- A supraventricular tachycardia with a ventricular response of less than 150 is unlikely to cause failure.
- A broad complex tachycardia is almost always ventricular in a patient with ischaemic heart disease.

TIME OUT 6.1

Ensure that you have a sound understanding of this protocol (Figure 6.2). If necessary take five minutes and copy the tachydysrhythmia management flow diagram to reinforce your knowledge.

Dysrhythmia – bradycardia

This is treated according to UK and European resuscitation committee guidelines (Figure 6.3).

TIME OUT 6.2

In a patient with a bradycardia, what are the risk factors for asystole?
If you cannot answer this question copy the bradycardia management flow diagram (Figure 6.3) to reinforce your knowledge.

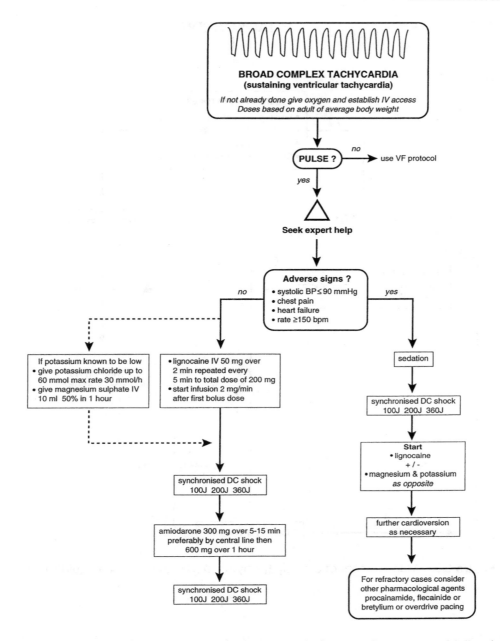

Figure 6.2 Management of a tachydysrhythmia (UK and European guidelines)

Pulmonary embolus

The minimum immediate management comprises high flow oxygen and anticoagulation. More comprehensive treatment details are provided in Chapter 10.

Cardiac tamponade

If this diagnosis is suspected clinically, then intravenous fluid should be administered to raise the end diastolic pressure and volume in order to maintain the cardiac output. This is only a temporising procedure and immediate cardiological referral is required for echocardiography and pericardiocentesis.

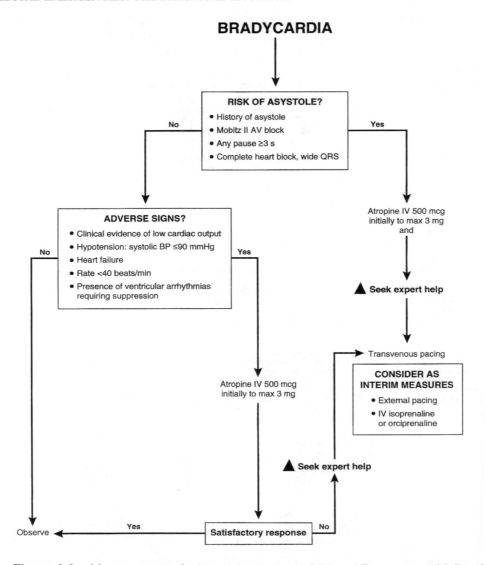

Figure 6.3   Management of a bradydysrhythmia (UK and European guidelines)

Investigations

Appropriate investigations at this stage include:

- a full blood count to exclude anaemia (possibly exacerbating left ventricular failure)
- urea and electrolytes for baseline values particularly in patients who are being treated with vasodilators, diuretics or inotropes
- cardiac enzymes
- arterial blood gases
- 12 lead ECG
- portable chest X-ray.

Key point
If the patient is still breathless and the cause remains in doubt a rapid reevaluation A, B and C is required
It is important to remember that hypovolaemia is an important cause of breathlessness

Once the patient's condition is stabilised then further information can be obtained from the secondary assessment.

TIME OUT 6.3

List the major causes of shock.

Summary

In the primary assessment, the immediately life threatening problems are:

- airway   obstruction
- breathing   acute severe asthma
  acute exacerbation of COPD
  pulmonary oedema
  tension pneumothorax
- circulation   shock

These conditions can be identified and differentiated clinically.
All patients require oxygen and intravenous access.

PERIPHERAL VENOUS CANNULATION

The antecubital fossa is the commonest site for peripheral venous cannulation.

The cephalic vein passes through the antecubital fossa on the lateral side and the basilic vein enters very medially just in front of the medial epicondyle of the elbow. These two large veins are joined by the **median cubital or antecubital vein**. The median vein of the forearm also drains into the basilic vein (Figure 6.4).

Although the veins in this area are prominent and easily cannulated, there are many other adjacent vital structures which can be easily damaged.

The most popular device for peripheral intravenous access is the cannula over needle, available in a wide variety of sizes, 12–27 gauge (g). It consists of a plastic (PTFE or similar material) cannula which is mounted on a smaller diameter metal needle, the bevel of which protrudes from the cannula. The other end of the needle is attached to a transparent "flashback chamber", which fills with blood indicating that the **needle** bevel lies within the vein. Some devices have flanges or "wings" to facilitate attachment to the skin. All cannulae have a standard luer-lock fitting to attach a giving set and some have a valved injection port attached through which drugs can be given.

Complications

- Failed cannulation is the most common, usually as a result of pushing the needle completely through the vein. It is inversely related to experience.
- Haematomata are usually secondary to the above with inadequate pressure applied to prevent blood leaking from the vein after the cannula is removed. They are made worse by forgetting to remove the tourniquet!
- Extravasation of fluid or drugs is commonly a result of failing to recognise that the cannula is not in the vein before use. Placing a cannula over a joint or prolonged use to infuse fluids under pressure also predisposes to leakage. The faulty cannula must be removed. Damage to the surrounding tissues will depend primarily on the nature of the extravasated fluid.

- Damage to other local structures is secondary to poor technique and lack of knowledge of the local anatomy.
- The plastic cannula can be sheared, allowing fragments to enter the circulation. This is usually a result of trying to reintroduce the needle after it has been withdrawn. The safest action is to withdraw the whole cannula and attempt cannulation at another site with a new cannula.
- The needle may fracture as a result of careless excessive manipulation with the finer cannulae. The fragment will have to be removed surgically.
- Inflammation of the vein (thrombophlebitis) is related to the length of time the vein is cannulated and the irritation caused by the substances flowing through it. High concentrations of drugs and fluids with extremes of pH or high osmolality are the main causes. Once a vein shows signs of thrombophlebitis, i.e., tender, red, and the flow rate is deteriorating, the cannula must be removed to prevent subsequent infection or thrombosis which may spread proximally.

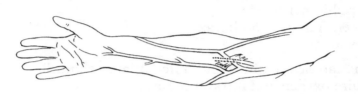

Figure 6.4   Veins of the forearm and antecubital fossa

SUMMARY

- Shock is the immediately life threatening condition diagnosed at the "circulation" assessment.
- A systematic A, B, C assessment is necessary for the treatment of shock.

CHAPTER

7

Disability assessment

OBJECTIVES

After reading this chapter you will be able to:

- describe the neurological examination in both the primary and secondary assessment phases.

PRIMARY NEUROLOGICAL ASSESSMENT

This is the D component as described in Chapter 3. This brief examination comprises:

- pupil size and response to light
- Glasgow Coma Scale.

SECONDARY NEUROLOGICAL ASSESSMENT

The most important component of the neurological examination is the history and this will follow the normal "phrased" format (see Chapter 3). Particular attention should be directed at the key features shown in the box.

Key neurological features

- Define the problem
- Describe the deficit
- Determine the   onset
                                    pattern
                                    extent and duration
- Associated symptoms   neurological
                                    other

A comprehensive neurological assessment is not required and so a screening examination will suffice. The components are listed in the box.

Components of the screening examination

- Higher mental function
- Speech
- Pupil response
- Visual fields
- Fundoscopy
- Eye movement
- Facial sensation
- Facial movement
- Movement of mouth, tongue and palate
- Motor:
  look for wasting and fasciculation
  test tone
  power
  reflexes
  coordination
- Sensation
  light touch and pin prick test

Often higher function and speech are assessed whilst taking the patient's history. Particular abnormalities that influence speech are shown in the box.

Important abnormalities affecting speech

- Deafness
- Dysphasia
- Dysarthria
- Dysphonia

The "four Ds" of speech can be easily assessed by remembering the following four questions.

Can the patient hear, understand, articulate, and vocalise?

Lack of comprehension as well as failure of thought or word generation implies a dysphasia, of which there are two major types. Expressive or motor aphasia is where the patient can understand either verbal or written information but has aphasia or non-fluent speech. In contrast poor comprehension and occasionally meaningless speech indicates receptive or sensory aphasia. These conditions are often referred to as Broca's or Wernicke's dysphasia and occur predominantly in the dominant hemisphere.

Broca's dysphasia is usually a lesion in Broca's area in the inferior frontal gyrus that can be associated with a hemiplegia. In contrast Wernicke's area (upper part of the temporal lobe and supramarginal gyrus of the parietal lobe) is often associated with a visual field defect. Total aphasia is a lesion of the dominant hemisphere that affects both Broca's and Wernicke's areas.

> **Key points in assessing aphasia**
>
> - Establish whether the patient is right or left handed
> - Discover the first language
> - Ask the patient simple questions initially with "yes/no" answers
> - Increase complexity of questions with simple commands such as "touch your right ear with your left index finger"
> - Always ensure that the patient has understood your instructions

Dysarthria is a failure of articulation that normally requires the coordination of breathing with movement of the vocal cords, larynx, tongue, palate, and lips. When taking the history listen for slurring and the rhythm of speech along with the words or sounds which cause the greatest difficulty.

> **Types of dysarthria**
>
> - Spastic – slurred, like "Donald Duck" speech
> - Extrapyramidal – slurred and monotonous, e.g., in Parkinson's disease
> - Cerebellar – slurred, disjointed, scanning or staccato (equal emphasis on each syllable) seen in alcohol intoxication and disseminated sclerosis

Lower motor neurone lesions affecting speech include:

- facial (VII) – difficulty with the letters P, B, M, and W
- palate (IX) – nasal speech (like nasal congestion)
- tongue (XII) – distorted speech with difficulty with T, S and D.

Dysphonia is a disturbance of voice production that may indicate laryngopharyngeal pathology or an abnormality of the vagus. Dysphonia is really not formally assessed unless the patient is unable to produce a normal volume of sound or speaks in a whisper.

Higher mental function tests

Whilst the clinical assessment of higher mental function is necessary for a comprehensive neurological examination, a full examination is rarely done in the first 24 hours of admission. A brief assessment of the Mini Mental State Examination, as described in Chapter 3, will often suffice.

When to test higher mental function?
Usually when a doctor is suspicious that there is an underlying abnormality or occasionally if a concern is expressed by the patient or, more particularly, the family.

How to test?
Explain that you are going to ask a few questions and ask the patient to perform some tests. Whilst these may seem very simple they yield extremely valuable results. The tests should not be regarded as condescending or derogatory.

Why test?
To provide some evidence that will facilitate differentiation of global and focal neurological disorders.

What to test?

There are many ways of assessing the mental state. A variation is shown in the box. The total score is out of 30 and cognitive impairment is defined as a score of less than 23.

Formal assessment of mini mental state

Orientation – time, date, day, month, year	Maximum score 5
Name of ward, hospital, district, town or country	Maximum score 5
Registration, ask the patient to name three objects	Maximum score 3
Patient to repeat the names of the three objects in the above test after five minutes	Maximum score 3
Attention can be assessed using the serial 7s or the 1 tap–2 tap test (an explanation of this test is given in Chapter 20)	Maximum score 5
Language – name two objects	Maximum score 2
Repeat a sentence	Maximum score 1
Three stage command	Score 3
Write command and see if the patient obeys correctly	Maximum score 1
Ask the patient to write a sentence which includes a verb	Maximum score 1
Draw diagram and ask the patient to copy	Maximum score 1

This is quite a comprehensive test and a quick overview can be obtained by assessing the patient's orientation, memory, ability to calculate, assess abstract thought and perception.

- Orientation — Time, place, person.
- Memory — *Short term.* Give the patient an address that is familiar to you and ask them to repeat it. Repeat the test after a further five minutes. Also note the number of attempts before the patient has repeated the address correctly.
  Long term. This will depend upon the patient's age, culture, and background, but questions related to things such as World War dates or important sporting events will often suffice.
- Calculation — Serial 7s or doubling 3s.
- Abstract thought — Interpretation of proverbs.
- Perception — *Spatial.* Ask the patient to draw a clock face and add the numbers and hands at a given time or ask the patient to draw a five pointed star.
  Body. Ask the patient to follow instructions such as to touch their left ear with their right index finger or to close their eyes and identify either an object in their palm (stereognosis) or numbers drawn on their palm (graphaesthesia).

These simple tests provide valuable information that can be interpreted as follows:

Orientation impaired	Acute – confusion
	Chronic – dementia
Memory impairment	Short term – (alert patient) lesion, encephalopathy, temporal lobe, Korsakoff's psychosis
	Long term – encephalopathy or dementia
	Solely – encephalopathy
Calculation impaired	With finger and left/right agnosia, astereognosis and dysgraphaesthesia – dominant parietal lobe lesion
Abstract thought interpretation impaired	Encephalopathy
Perception impaired	Spatial – parietal lobe lesion
	Body – parietal lobe lesion

Summary

Interpretation of higher mental functions can provide evidence of diffuse abnormalities, as found with encephalopathy or dementia, or focal lesions, for example stroke, neoplasm or abscess.

Pupil response

Check the pupils for symmetry and reaction to both light and accommodation.

Remember that the afferent pathway for light reaction is the optic nerve whilst the efferent pathway is the parasympathetic component of the third nerve. In contrast the accommodation reaction afferent pathway arises with the frontal lobe but the efferent pathway remains the parasympathetic component of the third nerve bilaterally.

A summary of pupillary abnormalities is given in the box.

	Pupillary response	**Cause**
Equal pupils	– small + reactive	– metabolic encephalopathy
		– midbrain herniation
	– pinpoint + fixed	– pontine lesion
		– opioids, organophosphates
	– dilated + reactive	– metabolic cause
		– midbrain lesion
		– ecstacy, amphetamines
	– dilated + fixed	– peri ictan
		– hypoxaemia
		– hypothermia
		– anticholinergics
Unequal pupils	– small + reactive	– Horner's syndrome
	– dilated + fixed	– uncal herniation
		– IIIrd nerve palsy

Visual fields

These should be tested to confrontation which will identify any gross field defects. Central vision is colour (cones) whilst peripheral is monochrome (rods). Thus a white hat pin should be used to provide further detail of peripheral fields defects. In contrast, red pins should be used to investigate defects of central vision.

Key points when assessing visual fields

- Screen for gross defects using finger movements
- Ensure that the patient cannot see either your finger or the pin before it is brought into the field of vision
- Slowly bring your finger or pin in a smooth arc to finish an equal distance between your eye and the patient's eye
- Ensure that the patient continues to look directly into your eye

The visual pathway with associated lesions is demonstrated in Figures 7.1 and 7.2.

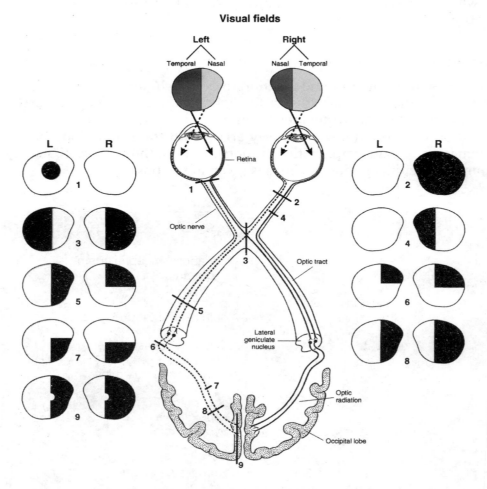

Figure 7.1 Visual pathway with associated lesions

Interpretation

Monocular defects   These usually indicate ocular, retinal or optic nerve pathology.

Key point

In monocular blindness due to a complete lesion of the optic nerve, the direct pupillary response to light is lost but the consensual response is retained.

- Tunnel vision –the size of the constricted field remains the same irrespective of the distance of the test object from the eye – usually hysterical.
- Constricted field –the field is reduced but is less marked as the object moves away from the eye; seen with chronic papilloedema or glaucoma.
- Scotoma – a hole in the visual field, disseminated sclerosis or neuropathy (toxic or ischaemic), retinal haemorrhage/infarct.

Binocular defects   These indicate a lesion at or behind the optic chiasm or very rarely bilateral lesions in front of the chiasm.

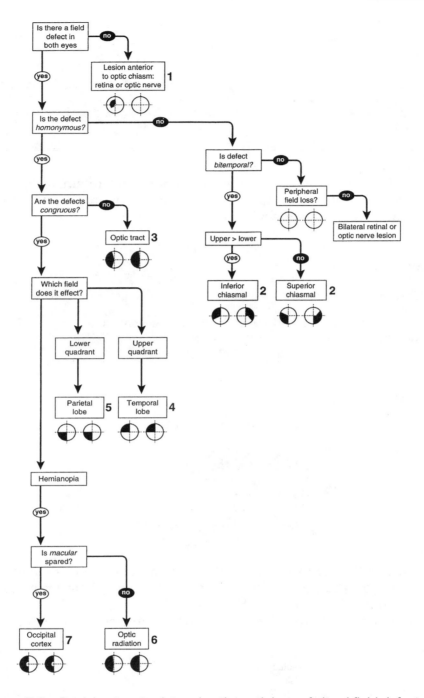

Figure 7.2 Decision tree to determine the aetiology of visual field defects.

- Homonymous hemianopia – a lesion anywhere along the optic tract including the occipital cortex where macular sparing may be evident.
- Homonymous quanorantanopia – upper = temporal lobe lesion
  – lower = parietal lobe lesion.
- Bitemporal hemianopia – indicates a chiasmal lesion, usually a pituitary adenoma.

Fundoscopy

It is important to have a system when examining the fundus. Key features are shown in the box.

Key features when examining the eye

- Optic disc – colour, cup, and margins
- Blood vessels – arteries, arteriovenous junctions, vascular patterns. Remember that arteries are approximately two thirds the diameter of veins
- Background – follow the four groups of vessels from the disc and examine each quadrant systematically

Papilloedema is often sought. Usually the patient will retain normal vision but the optic disc will appear pink with indistinct margins. It is important to remember that papilloedema can be absent even with raised intracranial pressure.

Causes of papilloedema

- Raised intracranial pressure
- Arterial hypertension
- Raised venous pressure due to obstruction of cerebral venous drainage
- Others including hypercarbia and severe anaemia

Eye movement

There are three control centres for eye movement.

Control centres for eye movement

- Frontal lobe – command
- Occipital lobe – pursuit
- Cerebellar/vestibular nuclei – positional

The pathways from these three key centres are integrated in the brain stem to ensure that the eyes move together. In addition the centre for lateral gaze is within the pons and the medial longitudinal fasciculus (MLF). This links the third, fourth and sixth nerve nucleii and these in turn control the external ocular muscles (see Figure 7.3).

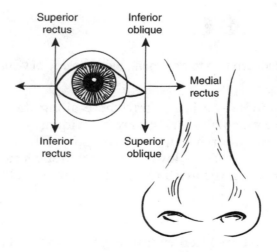

Figure 7.3 External ocular muscles

Nystagmus must also be actively sought.

The commonest form of nystagmus is horizontal and this can be:

- ataxic nystagmus, which is greater in the abducting than the adducting eye and is caused by disseminated sclerosis and cerebral vascular disease
- multidirectional gaze evoked nystagmus which occurs in the direction of gaze, occurring in more than one direction. This is often seen in cerebellar syndromes, associated with drugs, alcohol or disseminated sclerosis
- unidirectional nystagmus, second or third degree horizontal nystagmus usually implies a cerebellar syndrome or central vestibular syndrome
- contrasting vertical horizontal nystagmus may be central or peripheral. If it is the latter it is usually associated with fatigue and vertigo.

Facial sensation

Test for gross deficit using the finger tip in all three divisions of the trigeminal nerve.

Facial movement

After checking for symmetry, ask the patient to whistle, show their teeth, and shut their eyes against resistance.

There are two points to remember: (1) ptosis is not due to a seventh nerve lesion. (2) corneal reflex usually has the ophthalmic branch of the trigeminal nerve as the afferent pathway whilst the efferent pathway uses the seventh nerve. Therefore, when eliciting the corneal reflex, it is important to touch the cornea and not the conjunctiva. Further problems can be incurred if the patient wears contact lenses or if the cotton wool is brought towards the eye as this will act as a threat reflex inducing blinking. In response to corneal stimulation, failure of one side to contract indicates a seventh nerve lesion whilst failure of both sides to contract indicates a lesion affecting the first division of the fifth nerve.

Movement of the mouth, palate, and tongue

Clues to problems in these three areas may have been elicited when testing the integrity of the fifth nerve and the patient's speech.

Common abnormalities are shown in the box.

Abnormalities when examining the mouth

- Small tongue with fasciculation – lower motor neurone lesion
- reduced range of tongue movement – bilateral upper motor neurone lesion often associated with labile emotions and pseudobulbar palsy
- Tongue deviates to one side (with normal bulk) – unilateral upper motor neurone weakness associated with a stroke (common)
- Unilateral wasting or fasciculation of tongue – unilateral lower motor neurone lesion (rare)
- Uvula does not move on saying "ah" or gag – bilateral palatal muscle paresis
- Uvula moves to one side – contralateral upper or lower motor neurone lesion of the vagus nerve

---

Summary

A brief examination of cromal nerves (II to III and IX to XII) will identify abnormalities and guide further examination.

Motor system

Examination of the motor system is designed to detect muscular weakness. The five categories are given in Table 7.1.

Table 7.1   Classification of muscular weakness

Type of weakness	Clinical features
Upper motor neurone lesion (UMN)	Increased tone, increased reflexes, pyramidal pattern of weakness, i.e., weak arm extensors and leg flexors
Lower motor neurone lesion (LMN)	Wasting, fasciculation, decreased tone, absent reflexes
Neuromuscular junction	Fatiguable weakness, normal or decreased tone, normal reflexes
Muscle disease	Wasting, decreased tone, impaired or absent reflexes
Functional weakness	No wasting, normal tone, normal reflexes variable, inconsistent power

Thus the sequence of your examination should include:

- **observation** for wasting, fasciculation, posture
- **tone**. Ensure that the patient is either relaxed or distracted by conversation but remember that telling the patient to relax often has the opposite effect. Common abnormalities in tone are listed in the box.

Common abnormalities in tone

- Increased spasticity – upper neurone lesion
- Increased rigidity, including cogwheel extrapyramidal syndromes, e.g. Parkinson's disease

---

- **Power**. When assessing any component of the nervous system patient cooperation is vital. Instructions such as "pull your foot towards your bottom" can seem complex and difficult to understand, especially when the patient is anxious. It is, therefore, recommended that you not only explain to the patient what you are going to do and what you would like them to do but also show them. This demonstration can save a lot of time and frustration.

Before formally testing power, ask the patient to hold their arms out in front of their chest with palms uppermost and close their eyes. Watch the position of the arms as this will give you a clue as to underlying abnormalities, for example, pyramidal weakness will cause the arm to pronate and drift downwards. Muscular weakness, which may occur bilaterally, may make the arms drift downwards irrespective of whether the patient's eyes are open or closed. With cerebellar disease, the arm may raise spontaneously or a sharp tap on the back of the hand will cause exaggerated displacement with excessive compensatory return and overshoot. Disorders of joint position sense are manifested by the fingers moving up or down or the arm drifting particularly when the eyes are closed.

The key movements to be tested are listed in Table 7.2, along with the muscle and root value and associated nerve.

Table 7.2 Key movement of the upper limbs

Movement	Muscle	Nerve	Root value
Shoulder abduction	Deltoid	Axillary	C5
Elbow flexion	Biceps brachialis	Musculocutaneous	C5 C6
Elbow extension	Triceps	Radial	C6 C7
Finger extension	Extensor digitorum	Posterior interosseous	C7
Finger flexion	Flexor digitorum superficialis and profundus	Median and ulnar	C8
Thumb abduction	Abductor pollicis brevis	Ulnar	T1
Thumb adduction	First dorsal interosseous	Ulnar	T1
Finger adduction	Second palmar interosseous	Ulnar	T1

The radial nerve supplies all the extensors in the arm. The ulnar nerve supplies all the intrinsic hand muscles except for the lateral two lumbricals, opponens policis abductor policis brevis and flexor policis brevis. These muscles are supplied by the median nerve and can often be remembered by the acronym LOAF. Remember that all intrinsic hand muscles are innervated by T1.

Once the muscles in the arms have been tested it is easier to assess power in the legs rather than sensation in the arms. The reason for that will become apparent. The key movements and the appropriate muscles, nerves and root values for the lower limbs are listed in Table 7.3.

Table 7.3 Key movement of the lower limbs

Movement	Muscle	Nerve	Root
Hip flexion	Iliopsoas	Lumbar plexus	L1, 2
Hip extension	Gluteus maximus	Inferior gluteal	L5, S1
Knee extension	Quadriceps femoris	Femoral	L3, 4
Knee flexion	Hamstrings	Sciatic	L5, S1
Foot dorsiflexion	Tibialis anterior	Deep peroneal	L5
Foot plantarflexion	Gastrocnemius	Posterior tibial	S1
Big toe extension	Extensor digitorum longus	Deep peroneal	L5

The root values for each of the previously described movements are summarised in the following box. When testing muscle power always:

- ensure the joint is pain free
- allow the patient to move the joint through the full range before testing power
- compare the strength of right side with left side
- grade your findings according to the MRC scale.

Power grading – MRC scale

5 = normal power
4 = moderate movement against resistance
3 = movement against gravity but not resistance
2 = movement with gravity eliminated
1 = flicker
0 = no movement

- **Reflexes**. Remember that tendon reflexes are increased in upper motor neurone lesions and decreased with abnormalities in lower motor neurones and muscles. Reflexes are graded.

> **Grading reflexes**
>
> 4 = clonus
> 3 = increased
> 2 = normal
> 1 = diminished
> 0 = absent

- When eliciting a tendon reflex first palpate to ensure that the tendon is present and not tender.
- Make sure that the patient is relaxed.
- Use the whole length of the patella hammer and swing through a gentle arc.
- Use reinforcement if a reflex is directly unobtainable. The major reflexes are listed in Table 7.4.

Table 7.4 Major reflexes

Muscle	Nerve	Root
Triceps	Radial	C7
Brachioradialis (Supinator reflex)	Radial	C6
Biceps	Musculocutaneous	C5
Knee	Femoral	L3, 4
Ankle	Tibial	S12

In the presence of increased reflexes check for ankle and patella clonus. Reflex abnormalities are listed in Table 7.5.

Table 7.5 Reflex abnormalities

Reflex response	Interpretation
Increased, clonus	Motor neurone lesion
Absent, generalised	Peripheral neuropathy
Isolated	Lesion of either peripheral nerve or nerve root
Pendular	Cerebellar disease
Slow relaxing	Hypothyroid

Reflexes can be absent in the early stages of a severe upper neurone lesion. This is often, inappropriately, referred to as spinal shock. There is no evidence of shock but the nerves have been in effect stunned. The classic features of an upper motor neurone lesion will develop subsequently.

The plantar or Babinski response completes the assessment of the major reflexes. It is important to be aware of the following.

- A positive Babinski response is manifested by extension of the big toe and spreading of the adjacent digits.
- A negative Babinski response may be found in an upper motor neurone lesion.

- A positive Babinski response that does not fit in with other neurological features should be interpreted with caution.

Summary

- Examine the motor components in a logical, systematic fashion.
- An isolated abnormality should be interpreted with caution.
- Neurological problems are associated with a well described pattern of clinical features.
- Motor abnormalities are defined in the box.

Type of weakness	Clinical features
Upper motor neurone lesion (UMN)	Increased tone, increased reflexes, pyramidal pattern of weakness, i.e., weak arm extensors and leg flexors
Lower motor neurone lesion (LMN)	Wasting, fasciculation, decreased tone, absent reflexes
Neuromuscular junction	Fatiguable weakness, normal or decreased tone, normal reflexes
Muscle disease	Wasting, decreased tone, impaired or absent reflexes
Functional weakness	No wasting, normal tone, normal reflexes variable, inconsistent power

Sensation

The five basic types of sensation are shown in Figure 7.4. It is important to remember that on entry to the cord, the spinothalamic tract will cross within one or two segments. In contrast the posterior columns remain ipsilateral until they cross in the medulla. Pin prick and light touch are rarely lost without discernible symptoms. As the different sensory modalities are carried predominantly in two tracts, the preliminary sensory examination should focus on pin prick and joint position sense.

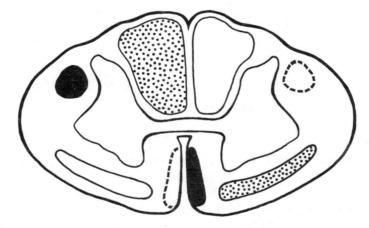

Figure 7.4   Cross section of the spinal cord

The sensory examination is used:

- as a screening test
- for assessment of symptomatic patients
- to confirm signs detected on an examination of the motor system.

There are several key points to consider when examining sensation. These are listed in the box.

Key points for sensory examination

- Explain to the patient what you are going to do
- Demonstrate to the patient what you want them to do
- Always ensure that the patient can appreciate that the sensory modality will be tested appropriately
- Assess dermatomes in a sequential fashion. The relevant dermatomes are shown in Figure 7.5.

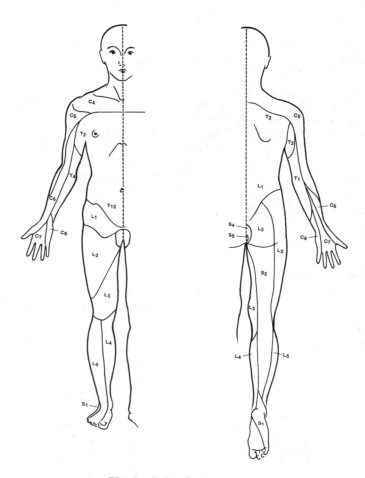

Figure 7.5   Dermatomes

Joint position sense
It is important to remember that Romberg's test assesses joint position sense.

Pin prick
Use a "neuro tip" or broken orange stick. Check intermittently using a blunt stimulus that the patient has recognised the "pin" appropriately. During sensory assessment, test the integrity of each dermatome and whether there is any difference when comparing left and right hand sides of the body. It is also convenient at this time to test whether the patient can distinguish between two stimuli applied simultaneously to the left and right side. Failure to do this indicates sensory inattention and therefore a parietal lobe lesion (most commonly non-dominant). Do not forget to test sacral sensation. Whilst this is not part of the screening test, it must be done in patients who have any of the following features:

- urinary or bowel symptoms
- bilateral leg weakness

- sensory loss in both legs
- suspicion of a conus medullaris or cauda equina lesion.

Types and causes of sensory loss
Patterns of sensory loss fall into three broad categories:

- peripheral nerves
- spinal cord
- brain.

The major abnormalities for each category are listed in Tables 7.6 and 7.7.

Table 7.6 Peripheral nerve abnormalities

Lesion	Sensory loss	Cause
Single nerve lesions	Within the distribution of a single nerve	Entrapment neuropathy, diabetes mellitus, rheumatoid disease
Multiple single nerve lesions	Distribution of relevant nerves	Vasculitis or more diffuse neuropathy
Root lesion	Confined to single root or number of roots in close proximity	Prolapsed intervertebral disc
Peripheral nerve	Glove and stocking distribution	Diabetes mellitus, alcohol, thiamine deficiency

Table 7.7 Spinal cord sensory loss

Lesion	Sensory loss	Cause
Complete transverse lesion	Loss of all modalities a few segments below the lesion	Trauma, spinal cord compression by tumour, cervical spondylitis, transverse myelitis
Hemisection	Ipsilateral loss of joint position sense, contralateral loss of pain and temperature a few segments below the lesion. Posterior column loss. Loss of joint position sense and vibration only	As with complete transection plus subacute combined degeneration of the cord and tabes dorsalis
Central cord	Loss of pain and temperature sensation at the level of the lesion	Syringomyelia
Anterior spinal syndrome	Loss of pain and temperature below the level of the lesion	Anterior spinal artery lesions
Brain stem	Loss of pain and temperature sensation in the face (ipsilateral) and body (contralateral)	Demyelination, lateral medullary syndrome
Thalamic	Hemicentral loss of all modalities	Stroke, tumour or disseminated sclerosis
Cortical parietal lobe dysfunction	The patient recognises all sensory modalities but localises them poorly. In addition there is loss of sensory attention and loss of two point discrimination astereognosis	Stroke, cerebral tumour, disseminated sclerosis

A bizarre distribution of sensory loss which does not conform to an anatomical distribution is suggestive of a dysfunctional disorder. This, however, is a difficult diagnosis to make.

Coordination

This requires integration of sensory feedback and motor output. Thus it is logical to assess coordination after any sensory motor abnormalities have been identified. The cerebellum is responsible for integrating information related to coordination. A clue to an underlying abnormality is often present during examination of the motor system. Watch for the exaggerated response when the patient has outstretched arms and you tap the back of their hands. Tests for demonstrating coordination are complex activities. It is therefore important to tell the patient what you are going to do as well as demonstrate the movement required. Assess the finger, nose, and heel to shin test as well as the presence of truncal ataxia. Other signs indicating cerebellar dysfunction are shown in the box.

Signs of cerebellar dysfunction

- Slurred speech
- Scanning speech
- Staccato speech
- Nystagmus
- Pendular reflexes
- Truncal ataxia
- Intention tremor
- Hypotonia

Interpretation
The presence of unilateral incoordination suggests ipsilateral cerebellar disease, such as demyelination or vascular disease. In contrast bilateral signs usually reflect alcohol, drugs or demyelination. The presence of truncal ataxia and/or gait ataxia without limb coordination indicates a midline (vermis) lesion.

Summary
Test coordination after motor and sensory assessment.

- Clues to the presence of cerebellar disease are obtained from other parts of the examination before coordination is assessed.

TIME OUT 7.1

- Draw an outline of a man and label the appropriate dermatomes.

SUMMARY

This chapter has provided an overview of the key components of a screening neurological examination. Although there are many other tests that may be relevant to comprehensive neurological assessment, the framework provided in this chapter will enable detection of neurological emergencies. One other skill that requires further mention is the ability to elicit meningeal irritation. This will be discussed in Chapters 11 and 14. Kernig's test and to a lesser extent Brudzinski's form a vital component of the screening in the neurological examination.

- The history is the most important component of neurological assessment. It is important to develop a simple common personalised structure to neurological assessment. A screening neurological examination is the minimum that should be done.
- Unlike other components of the physical examination, the nervous system is often not examined as there are no clinical indications. It is therefore important to take every opportunity to hone your clinical neurological skills.

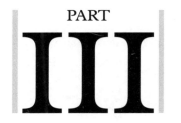

PART

III

PRESENTING COMPLAINTS

CHAPTER

8

The patient with breathing difficulties

OBJECTIVES

After reading this chapter you will be able to:

- describe a structured approach to the breathless patient
- understand why a structured approach is important in the management of such patients
- differentiate between the immediately life threatening and potentially life threatening causes of breathlessness
- describe the immediate management of these patients and appropriate definitive care.

INTRODUCTION

Acute breathlessness is a common emergency condition. The effort required for breathing makes it virtually impossible for the patient to provide any form of medical history and questioning may only make the situation worse. The clinician's skills will help to determine the underlying cause and dictate appropriate management.

Immediately life threatening causes of breathlessness

Airway
- Obstruction

Breathing
- Acute severe asthma
- Acute exacerbation of chronic obstructive pulmonary disease
- Pulmonary oedema
- Tension pneumothorax

Circulation
- Acute severe left ventricular failure
- Dysrhythmia
- Hypovolaemia
- Pulmonary embolus
- Cardiac tamponade

Key point
It is important to remember that the breathless patient does not always have pathology affecting the respiratory or cardiovascular systems

PRIMARY ASSESSMENT AND RESUSCITATION

Airway

Assessment
This has been described in Chapter 4 and is summarised in the box below.

Summary of airway assessment

- Look   – respiratory – rate
                         – effort
                         – symmetry
- Feel   – expired air
           – trachea
- Listen   – 'count to 10'
             – breath sounds

Treatment
High flow oxygen ($FiO_2 = 0.85$) may relieve some of the patient's distress. If airway obstruction is suspected, request immediate review by a specialist. If a foreign body has been inhaled attempt a Heimlich or modified Heimlich manoeuvre.

Breathing

Assessment
This is summarised in the box.

Summary of breathing assessment

- **Look**   colour, sweating
                      posture
                      respiratory – rate
                                     – effort
                                     – symmetry
- **Feel**   tracheal position
                      tracheal tug
                      chest expansion
- **Percuss**
- **Listen**

Treatment
Irrespective of the underlying cause of the bronchospasm, treat patients with nebulised bronchodilators whilst clues to the underlying diagnosis are sought.

Immediate management of a tension pneumothorax is needle thoracentesis followed by intravenous access and then chest drain insertion.

TIME OUT 8.1

Take 30 seconds to mentally rehearse the key components of the assessment so far.

Circulation

Assessment

This has been described in Chapter 6 and is summarised in the box.

Summary of circulatory assessment

- **Look:** pallor, sweating, venous pressure
- **Feel:** pulse – rate, rhythm and character
  capillary refill time
  blood pressure
  apex beat
- **Listen:** heart sounds, extra sounds

Treatment

All patients should receive high flow oxygen, be treated in a seated position and have their oxygen saturation, pulse, blood pressure, and cardiac rhythm monitored. Intravenous access is necessary and at least one large venflon (12–14 gauge) is required in the antecubital fossa.

The management of the "shocked" patient will depend on the underlying cause. Treatment options are summarised in the box.

Treatment of shock

Cause	Treatment
Acute, severe, left ventricular failure	Inotropes
Dysrhythmia – tachycardia – bradycardia	Cardioversion Atropine Inotropes Pacing
Hypovolaemia	Fluid challenge
Pulmonary embolus	Anticoagulation Thrombolysis Fluids
Sepsis	Fluids Antibiotics Inotropes
Anaphylaxis	Adrenaline Fluids Chlerpheniramine Hydrocortisone
Cardiac tamponade	Fluids Pericardiocentesis

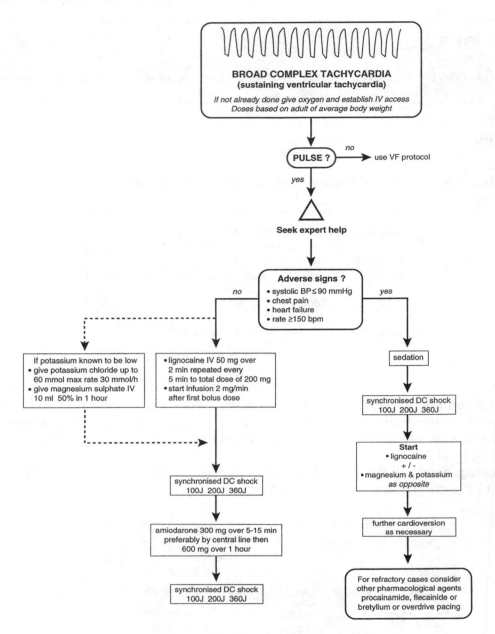

Figure 8.1 Broad complex tachycardia

Key points
If the patient is still breathless and the cause remains in doubt, a rapid reevaluation of the ABC is required
It is important to remember that hypovolaemia is an important cause of breathlessness

Once the patient's condition is stabilised then further information can be obtained from the secondary assessment.

Summary

In the breathless patient, the immediately life threatening problems are:

- Airway   obstruction
- Breathing   acute severe asthma
  acute exacerbation of COPD
  pulmonary oedema
  tension pneumothorax
- Circulation   acute severe left ventricular failure
  dysrhythmia
  hypovolaemia
  pulmonary embolus
  cardiac tamponade

These conditions can be identified and differentiated clinically.
All patients require oxygen and intravenous access.

TIME OUT 8.2

Mentally rehearse your approach to the patient with breathing difficulties. Then list the major components of the primary assessment. Armed with this structure read the following information and then answer the associated questions.

A 64 year old man with known ischaemic heart disease was admitted to the coronary care unit after becoming acutely breathless. He denied any chest pain or cough. The following physical signs were elicited:

- respiratory rate 26/minute
- fine inspiratory crackles were heard at both bases
- pulse rate 140/minute and regular
- blood pressure 80/50
- peripherally shut down
- no other relevant features

a. What would be your immediate management?
b. What investigations would you request?

SECONDARY ASSESSMENT

Many patients with breathlessness will be able to give a history, albeit fragmented. The conditions diagnosed in this assessment phase are shown in the box.

Potentially life threatening causes of breathlessness

Severe asthma
Acute chronic respiratory failure
Pulmonary oedema
Simple pneumothorax
Pneumonia
Pleural effusion
Pulmonary embolus
Metabolic acidosis – diabetic ketoacidosis, salicylate overdose
Pontine haemorrhage

SPECIFIC CONDITIONS

Asthma

Asthma is a chronic inflammatory condition resulting in reversible narrowing of the airways. It affects approximately 5% of the population and can occur for the first time at any age with a male predominance in childhood and females in later life. Asthma in children is usually associated with atopy, whilst in adults it is more commonly non-atopic. Both, however, have an inherited component.

Although there are many potential triggers, asthma is characterised by wheezing due to widespread narrowing of the peripheral airways. There may be an associated increase in sputum volume and viscosity. Occasionally a nocturnal cough will be a prominent symptom and patients may describe tightness in the chest or a sensation of choking rather than wheezing. Furthermore, exposure to external stimuli like cold air, cigarette smoke and paint fumes may induce an acute "asthmatic" attack. This does not indicate an allergic response but demonstrates that the airways are hyperreactive and produce an exaggerated response to non-specific irritants.

Pathophysiology

Acute attacks of bronchospasm may be precipitated by IgE mediated mast cell degranulation. In contrast, when exposed to environmental factors, e.g. allergens and pollutants, the airways of known asthmatics are susceptible to chronic inflammation characterised by eosinophil and T lymphocyte infiltration. These cells are responsible for liberating inflammatory mediators that evoke a variety of responses (see next box) culminating in airways narrowing and hence increased airflow resistance. Since resistance is inversely proportional to the fourth power of the radius (Poiseulle's law) a small increase in airways thickness will have a marked effect on airways resistance and therefore reduce airflow. The change in airway radius is usually due to bronchial muscle contraction, but in the asthmatic this is exacerbated by mucosal oedema, increased mucus production and epithelial cell damage. In addition, the chronic inflammatory response reduces elastic recoil of the airways, further exacerbating the narrowing (Figure 8.2).

> **Inflammatory mediator induced changes in asthma:**
>
> - disrupt the functional and structural integrity of the epithelium
> - stimulate   mucus secretion
>   oedema formation
>   smooth muscle contraction
> - induce collagen deposition under the basement membrane

This disturbed and decreased airflow is manifest clinically as audible wheeze, reduced forced expiratory volume in one second (FEV_1) and peak expiratory flow rate (PEFR), along with increased functional residual capacity (FRC) due to air trapping, with no change in the total lung capacity (TLC). Thus, because of increased airways resistance the work of breathing is increased and the patient feels breathless.

In an acute asthmatic attack some of the airways become blocked by mucus plugs resulting in hypoxia due to ventilation perfusion (V/Q) mismatch. This further increases the work of breathing, causing hyperventilation in an attempt to reverse the hypoxaemia.

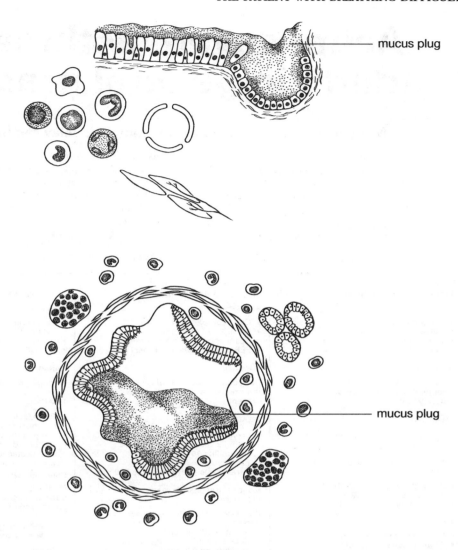

mucus plug

mucus plug

Figure 8.2   Diagrammatic representation of the pathophysiology of asthma: (a) longitudinal section (b) cross section.

> **Key point**
> Failure to sustain this increased respiratory effort, usually in a severe exacerbation, will be manifest by a silent chest, hypoxaemia and a rising $PaCO_2$

Management

> **Key point**
> Preventable deaths from acute asthma still occur due to treatment delay

Management is summarised in Figure 8.3, the British Thoracic Society guidelines.

Acute severe asthma in adults in general practice

Many deaths from asthma are preventable: delay can be fatal

Factors include:

- Doctors failing to assess severity by objective measurement
- Patients or relatives failing to appreciate severity
- Underuse of corticosteroids

Regard each emergency consultation as for acute severe asthma until it is shown otherwise.

Assess and record:

- Symptoms and response to self treatment
- Heart and respiratory rates
- Peak expiratory flow (PEF)

Caution:
Patients with severe or life threatening attacks may not be distressed and may not have all these abnormalities. The presence of any should alert the doctor.

Uncontrolled asthma

ASSESSMENT

- Speech normal
- Pulse < 110 beats/min
- Respiration < 25 breaths/min
- PEF > 50% predicted or best

MANAGEMENT

Treat at home but response to treatment MUST be assessed before you leave

TREATMENT

Nebulised salbutamol 5 mg or terbutaline 10 mg

MONITOR RESPONSE 15–30 MIN AFTER NEBULISER

If PEF > 50–75% predicted/best
- Give prednisolone 30–60 mg
- Step up usual treatment

or

If PEF > 75% predicted/best
- Step up usual treatment

FOLLOW UP

- Monitor symptoms and PEF on PEF chart
- Self management plan
- Surgery review ≤ 48 hours
- Modify treatment at review according to guidelines for chronic persistent asthma

CRITERIA FOR HOSPITAL ADMISSION

- Any life threatening features
- Any features of acute severe asthma present after initial treatment, especially PEF < 33%

LOWER THE THRESHOLD FOR ADMISSION IF:

Attack is in afternoon or evening, recent nocturnal symptoms etc, recent hospital admission, previous severe attacks, patient unable to assess own condition, concern over social circumstances

Acute severe asthma

ASSESSMENT

- Can't complete sentences
- Pulse ≥ 110 beats/min
- Respiration ≥ 25 breaths/min
- PEF ≤ 50% predicted or best

MANAGEMENT

Seriously consider admission if more than one feature above present

TREATMENT

- Oxygen 40–60% if available
- Nebulised salbutamol 5 mg or terbutaline 10 mg
- Prednisolone 30–60 mg or intravenous hydrocortisone 200 mg

MONITOR RESPONSE 15–30 MIN AFTER NEBULISER

If any signs of acute severe asthma persist
- Arrange admission
- Repeat nebulised β agonist plus ipratropium 0.5 mg or give subcutaneous terbutaline or give intravenous aminophylline (slowly) while awaiting ambulance

or

If good response to first nebulised treatment (symptoms improved, respiration and pulse settling, and PEF > 50%):
- Step up usual treatment and continue prednisolone

FOLLOW UP

- Monitor symptoms and PEF
- Self management plan
- Surgery review ≤ 24 hours

Modify treatment at review according to guidelines for chronic persistent asthma

Life threatening asthma

ASSESSMENT

- Silent chest
- Cyanosis
- Bradycardia or exhaustion
- PEF < 33% of predicted or best

MANAGEMENT

Arrange immediate ADMISSION

TREATMENT

- Prednisolone 30–60 mg or intravenous hydrocortisone 200 mg immediately
- Oxygen driven nebuliser in ambulance
- Nebulised β agonist and ipratropium or subcutaneous terbutaline or intravenous aminophylline (250 mg slowly)

Stay with patient until ambulance arrives

NB If there is no nebuliser give 2 puffs of β agonist via a large volume spacer and repeat 10–20 times

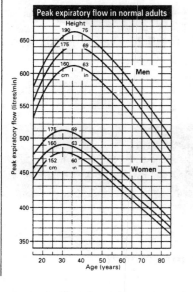

From: Gregg I, Nunn AJ. BMJ 1989; 298: 1068–70

NATIONAL **ASTHMA** CAMPAIGN
conquering asthma

Working for Healthier Lungs

in association with the General Practitioner in Asthma Group, the British Association of Accident and Emergency Medicine, the British Paediatric Respiratory Society and the Royal College of Paediatrics and Child Health

Adapted from poster designed by Business Design Group

Figure 8.3 The British Thoracic Society guidelines for asthma treatment

Life threatening asthma

Assessment   This is characterised by:

- airway   – normally patent but can be compromised by exhaustion
- breathing   – cyanosed, exhausted, minimal respiratory effort and a silent chest
- circulation   – tachycardia greater than 130 beats per minute, brachycardia, hypotension.

In addition the peak expiratory flow is less than 33% of the predicted or the patient's best.

Key point

A silent chest is a life threatening sign as it means there is insufficient air being moved (in and out of the chest) to generate a wheeze

---

Immediate treatment   See Figure 8.4. It is important to remember that acute breathlessness in an asthmatic is usually due to bronchospasm. However, because of "gas trapping" there is an increase in positive end expiratory pressure. This increases the potential to develop a pneumothorax that can further embarrass the respiratory system. Always be alert to this possibility in asthmatics who either fail to respond to treatment or become acutely breathless. Regular reassessment and an urgent chest X-ray are required.

Intravenous fluids should be administered as most patients have coexisting dehydration. Adequate hydration also helps to render the sputum less tenacious. In addition, hypokalaemia can occur as a consequence of either asthma or coexistent with β_2 agonist therapy. Thus, careful monitoring and appropriate replacement therapy are required.

The patient's clinical response to treatment (as described earlier) should be monitored continuously and arterial blood gases should be performed regularly.

If the patient either becomes exhausted, retains CO_2 or adequate oxygenation is not possible then intermittent positive pressure ventilation will be required (see box). Early liaison with the anaesthetist/intensivist is vital.

Indications for intensive care

Hypoxia ($PaO_2 < 8$ kPa despite $FiO_2 > 0.6$)
Hypercapnia ($PaCO_2 > 6$ kPa)
Exhaustion
Altered conscious level (confused, drowsy, unconscious)
Respiratory arrest

Please also see Figure 8.4 for the assessment and management of patients with acute asthma that is not immediately life threatening.

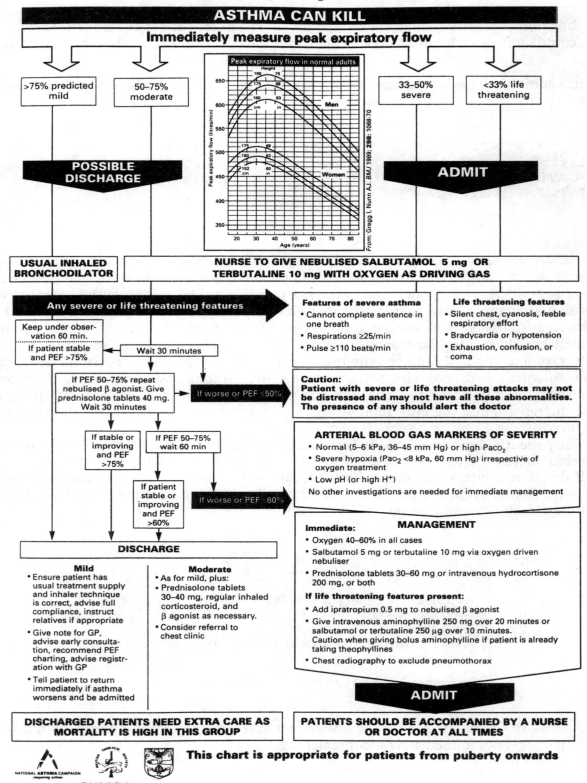

Figure 8.4 British Thoracic Society's Guidelines for Asthma Treatment

---

TIME OUT 8.3

Have a five minute break, then answer the following questions.

a. What type of condition is asthma?
b. List the major components of this response.
c. What is the overall effect of this process?
d. How does this affect pulmonary physiology?
e. Describe how you would manage life threatening asthma
f. What are the indications for ventilation?

Acute on chronic respiratory failure

This is an important cause of breathlessness and is considered in detail in Chapter 19 on organ failure.

Pulmonary oedema

This is an important cause of breathlessness and is considered in detail in Chapter 19.

Pneumothorax

A pneumothorax results from gas entering the potential space between the visceral and parietal pleura. This may arise spontaneously from the rupture of a bulla or cyst on the lung surface or following penetrating trauma. Underlying lung disease is therefore an important predisposing factor in the development of a pneumothorax. However, there are a number of invasive procedures such as subclavian vein catheterisation that can also be responsible (see box).

Iatrogenic pneumothoraces

Attempted internal jugular/subclavian vein access
Pleural aspiration/biopsy
Percutaneous lung/liver biopsy
Transbronchial biopsy
Intermittent positive pressure ventilation (IPPV)

Pathophysiology

The outward recoil of the chest and inward elastic retraction of the lung produces a negative pressure in the potential space between the visceral pleuro and parietal pleura. This pressure, with respect to atmosphere, becomes more negative during inspiration. Following a breach of the visceral pleura, air preferentially moves from the alveolus into the pleural space until these pressures equilibrate – hence the lung collapses, resulting in a simple pneumothorax. If, however, the breach in the pleura acts as a one-way valve then air will preferentially enter the pleural space during inspiration and not return during expiration. Thus the pressure in the intrapleural space rises above atmospheric pressure. The resulting hypoxaemia acts as a respiratory stimulus causing deeper inspiratory efforts which in turn further increase the intrapleural pressure. This produces a tension pneumothorax. If untreated, mediastinal shift occurs, causing kinking of the great vessels, impairing venous return, and compressing the opposite lung. This process exacerbates hypoxia and eventually causes pulseless electrical activity (electromechanical dissociation).

> **Key point**
> Tension pneumothorax is a clinical diagnosis. Needle thoracocentesis is the immediate management

Primary pneumothorax

This condition is relatively uncommon (affecting about 9/100 000 patients with a male to female ratio of approximately 4 : 1). It occurs in previously normal lungs and is attributed to rupture of a surface bulla or cyst which is often at the apex. About 20% of patients will have recurrent pneumothoraces on both the ipsilateral and the contralateral sides.

Secondary pneumothorax

This condition is associated with preexisting lung disease (see next box) and medical procedures (see previous box).

> **Preexisting lung conditions associated with pneumothoraces**
>
> Emphysema
> Chronic obstructive pulmonary disease
> Acute exacerbations of asthma
> Infections: empyema
>   staphylococcal pneumonia
>   tuberculosis
> Malignancy
> Cystic fibrosis

Assessment

Simple pneumothorax

Symptoms and signs may be absent but commonly the patient will present with breathlessness and pleuritic chest pain localised to the affected side. Breathlessness may be related to pain, size of pneumothorax and preexisting lung disease.

> **Key point**
> In a patient with preexisting lung disease even a small pneumothorax can produce acute respiratory failure

Clinical signs are difficult to detect when the pneumothorax is small or when there is coexistent emphysema. Often there is reduced chest expansion on the affected side (usually due to pain) and the percussion note is typically resonant. Hyperresonance is very difficult to detect even when comparing with the non-affected side. The most consistent sign is a reduction in breath sounds over the pneumothorax.

Tension pneumothorax

This presents as acute respiratory distress. Initially there may be increased respiratory rate and effort with reduced absence of movement, a hyper-resonant percussion note and reduced absent breath sounds on the affected side. Tracheal deviation, jugular venous distension and cyanosis are late, often preterminal, manifestations.

Management

Simple pneumothorax

Spontaneous resolution will occur in an asymptomatic patient with only partial lung collapse (and no deterioration for 24 hours) at approximately 1·25% of the volume of the hemithorax per day. Occasionally pain relief is required in the form of non-steroidal anti-inflammatory analgesics. Do not forget to reassure the patient!

Guidelines for the management of a confirmed and treated pneumothorax are shown in Figure 8.5.

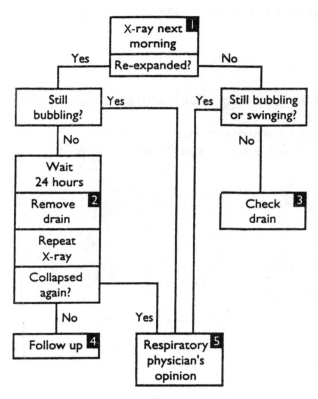

consider premedication as above. After removing the suture that holds the drain in place, withdraw the tube while the patient holds his or her breath in full inspiration. Use the two remaining sutures to seal the wound.

3 Check chest drain

If the lung has not reinflated but there is no bubbling in the underwater bottle, then the tube is blocked or kinked—this can be corrected; or else the tube has become displaced—a replacement must be inserted through a clean incision.

4 Follow up

Arrange for a chest clinic appointment in 7–10 days. The patient must be given a discharge letter and told to attend again immediately in the event of noticeable deterioration. Air travel should be avoided until changes seen on radiographs have resolved.

5 Respiratory physician's opinion

Should advice from a specialist be required, transfer of continuing care is advisable. Important considerations in management are:

- assessing why reexpansion has not been achieved (for example, air leaking around the drain site, tube displaced or blocked, large persistent leak);

- the use of suction to reexpand the lung (this can be lengthy, requires appropriate equipment and pressure settings, influences how and where confirmatory radiographs are taken, and involves care from experienced nursing staff);

- whether early thoracic surgery would be appropriate (for example, failure of conservative measures, need to prevent recurrence);

- consideration of chemical pleurodesis in certain cases;

- management of surgical emphysema.

Explanatory notes

1 Chest X-ray

If the underwater seal is *always* kept below the level of the chest, clamping is unnecessary and potentially dangerous. As far as possible, an X-ray film should be taken in the department, rather than on the ward with a portable machine; an expiration film is unnecessary.

2 Removal of chest drain

Bubbling should have stopped for at least 24 hours.

Since some patients find tube removal unpleasant,

Figure 8.5 Management of chest drain

95

Aspiration is a simple technique with negligible morbidity even when done by relatively junior staff. If successful it produces rapid resolution of breathlessness and chest discomfort.

Tension pneumothorax
Immediate thoracocentesis is needed. This will relieve the tension and the acute problems, but formal chest drain insertion is still required after securing intravenous access. This is a precaution because occasionally pneumothoraces can be complicated by a haemothorax, possibly due to tearing of a pleural lesion or from an adjacent necrotic tumour.

Investigation

Radiological confirmation of a simple pneumothorax is important and will guide appropriate therapy. In contrast, tension pneumothorax is a clinical diagnosis and an X-ray is only needed after chest drain insertion.

Potential problems
- Imminent air travel for the patient
- Lung fails to reexpand after intercostal drain insertion – liaise with respiratory physician regarding use of low pressure suction
- Recurrent pneumothoraces – liaise with cardiothoracic surgeon regarding chemical or surgical pleurodesis. Surgical advice should also be sought if there are bilateral pneumothoraces.

TIME OUT 8.4

A 72 year old lady, who has COPD presents with acute breathlessness. She has a respiratory rate of 28 per minute, a hyperexpanded chest with scattered wheezes and a prolonged expiratory phase. Her SaO_2 is 72% on 28% oxygen. What is your immediate management?

PNEUMONIA

Pneumonia is a general term used to describe inflammation of tissues involved with gaseous exchange in the lung. Traditionally pneumonia has been described according to its radiological appearance, i.e. lobar, lobular or broncho pneumonia. Unfortunately these do not help in either the diagnosis or the management. In contrast, the circumstances of the illness and the clinical background of the patient, as described in the box, provide helpful clues to aid investigation, management, and treatment.

Classification of pneumonia

Community acquired
Hospital acquired
Aspiration and anaerobic
Recurrent
Immunosuppression associated
Travel related

Management principles – check list

Diagnosis

- History
- Examination
- Investigations: chest X-ray   – PA
                    arterial blood gases
                    venous blood   – cultures
                                            – full blood count and film
                                            – electrolytes, glucose and liver profile
                                            – initial serology: *Mycoplasma, Legionella, Chlamydia*
                    sputum   – culture and sensitivity
                                            – microscopy
                                            – acid and alcohol fast bacilli
                                            – cytology

Treatment

- Oxygen – unless the patient is not breathless or blood gases are normal
- Antibiotic – see Figure 8.5.
- Fluid replacement, either oral or intravenous according to clinical picture
- Analgesia if required
- Consider early liaison with clinical microbiologist/respiratory physician

Community acquired pneumonia

This is a common cause of acute hospital admission and often occurs in the winter months. Community acquired pneumonia can affect previously healthy individuals or patients with coexistent lung disease. The age of the patient is likely to influence the pathogen involved.

Modes of infection transmission

Extension of bacteria colonising respiratory tract
Droplet, e.g., respiratory viruses from infected individuals
Animals, e.g., *Chlamydia psittaci*
Water droplet, e.g., *Legionella pneumophilia*

The organisms likely to cause community acquired pneumonia in the UK are shown in the box.

Organisms causing community acquired pneumonia

Streptococcus pneumoniae
Haemophilus influenzae
Staphylococcus aureus
Influenza virus
Mycoplasma pneumoniae
Chlamydia psittaci/Q fever
Legionella species

Streptococcus pneumoniae (pneumococcal pneumonia) is the major pathogen involved, whilst influenza is the commonest viral infection. It is important to realise that viral infections caused by influenza, parainfluenza and respiratory syncytial virus are usually associated with supraadded bacterial infection.

Assessment
The clinical features are very variable.

Respiratory symptoms

Clinical:	cough	Prodromal:	pyrexia
	sputum production		malaise
	breathlessness		anorexia
	pleuritic pain		sweating
	haemoptysis		myalgia
			arthralgia
			headache

On examination most patients appear flushed and unwell with tachypnoea and/or tachycardia. The temperature can exceed 39·5°C and rigors are not uncommon in young people. In contrast, elderly patients may remain afebrile. Herpes simplex labialis is present in approximately one third of patients having pneumococcal pneumonia. Often chest movement is reduced on the affected side, especially if pleuritic pain is present. Inspiratory crackles are the commonest sign and bronchial breathing is infrequent. A pleural rub can be heard even when pleuritic pain is absent. **Occasionally the physical examination is entirely normal;** therefore a chest X-ray is necessary.

It is important to realise that non-respiratory symptoms may predominate; for example, a patient with a lower lobe pneumonia may present with abdominal pain and peritonism. Confusion may be due to hypoxia and/or metabolic derangement. In addition, *Legionella pneumophila* is also associated with severe headache, cerebellar dysfunction, and amnesia. Vomiting and diarrhoea may occur as a direct manifestation of the illness or related to antibiotic therapy.

Unfortunately the mortality from severe pneumonia remains high. Clinical features associated with severe pneumonia are listed in the box and their presence indicates a poor prognosis. Early liaison with an anaesthetist/intensivist is needed if **two** or more are present.

High risk features in patients with pneumonia

Clinical	**Investigations**
Confusion	Blood urea > 7 mmol/l
Respiratory rate > 30 per minute	White cell count $< 4 \times 10^9$ or $> 20 \times 10^9$
Diastolic blood pressure < 60 mm Hg	$PaO_2 < 8$ kPa (60 mm Hg)
Recent onset atrial fibrillation	Serum albumin < 25 g/l
	Multilobe involvement on chest radiograph

Management
Not all patients require admission to hospital. All patients should be managed in bed; treat fever and pleuritic pain with appropriate non-steroidal anti-inflammatory drugs.

Correction of hypoxia and fluid balance is very important as described above. Chest physiotherapy is rarely helpful in the acute phase.

Specific treatment   When the patient presents acutely the microorganism responsible for the pneumonia is not usually known. Therefore, the choice of antibiotic is made according to the limited number of organisms that cause community acquired pneumonia. Most hospitals have devised specific antibiotic policies.

- **Severe** pneumonia. This can affect even previously fit individuals. As the mortality is high parenteral antibiotics must be given immediately. Considering the potential organisms that may be responsible (see earlier) a combination of ceftriaxone 2 g combined with clarithromycin 1 g daily is advised. The duration of intravenous therapy is based on the patient's clinical response.
- **Mild** pneumonia. In most previously fit people the likely organism is *Streptococcus pneumoniae* or occasionally *Mycoplasma pneumoniae*, *Chlamydia* species, *Legionella* species or *Coxiella burnetii*. The combination of amoxycillin and erythromycin is both cheap and effective. Erythromycin alone is appropriate for patients who are allergic to penicillin or if an atypical organism, is suspected e.g. *Mycoplasma*, *Chlamydia*, *Legionella*. If the patient fails to respond to this combination, then either ciprofloxacin or co-amoxiclav should be substituted.

TIME OUT 8.5

Factual overload? Take a five minute break and then answer the following questions.

a.   What is the major pathogen responsible for community acquired pneumonia?
b.   What are the clinical features?
c.   How would you manage a patient with severe community acquired pneumonia?
d.   List the high risk features in patients with pneumonia.

Hospital acquired pneumonia

This is defined as pneumonia developing more than 48 hours after hospital admission, irrespective of the reason.

Pathophysiology
Bacterial colonisation of the nasopharynx changes markedly in hospital patients, particularly those who receive broad spectrum antibiotics and are severely ill. These bacteria arise either from the hospital environment or the patient's gastrointestinal tract. Such pathogens are likely to be aspirated in patients who are ill, bed bound or who have impaired consciousness for whatever reason. This may be exacerbated by an inability to clear bronchial secretions after a general anaesthetic or where coughing is impaired due to thoracic or abdominal surgery. The risk of postoperative pneumonia is associated with increasing age, smoking, obesity, underlying chronic illness, and prolonged anaesthesia. Pathogens may also be spread from contaminated equipment such as nebulisers, ventilators, suction equipment or even from the hospital staff.

   A host of pathogens are responsible for hospital acquired pneumonia (see box). Gram negative bacilli are commonly implicated and to a lesser extent Gram positive bacteria, especially *Staphylococcus aureus*, except if the host is immunocompromised.

Hospital acquired pneumonia in specific circumstances

Streptococcus pneumoniae	Early postelective surgery, especially if chronic chest pathology
Haemophilus influenzae	Contaminated respiratory equipment
Pseudomonas	
Klebsiella	
Pseudomonas	Aspiration
Klebsiella	
Bacteroides	
Clostridium	
Legionella	Contaminated water (cooling towers, heating and showers)

Specific treatment

As there are a wide range of potential organisms responsible for hospital acquired pneumonia initial therapy will include either ceftriaxone or a combination, e.g. ciprofloxacin plus an aminoglycoside (gentamicin). An alternative combination is recommended for anaerobic infections, i.e. ceftriaxone and metronidazole. If a pseudomonal infection is suspected then an appropriate penicillin derivative such as ticacillin should be used. Early liaison with a clinical microbiologist is advised.

Antibiotic therapy can be tailored according to the results of investigations.

Ideally, treatment should be proactive in preventing such infections by scrupulous hygiene retention, appropriate infection control and preoperative advice for the patient.

TIME OUT 8.6

a. Define the term hospital acquired pneumonia.
b. List those patients at risk.
c. How would you manage a patient with hospital acquired pneumonia?

Aspiration and anaerobic pneumonia

This is commonly associated with impaired conscious and/or dysphagia. Infection is usually with either *Pseudomonas aeruginosa* or an *Enterobacter* species in the hospital environment. Treatment usually comprises intravenous ceftriaxone 1 g daily and oral metronidazole 400 mg t.d.s.

Recurrent pneumonia

If a patient experiences three or more pneumonic episodes, the following should be considered.

- Localised bronchiectasis
- Bronchial obstruction, e.g. foreign body, carcinoma or external compression
- A generalised respiratory disorder if the pneumonia recurs in different sites
- COPD with or without bronchiectasis
- Aspiration of oesophagogastric contents in patients with, e.g. motor neurone disease, disseminated sclerosis, achalasia, epilepsy, alcoholism, and drug/substance use
- Consider chronic organising pneumonia (bronchiolitis obliterans organising pneumonia)

Immunosuppression associated pneumonia

An in-depth discussion on this topic is well beyond the scope of this book. However, the following practical guidelines are suggested.

Pneumonia of acute onset and rapid progression suggests bacterial origin. Therefore initial treatment should include a combination of ceftriaxone and gentamicin to ensure adequate cover against *Streptococcus pneumoniae*, *Haemophilus influenzae*, *Staphylococcus aureus* and many other Gram negative species. If the patient fails to respond or the pace of the illness is less acute then specialist help should be sought early.

Travel related pneumonia

With the increase in worldwide travel, a variety of unexpected respiratory infections may be seen and/or enter into the differential diagnosis of pneumonia. This subject is too extensive to be covered here, but do not forget to:

- take a full travel history
- consider bacterial, viral and fungal infections
- consider an esoteric infection if the patient fails to respond appropriately
- liaise **early** with a consultant in infectious diseases/clinical microbiology/respiratory medicine.

TIME OUT 8.7

Pneumonia is a common condition. You have already boosted your knowledge by reading this section and answering the associated questions. To complete your understanding review the management of pneumonia as shown in Figure 8.6.

PLEURAL EFFUSION

Pathophysiology

The pleural surfaces are lubricated by a thin layer of fluid that allows the lung and chest wall to move with minimum energy loss. The volume of pleural fluid is a balance between production by the parietal pleura and absorption by the visceral pleura. The increase in hydrostatic pressure within the capillaries of the parietal pleura ensures that fluid passes into the pleural space. Thus, the parietal pleura acts like a plasma ultrafiltrator. In comparison, the pressure within the capillaries of the visceral pleura is lower ensuring that fluid is absorbed. Lymphatic drainage also facilitates removal of fluid and protein from the pleural space.

A pleural effusion results from an excessive accumulation of fluid within the pleural space. Considering the normal production of pleural fluid, as described earlier, the potential factors involved in the production of excess fluid are summarised in the box.

Factors involved in the production of excess pleural fluid

An imbalance between the hydrostatic and oncotic pressures
Alteration in pleural capillary permeability
Impaired lymphatic drainage
Disruption of structural integrity
Transdiaphragmatic passage of fluid

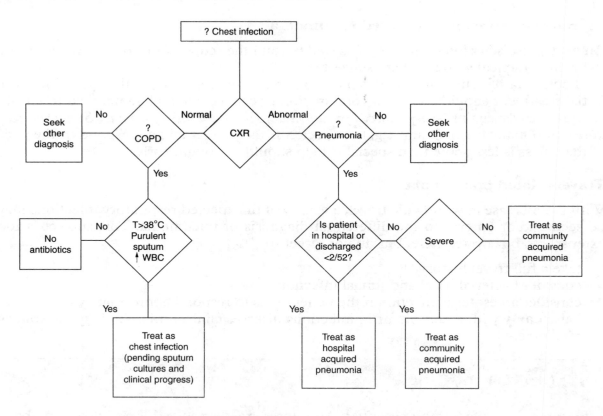

Figure 8.6 Pneumonia management algorithm

More than one of these factors may be involved in the production of pleural fluid according to the underlying disease process as described below.

Causes of pleural effusion

Some of the reasons why a patient may develop a pleural effusion are listed in the box. The estimated "chance" of meeting these causes is given in brackets.

Specific pleural effusions

Transudate

These are characterised by low protein concentrations. Excess fluid forms when there is an increase in pleural hydrostatic pressure, for example, in congestive cardiac failure, or when there is a reduction in colloidal osmotic pressure, for example, with hypoalbuminaemia associated with nephrotic syndrome or liver disease.

Small effusions can be associated with failure of either the left or right or both ventricles. Elevated left heart pressures will be transmitted to the pulmonary circulation and hence result in reduced fluid absorption from the visceral pleura. In contrast, increased pressure from the right heart is transmitted to the systemic capillaries and this leads to increased production of fluid from the parietal pleura. Resolution occurs with treatment of heart failure, but unilateral effusions that fail to respond to this treatment require further investigation.

Hypoalbuminaemia, as listed earlier, is a major contributory factor in the development of generalised oedema. Thus, both pleural effusions and ascites are common. Formation of pleural fluid is due to a reduction in colloidal osmotic pressure combined with the transdiaphragmatic passage of fluid.

Causes of pleural effusion

(a) Transudate
Cardiac failure (D)
Hypoalbuminaemia   nephrotic syndrome (W)
         cirrhosis (W)
         malabsorption (W)
Peritoneal dialysis (M)
Myxoedema (O)

(b) Exudate
Infective   pneumonia (D)
         subphrenic abscess (M)
         tuberculosis (A)
Inflammatory   pancreatitis (W)
         connective tissue disease (M)
         Dressler's syndrome (O)
Neoplastic   metastatic carcinoma (D)
         lymphoma (A)
         mesothelioma (A)
         Meigs' syndrome (O)
Haemothorax   pulmonary emboli (M)
         trauma (M)
         spontaneous bleeding disorders (A)
Chylothorax   trauma (A)
         carcinoma (A)
         lymphoma (A)

D, daily; W, weekly; M, monthly; A, annually; O, only in examinations.

Exudate

Malignancy The commonest cause of a large pleural effusion is malignant involvement of the pleura. This can occur as:

- direct spread from an adjacent bronchogenic carcinoma
- metastatic spread via the lymphatics, e.g. from breast malignancy
- haematogenous spread from the gastrointestinal tract.

In contrast, primary pleural tumours (mesotheliomas) are rare.
 Excess pleural fluid is formed by a combination of mechanisms, including:

- disruption of the integrity of the pleura
- an associated adjacent inflammatory response
- the tumour secreting fluid
- infiltrating malignancy causing haemorrhage
- interference with lymphatic drainage.

Initial treatment is symptomatic and referral to an oncology specialist may be prudent.

Connective tissue diseases Pleural involvement is common in patients with systemic lupus erythematosus but to a much lesser extent in those who have rheumatoid disease.

Haemothorax As an acute medical emergency this is rare because most cases occur in association with penetrating or non-penetrating trauma. However, it can occur after:

- attempts at central venous access due to disruption of associated arteries or veins
- percutaneous biopsy of the pleura and liver secondary to intercostal vessel damage.

Haemothorax is a rare sequel to either bleeding diatheses, overanticoagulation or following a dissection/rupture of the thoracic aorta.

Chylothorax This is rare. It is associated with trauma to, or malignant invasion of, the thoracic duct. This structure can also be damaged during an oesophageal resection or mobilisation of the aortic arch. It is important to differentiate a chylothorax from a pyothorax. A chest drain is the initial management of choice.

Assessment

Symptoms

Pain and breathlessness are the cardinal symptoms of pleural disease. Their presence will, however, vary according to the underlying pathology. Pleuritic pain, which is worse on deep inspiration or coughing, is typical of dry pleurisy. As fluid accumulates, however, the pain spontaneously improves. Breathlessness, as described earlier, only becomes apparent if the pleural effusion is either large or rapidly expanding or there is significant underlying pulmonary pathology.

Signs

Physical signs are often absent unless the effusion is large. Tachypnoea and tachycardia may be present. Chest wall movement and expansion are often reduced on the affected side. The percussion note is "stoney dull" and both vocal resonance (or tactile vocal fremitus) and breath sounds will be diminished or absent. Above the effusion, however, the lung may collapse with signs of consolidation, i.e. bronchial breathing and increased vocal resonance. Remember that consolidated lung tends to filter out low frequency sounds; thus high pitched bronchial breathing is prominent. Furthermore, vocal sounds, i.e. "99" or "11" are transmitted by normal lung and, in particular, solid lung but not by air space or fluid.

Specific management

Frequently all that is required, initially, is a sample of pleural fluid for laboratory investigations.

Immediate drainage of pleural fluid is only required if the patient is breathless. This usually occurs if pleural effusion is massive, rapidly accumulating or there is underlying pulmonary disease. Insertion of a chest drain is described in Chapter 30.

Transudates rarely require direct treatment as they usually resolve with improvement in the underlying condition. In contrast, the management of an **exudate** is governed by the results of investigations. A chest drain may be required for the reasons listed earlier and in the presence of an empyema or pyopneumothorax. The latter should alert the clinician to the presence of either necrotic lung tissue or oesophageal rupture. Antibiotic treatment with intravenous ceftriaxone and per rectum metronidazole is advocated.

Investigation of pleural effusion

Radiology

Chest radiographs are of limited value in identifying the cause of a pleural effusion. In contrast, ultrasound can help confirm the site and presence of an effusion. It is especially useful when a drain has to be placed into loculated fluid.

Examination of pleural fluid

Macroscopic appearance

- Straw coloured fluid, which does not clot on standing, typifies a transudate.
- Turbid fluid is usually due to the increased protein content which often reflects an exudate.
- Bloodstained fluid is likely to be associated with an underlying malignancy or pulmonary embolus.
- Chyle is odourless and milky in appearance.
- Empyema fluid is often very viscous, yellow and frequently foul smelling.

Microscopic and cytological examination

- Transudate cell count less than 100 per mm^3
  - often mixed cells, i.e. lymphocytes, neutrophils, and mesothelial cells.
- Exudate has high white cell count
  - neutrophil leucocytosis often indicative of bacterial infection
  - lymphocytosis suggests tuberculosis or lymphoma.

The presence of malignant cells is likely to be diagnostic though on occasion the precise cell of origin may be difficult to determine.

Microbiology Fluid should be sent for Gram stain, culture and acid and alkali-fast bacillus identification.

Biochemistry Pleural fluid has been described as either a transudate or an exudate based on the protein concentration of less than or greater than 30 g per litre, respectively. Unfortunately this is only a rough guide. A better assessment can be obtained by comparing the pleural fluid concentrations of protein and lactate dehydrogenase with those of blood as shown in the box.

> **Criteria for identifying an exudate**
>
> Total protein pleural fluid to serum ratio greater than 0·5
> Lactate dehydrogenase concentration in pleural fluid greater than 200 IU
> Lactate dehydrogenase serum to pleural fluid ratio greater than 0·6

Other important investigations include:

- glucose – which is consistently low in rheumatoid associated effusions as well as malignancy, empyema, and tuberculosis
- amylase – as pancreatitis can result in a pleural effusion which is most frequently on the left

Pleural biopsy
This is only indicated when pleural fluid analysis fails to establish a diagnosis and ideally should be done at thoracoscopy.

PULMONARY EMBOLISM

Pulmonary embolism is an important condition because it is potentially fatal, often preventable, and sometimes treatable. The majority of pulmonary emboli originate in the deep veins of the legs and pelvis. Occasionally, however the right side of the heart can be the source of emboli, e.g. atrial fibrillation, right ventricular infarction or a dilated right ventricle. Major risk factors of pulmonary embolism are shown in the box.

Risk factors for pulmonary embolism and the "chance" of meeting this factor

Recent surgery	Daily
Immobility for greater than four days	Daily
Age over 40 years	Daily
Previous venous thrombosis/embolism	Daily
Malignant disease	Daily
Sepsis	Daily
Obesity	Daily
Varicose veins	Daily
Pregnancy/oral contraceptive pill	Daily
Nephrotic syndrome	Weekly
Diabetic ketoacidosis	Weekly
Resistance to activated protein C	Annually
Deficiency of antithrombin III	Annually
Deficiency of protein C and S	Only in examinations
Paroxysmal nocturnal haemoglobinuria	Only in examinations
Behçet's disease	Only in examinations

Pathophysiology

One of the normal functions of the lungs is to filter out small blood clots. This process occurs without any symptoms. However, emboli blocking larger branches of the pulmonary artery provoke a rise in pulmonary arterial pressure and rapid shallow respiration. The rise in pressure is believed to be due, in part, to reflex vasoconstriction via the sympathetic nerve fibres and also hypoxia. Tachypnoea is a reflex response to the activation of vagal innervated luminal stretch receptors and interstitial J receptors within the alveolar and capillary network. Furthermore, the release of vasoactive substances suggests that 5-hydroxytryptamine and thromboxane released from activated platelets may enhance vasoconstriction and neurotransmission.

Key point
The effect on haemodynamics will be related to the size of the embolus

---

For clarity, pulmonary embolus will be classified as massive, moderate, and repeated minor emboli.

Massive pulmonary embolism
This usually follows an acute obstruction of at least 50% of the pulmonary circulation. An embolus in the main pulmonary trunk or at the bifurcation of the pulmonary artery (saddle embolus) can produce circulatory collapse, i.e. pulseless electrical activity (PEA or electromechanical dissociation) and death. However, an identical clinical picture may

arise with lesser degrees of obstruction when there has been previous cardiorespiratory dysfunction. An acute massive pulmonary embolus, without immediate death, excites the haemodynamic response as described earlier. The acute increase in pulmonary vascular resistance and thus right ventricular afterload causes a sudden rise in end diastolic pressure and hence dilatation of the right ventricle. This may be manifest clinically as an elevated jugular venous pressure and tricuspid regurgitation. The dilated right ventricle and rise in pulmonary arterial pressure cause a marked fall in systemic arterial pressure by the following mechanisms.

- A fall in left ventricular stroke volume. Dilatation of the right ventricle and increased pulmonary artery pressure ensures that the right ventricular stroke work is depressed. This results in delayed emptying of the right ventricle, and hence a fall in left ventricular stroke volume.
- Interventricular septum displacement. The dilated right ventricle and associated increased pressure cause displacement of the interventricular septum into the left ventricular cavity (the reverse Bernheim effect) reducing left ventricular volume.

These processes culminate in a fall in systemic stroke volume which to some extent is offset by the sympathetic mediated increase in systemic (peripheral) vascular resistance. Thus, the patient with a massive pulmonary embolus can present with the features of "shock" (see Chapter 9).

Moderate pulmonary emboli

Whilst the pathophysiology is identical to that described above, the effect on pulmonary arterial resistance and hence right ventricular function is minimal. The mechanisms underlying breathlessness have already been described. Infarction of the pulmonary parenchyma and associated pleura induces inflammation, both processes culminating in haemoptysis and pleuritic pain.

Minor emboli

These will often go unnoticed but repeated attacks can result in progressive breathlessness, hyperventilation, and possibly effort-induced syncope. If this problem remains undiagnosed pulmonary hypertension will develop leading to hypertrophy and subsequently failure of the right ventricle.

Assessment

The different sites of pulmonary emboli are shown in Figure 8.7.

Differential diagnosis

Acute circulatory collapse is a cardinal feature of massive pulmonary embolism. The differential diagnosis of this shocked state is considered in detail in Chapter 10. However, specific conditions that warrant mention here in the context of acute breathlessness, hypotension, central chest pain, and unconsciousness are acute ventricular failure, myocardial infarction, and cardiac tamponade. All of the major features are related to diminished cardiac output and hence hypoxia and relative hypovolaemia. The differential diagnosis of these conditions, in the acutely ill patient, can be difficult but there are several key features that can help (Table 8.1).

As with all shocked patients high flow oxygen ($FiO_2 = 0.85$) is required. More comprehensive details regarding the management of the shocked patient are provided in Chapter 9.

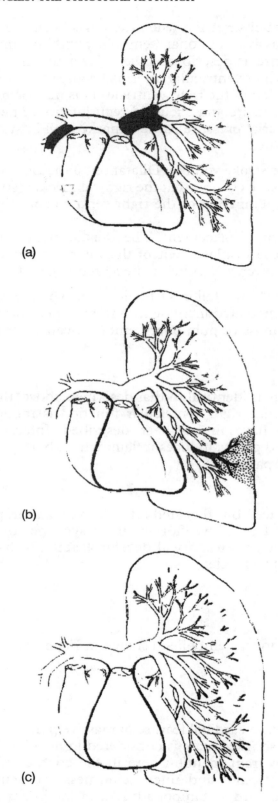

(a)

(b)

(c)

Figure 8.7 The different sites of pulmonary emboli: (a) main trunk (b) third division vessel (c) multiple peripheral

Table 8.1 Key features in the differential diagnosis of breathlessness

Symptoms/signs	PE	LVF	RVF	MI	Tamponade
Breathlessness improves with sitting	No	Yes	No	No	No
Pulmonary oedema	No	Yes	No	No	No
Pulsus paradoxus	Yes	No	No	No	Yes
Raised venous pressure	+++	+	+++	No	+++ (Kussmaul's)
Palpable apex beat	Yes	Yes	Yes	Yes	No
Heart sounds	+ S3/S4	+ S3	+ S3	+ S4	Quiet

PE, pulmonary embolus; LVF, left ventricular failure; RVF, right ventricular failure; MI, myocardial infarction.

Investigations are required to differentiate between the remaining four conditions, of which left ventricular failure is the commonest.

Investigations

- ECG changes will occur in approximately 75% of all patients after a massive pulmonary embolus. However, these are non-specific changes and T wave inversion in the chest leads is the most frequent abnormality. In addition rhythm disturbances, usually a sinus tachycardia or atrial fibrillation, can occur along with manifestations of acute right heart strain ranging from the classic S1, Q111, T111 pattern to right bundle branch block and voltage criteria of right ventricular hypertrophy. Small complexes, possibly with electrical alternans, are suggestive of cardiac tamponade.

Key point
A normal ECG does not exclude either an acute pulmonary embolus or a myocardial infarction

- Chest X-ray is usually unhelpful in the diagnosis of acute pulmonary embolus. Occasionally the affected main pulmonary artery may be prominent or there may be loss of lung volume or rarely a "wedge" shaped defect. However, the chest radiograph will be helpful in the diagnosis of both pulmonary oedema and, to a lesser extent, cardiac tamponade.
- Arterial blood gases. Hypoxaemia and hypercapnia are common after massive or moderate pulmonary emboli. In contrast, a respiratory alkalosis/alkalaemia secondary to hyperventilation is compatible with recurrent small emboli.
- Plasma D-dimer (simply-red test). This is a breakdown product of cross-linked fibrin which is always detectable in thromboembolism. Therefore, its absence excludes a recent pulmonary embolus. This investigation may become widely used in the near future.
- Ventilation/perfusion scans. These remain the most useful screening test to rule out clinically important pulmonary emboli. A high probability of such pathology will be demonstrated in 41% of patients. However, it is not uncommon to receive a report stating "compatible with, but not diagnostic of PE". Under these circumstances, the doctor should treat the patient according to the clinical findings.
- Echocardiography. This will show right ventricular abnormalities in 40% of patients.

- Pulmonary angiography. This remains the gold standard.
- Spiral CT and MRI scans are increasing in popularity, but are not yet routinely available.

Specific treatment for acute pulmonary embolism

Irrespective of the results of investigations, if the clinical suspicion of a pulmonary embolus remains high then the patient should be treated appropriately.

If pulseless electrical activity (electromechanical dissociation) results from a massive pulmonary embolus then resuscitation should follow the European and UK guidelines. With the patient who is hypoxaemic and hypotensive, then immediate resuscitation should reduce hypoxaemia and maintain cardiac output. The major decision is medical versus surgical therapy. This will depend primarily upon:

- whether the patient has any contraindications to thrombolysis
- local surgical expertise.

Contraindications to thrombolysis are shown in the box.

Contraindications to thrombolysis

Prolonged cardiopulmonary resuscitation
Recent major surgery
Active bleeding from the gastrointestinal tract
Recent head injury or neurosurgery (14–17 days previously)
Preceding stroke
Previous streptokinase (greater than one week or less than one year ago)

Thrombolysis, usually in the form of streptokinase, is given intravenously with a loading dose of 250 000 units over one hour, followed by 100 000 units an hour for the first 24 hours. If thrombolysis can be given quickly, where facilities for pulmonary angiography are available, there is often no need for surgical intervention. Angiography has the potential advantages that disruption of the embolus may occur during catheterisation of the pulmonary artery and that thrombolytics can be given directly into the required area.

Most patients with a definitive or suspected diagnosis of pulmonary embolus are treated with intravenous heparin or a low molecular weight variant given subcutaneously. If unfractionated heparin is used, check the activated partial thromboplastic time (APTT) six hours after either starting or changing the dose.

TIME OUT 8.8

Take a five minute break and reflect on the previous section whilst you drink your tea or coffee and answer the following question.

Why do patients with pulmonary emboli become breathless?

NON-CARDIOPULMONARY CAUSES OF BREATHLESSNESS

The respiratory centre is under the influence of both chemical and neurogenic stimuli. Hypoxaemia, for example, at high altitude or acidaemia due to diabetic ketoacidosis or salicylate overdose may, therefore, stimulate the respiratory centre in an attempt to provide more oxygen or promote carbon dioxide excretion. Disruption of the integrity of this centre, for example by a brain stem haemorrhage, will also result in breathlessness.

> **Key point**
> Be wary of labelling people as "hysterical hyperventilators" unless underlying pathology has been excluded

SUMMARY

- Breathlessness is a common medical emergency.
- The structured approach will ensure that the immediately life threatening causes are identified and treated.
- Immediately life threatening causes of breathlessness are:

airway	obstruction
breathing	acute severe asthma
	acute exacerbation of COPD
	acute pulmonary oedema
	tension pneumothorax
circulation	acute severe left ventricular failure
	dysrhythmia
	hypovolaemia
	pulmonary embolus
	cardiac tamponade.

- The pathophysiology of these conditions has been linked to their diagnosis, investigation and management.
- A similar framework has been applied to non immediately life threatening conditions, in particular pneumonia and pleural effusion.

CHAPTER

9

The patient with shock

OBJECTIVES

After reading this chapter you will be able to understand the:

- definition and causes of shock
- underlying pathophysiology of shock
- importance of oxygen delivery and consumption
- structured approach to the shocked patient.

INTRODUCTION

Shock is the result of a series of physiological processes that differ according to the underlying cause. Nevertheless they culminate in a final common pathway that prevents tissues gaining enough oxygen and glucose.

Shock can therefore be defined as a clinical syndrome resulting from inadequate delivery, or utilisation, of essential substrates by vital organs.

It has many causes, but this chapter will concentrate on those giving rise to inadequate delivery of oxygen to the tissues. The other causes will be mentioned only briefly, but will be cross-referenced to more detailed descriptions elsewhere in this manual.

PATHOPHYSIOLOGY

Disruption of oxygen delivery and tissue perfusion are fundamental processes in the pathophysiology of shock. The mechanisms that maintain their integrity in the healthy state have been described in Chapters 5 and 6.

Summary

The body has a number of ways of ensuring that an adequate delivery of blood to vital tissues is maintained. For those who like to think in equations, it is also possible to link these factors as follows.

Delivery of oxygen to tissues = cardiac output × arterial oxygen content
= cardiac output × [(Hb × 1·34 × oxygen saturation) + (0·003 × PaO_2)]

Under normal circumstances using previously defined values the delivery of oxygen to the tissues approximately equals:

$$5000 \text{ ml/min} \times 19 \cdot 8 \text{ ml/100 ml}$$

To remove the effect of the patient's size the delivery index is used. This is the oxygen delivery divided by the surface area of the person.

$$\text{Delivery index} = \text{cardiac index} \times \text{arterial oxygen content} \times 10$$

(10 is added to the equation to convert O_2/100 ml to O_2/litre.)
In normal cases the delivery index approximately equals 500–700 ml/min/m².

Ability of the tissues to take up and use oxygen

At the tissue level, the partial pressure gradient of oxygen is opposite to that found at the alveolar/capillary interface. The capillary PO_2 is approximately 20 mm Hg (2·6 kPa) and cellular PO_2 is only 2–3 mm Hg (< 0·4 kPa). Furthermore, local factors also decrease the affinity of haemoglobin for oxygen (shifting the curve to the right), allowing O_2 to be released more readily. As mentioned earlier this occurs with an increase in:

- hydrogen ion concentration (i.e. fall in pH)
- $PaCO_2$
- 2,3-DPG
- temperature.

> **Tip**
> To help remember these effects, think of the athlete during a race. Active muscles require more oxygen than when they are at rest. With increased metabolism lactic acid, CO_2, and heat are generated. All of these facilitate the release of oxygen from haemoglobin. In addition they will also affect local autoregulatory mechanisms

COMPENSATORY MECHANISMS

When a body is under stress it does not immediately fall. Instead it has several compensatory mechanisms which attempt to maintain adequate oxygen delivery to the essential organs of the body.

Oxygen uptake

Although a sympathetically induced tachypnoea occurs, this does not produce any increase in oxygen uptake because the haemoglobin in blood passing ventilated alveoli is already 97·5% saturated. However, the clinician can help by increasing the inspired concentration of oxygen and ensuring there is adequate ventilation. The slight rise in PAO_2 due to the hypocapnia from hyperventilation only increases this value by around 1%.

Circulatory control

Pressure receptors in the heart and baroreceptors in the carotid sinus and aortic arch trigger a reflex sympathetic response via control centres in the brain stem in response to hypovolaemia. The sympathetic discharge stimulates many tissues in the body including the adrenal medulla which leads to an increased release of systemic catecholamines, enhancing the effects of direct sympathetic discharge, particularly on the heart. This response prevents or limits the fall in cardiac output by positive inotropic and chronotropic effects on the heart and by increasing venous return secondary to veno-constriction.

Furthermore, selective arteriolar and precapillary sphincter constriction of non-essential organs (e.g. skin and gut) maintains perfusion of vital organs (e.g. brain and heart). Selective perfusion also leads to a lowering of the hydrostatic pressure in those capillaries serving non-essential organs. This reduces the diffusion of fluid across the capillary membrane into the interstitial space, thereby decreasing any further loss of intravascular volume. It also has the effect of increasing the diastolic pressure and thereby reducing the pulse pressure.

Tip

Sympathetic stimulation can give rise to the common clinical presentation of shocked patients
- Sweaty and tachycardic – direct sympathetic stimulation
- Pale and cool – reduced skin perfusion
- Ileus – reduced gut perfusion
- Thready pulse – reduced pulse pressure

Any reduction in renal blood flow is detected by the juxtaglomerular apparatus in the kidney, causing renin release. This leads to the formation of angiotensin II and aldosterone. These, together with antidiuretic hormone released from the pituitary, increase the reabsorption of sodium and water by the kidney and reduce urine volume. In addition, the thirst centre of the hypothalamus is also stimulated. The overall result is that the circulating volume is increased. Renin, angiotensin II and antidiuretic hormone can also produce generalised vasoconstriction and so help increase the venous return. Furthermore, insulin and glucagon are also released to assist the supply and utilisation of glucose by the cells. In addition, the body attempts to enhance the circulating volume by releasing osmotically active substances from the liver. These increase plasma osmotic pressure and so cause interstitial fluid to be drawn into the intravascular space.

Key point

A fall in blood pressure will only take place when no further compensation is possible. It is therefore a **late** sign in shock

---

Tissue oxygen consumption

The total consumption of oxygen per minute (VO_2) for a resting healthy male is 100–160 ml/min/m^2. As the delivery of oxygen (DO_2) is 500–720 ml/min/m^2, the tissues use only 20–25% of the oxygen that is available. This is referred to as the **oxygen extraction ratio** (OER). This low value indicates that body tissues have a tremendous potential to extract more oxygen from the circulating blood.

The total consumption of oxygen per minute is constant throughout a wide range of oxygen delivery in a healthy subject (Figure 9.1). Under normal circumstances an increase in oxygen demand is met by increasing the oxygen delivery, usually from a rise in the cardiac output. However, should this not be possible, or inadequate, then VO_2 can

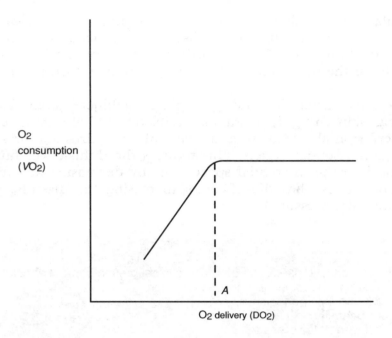

Figure 9.1   The relationship between oxygen delivery and consumption A is the critical level for DO_2. VO_2 below A depends directly on DO_2.

be maintained to a limited extent by increasing the oxygen extraction ratio. Should this also fail, then VO_2 will begin to fall because it is now directly dependent on the delivery of oxygen (Figure 9.1).

Increasing the oxygen extraction ratio leads to a fall in the venous oxygen saturation. This is difficult to detect clinically early on and its actual value varies from organ to organ. However, it can be measured from a mixed venous sample directly. This is done through a special port on the pulmonary artery flotation catheter that allows sampling of blood in the pulmonary artery. Under normal circumstances this is approximately 75%, with values below 70% indicating that global delivery of oxygen is becoming inadequate. An alternative method, albeit crude, is to calculate the difference in carbon dioxide content between central venous and arterial blood. When tissue oxygenation is adequate this difference is less than 6 mm Hg.

Key point
There is a chain of events that delivers oxygen to the tissues where it is utilised by the cells. Each part has a finite capacity to compensate when one or more links in the chain are defective

---

TIME OUT 9.1

a. Take a moment to list the 5 factors that influence the delivery of oxygen to tissues.
b. How does the sympathetic nervous system help to compensate for a defect in oxygen delivery?

CAUSES OF SHOCK

Many conditions can lead to an inadequate delivery of oxygen to vital structures of the body. An *aide-mémoire* can be categorised as.

- Decrease in oxygen uptake by the lungs
- Reduced venous return
- Impaired cardiac function
- Reduced arterial tone
- Impaired organ autoregulation
- Decreased oxygen uptake and utilisation by tissues

Each of these can be responsible alone or in combination as the cause of shock (Figure 9.2).

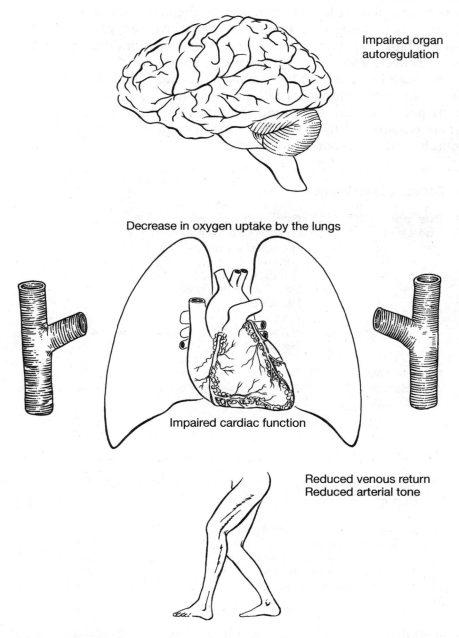

Impaired organ autoregulation

Decrease in oxygen uptake by the lungs

Impaired cardiac function

Reduced venous return
Reduced arterial tone

Figure 9.2   Diagrammatic representation of systems that cause shock

The first component represents 'A' and 'B' causes of shock whereas the next four are 'C' related. The final one usually follows poisoning.

Decrease in oxygen uptake by the lungs

The airway and pulmonary conditions leading to a fall in oxygen uptake are described in detail in Chapter 19.

Reduced venous return

This reduction in preload is commonly due to **hypovolaemia** or **interference with venous return**.

True hypovolaemia is associated with loss of either blood or plasma (see next box). Upper gastrointestinal sources are a common cause for haemorrhage in medical patients. In contrast excessive plasma loss is often seen at the extremes of age with gastroenteritis. However, there may be more than one mechanism involved, e.g. in diabetic ketoacidosis the fluid loss is related to a combination of hyperventilation, osmotic diuresis, decreased body sodium, vomiting and, possibly, the precipitating condition.

Many drugs cause hypotension by reducing preload. Though this effect may be beneficial to patients with left ventricular failure, it can lead to a marked fall in blood pressure particularly in patients with low blood volumes. The true hypovolaemia and hyponatraemia associated with Addison's adrenal insufficiency are attributed to the deficiency of both mineralo and gluco corticoid hormones.

Causes of hypovolaemic shock

True loss	Common examples
Blood loss	Gastrointestinal haemorrhage
	Ruptured aortic aneurysm
	Trauma
Plasma loss	Diarrhoea and vomiting
	Diabetic ketoacidosis
	Pancreatitis
	Osmotic diuresis
	Hyponatraemia and mineralocorticoid deficiency
	Burns
	Fistula and ostomies
Apparent loss	**Common examples**
Venodilators	Nitrates, opiates, intravenous loop diuretics
Hyponatraemia	Glucocorticoid deficiency

The common causes of impeding preload are shown in the box.

Common causes of reduced preload

- High mean airway pressure (e.g., high PPV)   Daily
- Acute asthma   Daily
- Massive pulmonary embolus   Weekly
- Tension pneumothorax   Monthly
- Cardiac tamponade   Annually

Blood returning to the heart depends on the pressure gradient created by the high hydrostatic pressure in the peripheral veins and low hydrostatic pressure in the right atrium of the heart. Any reduction in this gradient, e.g. by increasing right atrial pressure, will lead to a fall in venous return to the heart. External compression on the thorax or abdomen can have a similar action in obstructing the venous return. Consequently in the supine position, the gravid uterus can compress the inferior vena cava and impair venous return.

Impaired cardiac function

A variety of conditions can adversely influence ventricular function and lead to shock.

Summary of the cardiac causes of shock		
● Endocardial	Acute valve lesion	Infective endocarditis
		Papillary muscle rupture
● Myocardial	Ventricular failure/	Ischaemia/infarction
	conduction problems	Myocarditis
		Drugs
		Toxins
		Cardiomyopathy
● Epicardial	Acute tamponade	Ventricular wall rupture
		Malignancy
		Post surgery
	Constrictive pericarditis	Viral
		Tuberculosis
		Radiotherapy

It is important to remember that antiarrhythmic drugs being taken by the patient, or given acutely, may have a significant negative inotropic effect. The same effect is seen with certain drugs taken as an overdose, for example, tricyclic antidepressants. Myocardial function can also be impaired by infection (myocarditis), an underlying cardiomyopathy or toxins associated with the systemic inflammatory response syndrome (see later). Cardiac tamponade, in addition to its effect on venous return, also impedes ventricular filling.

As can be seen from the earlier description, several factors can interfere with the effectiveness of the cardiac pump. However, the term **cardiogenic shock** is reserved for patients who have an impaired cardiac performance resulting from 40%, or more, of the ventricular myocardium being affected. Consequently shock due to hypovolaemia, vasovagal reactions, arrhythmias and drug reactions must be excluded first.

> **Key point**
> In cardiogenic shock the compensatory sympathetic and catecholamine response, i.e., increased heart rate and systemic vascular resistance, only serve to raise the myocardial oxygen demand and exacerbate the degree of ischaemia

Impaired arterial tone

Anaphylactic shock
Anaphylaxis is an acute reaction to a foreign substance to which the patient has already been sensitised. This leads to an immunoglobulin E (IgE) triggered rapid degranulation of mast cells and basophils (see box). Anaphylactoid reactions have an identical clinical presentation but are not triggered by IgE and do not necessarily require previous exposure. Furthermore, they may not produce a reaction every time.

119

Common causes of anaphylaxis/anaphylactoid reactions

- Anaphylaxis — Drugs (protein and non-protein) – commonly penicillin or other β lactam drugs, blood products, and immunoglobulins
  Vaccines
  Food – especially nuts, shellfish
  Venoms – especially bees, wasps, and hornets
  Parasites
  Chemicals
  Latex
- Anaphylactoid — Complement activation
  Coagulation/fibrinolysis system activation
  Direct pharmacological release of mediators
  Exercise induced
  Idiopathic

Key point
The most common causes of anaphylactic fatalities are parenteral penicillin, bee stings and food-related reactions. Radio-contrast and non-steroidal anti-inflammatory medications are the most common anaphylactoid fatalities

The body's response to these stimuli is to release a collection of mediators from mast cells and basophils that have inflammatory, spasmogenic, and chemotactic actions. The inflammatory activators induce vasodilatation and oedema. The spasmogens cause bronchial smooth muscle contraction, increased mucus production and mucosal oedema. The chemotactic agents attract platelets and white blood cells to the affected area.

Systemic inflammatory response syndrome and septic shock
It has long been recognised that the physiological and clinical signs of sepsis can result from a variety of causes as well as infection (Figure 9.3). As a consequence the term systemic inflammatory response syndrome (SIRS) should be used when describing the inflammatory response and 'sepsis' reserved for SIRS patients with definite infection.

Systemic inflammatory response syndrome (SIRS) and sepsis

To avoid previous confusion and aid communication, the meanings of SIRS, sepsis and septic shock have been standardised (see box).

Recommended standard terminology

SIRS
Resulting from a variety of severe causes, SIRS is manifested by two of the following.
- Temperature greater than 38°C or less than 36°C
- Heart rate greater than 90/min
- Respiratory rate greater than 20/min or $PaCO_2$ less than 4·3 kPa (32 mm Hg)
- White blood count greater than 12 000 cell/mm³, less than 4000 cell/mm³ or greater than 10% immature forms

Sepsis
- SIRS resulting from documented infection

Septic shock
Sepsis associated with organ dysfunction and systolic BP less than 90 mm Hg (or a reduction of over 40 mm Hg from baseline) in the absence of other causes for hypotension and despite adequate fluid resuscitation.

When SIRS has an infective origin the circulating endotoxins (inflammatory mediators) have a negative inotropic effect, cause vasodilatation and impair energy utilisation at a cellular level; the source is usually Gram negative bacteria. Occasionally Gram positive bacteria release toxins causing the **toxic shock syndrome**. *Staphylococcus aureus* is the usual organism although some severe streptococcal infections can have a similar presentation.

Causes of toxic shock syndrome

- Retained tampon
- Abscess
- Empyema
- Surgical wound infection
- Osteomyelitis
- Cellulitis
- Infected burns
- Septic abortion

With SIRS, tissue hypoxaemia may occur even with normal or high oxygen delivery rates because the tissue oxygen demand is extremely high. In addition there is increased capillary permeability at the primary site of the infection/inflammation. Without treatment this becomes more generalised, allowing sodium and water to move from the interstitial to the intracellular space. Eventually hypovolaemia develops and the condition becomes indistinguishable from hypovolaemic shock.

Arteriovenous shunts develop in the tissues resulting in maldistribution of blood flow. This either increases the chances of or exacerbates tissue ischaemia. This situation may be aggravated by endotoxin (tumour necrosis factor) and other cytokines which act as negative inotropes on the myocardium.

In the late stages, septic shock will affect all parts of the circulatory system. Venous return is reduced as pro-inflammatory cytokines increase capillary permeability. Further cellular damage by endotoxins causes the release of proteolytic enzymes. These paralyse precapillary sphincters, enhance capillary leakage and increase hypovolaemia. The resultant loss of fluid and protein causes hypovolaemia which, combined with venodilatation, produces a fall in preload. The reduction in tissue blood flow resulting from decreased perfusion and the increased viscosity leads to platelet aggregation and clot formation. At the same time thromboplastins are activated. Consequently disseminated intravascular coagulation can result and lead to further falls in tissue perfusion.

Myocardial depression occurs, especially in severe sepsis. This is due to multiple factors including hypoxaemia, acidosis, myocardial oedema, and circulating negative inotropes. Tissue autoregulation is disrupted and there is marked peripheral arterial dilatation. In addition to all of these changes, tissue oxygen demand increases but uptake is impaired. It will not, therefore, be surprising to find that septic shock has an extremely high mortality rate (> 50%).

Key point
In the late stage of SIRS, there are several causes for the shocked state

---

Neurogenic shock

A spinal lesion above **T6** can impair the sympathetic nervous system outflow from the cord below this level. As a consequence both the reflex tachycardia and vasoconstriction responses to hypovolaemia are eliminated. The result is generalised vasodilatation, bradycardia and loss of temperature control. As neurogenic shock leads to a reduction in blood supply to the spinal column, it gives rise to additional nervous tissue damage.

Impaired autoregulation

The intrinsic properties of some vascular smooth muscle can be lost when the vessels become rigid, for example, with atheroma.

Consequently tissue flow will begin to fall at a higher perfusing pressure than normal and as the condition deteriorates there is paralysis of the smooth muscle in the small blood vessel walls. This allows flow to become pressure dependent and vessels, such as skin arterioles, will begin to distend. The latter can lead to blood going to non-vital areas at the expense of more clinically important tissues.

Microcirculatory changes in the late stages lead to stagnation of blood flow, sludging of red cells and a further impairment of tissue perfusion. In addition, the hydrostatic pressure within the capillaries increases because blood can still perfuse the capillaries but cannot escape. Consequently further intravascular fluid is lost as it diffuses through the capillary wall into the interstitial space.

Decreased oxygen uptake and utilisation by tissues

This occurs as a result of toxins released in sepsis as well as from poison such as carbon monoxide and cyanide.

TIME OUT 9.2

Describe how sepsis can lead to shock.

MANAGEMENT OF THE SHOCKED PATIENT

It follows that patients cannot remain permanently in a state of shock; they either improve or die. Indeed shock could be looked upon as a momentary pause on the way to death. Its detection depends on certain physical signs that are produced as a result of poor oxygen delivery. Similarly, the treatment of shock consists of restoration of an adequate delivery of oxygen and not simply the restoration of a normal blood pressure.

Airway

The first priority in any shocked patient is to clear and on occasion secure the airway and give oxygen at 15 l/min (see Chapter 4). Once the airway has been cleared, adequate ventilation with a high, inspired oxygen concentration is required. This is often difficult (in patients with active haematemesis), therefore early liaison with an anaesthetist is necessary.

Unconscious patients with grade IV shock should be intubated and ventilated with 100% oxygen.

Breathing

Record the respiratory rate and examine for signs of bronchospasm, pulmonary oedema, embolus or tension pneumothorax, and treat as appropriate.

Circulation

Look at the patient noting colour, sweating, distress, and the presence of distended or flat neck veins. Then **feel** the pulse for either a brady or a tachycardia. Is the patient vasodilated with a bounding pulse? Then check the position of the apex beat if it is palpable. Finish by **listening** for the presence of a third sound and/or heart murmur/s.

Follow this brief cardiovascular assessment by connecting the patient to an ECG and blood pressure monitor. Then obtain peripheral intravenous access with the largest cannula possible (ideally a 14 or 16 gauge) and take 20 ml of blood for laboratory tests. These include full blood count, urea and electrolytes, glucose and, if clinically appropriate, crossmatch, cardiac enzymes, amylase, blood cultures, and toxicology.

The antecubital fossa is the site of choice for venous access. With hypovolaemia it is important that fluid is infused quickly, therefore short, wide cannulae should be used because the flow of a liquid in a tube is directly related to its diameter and inversely proportional to the length (Table 9.1).

Table 9.1 Cannula size and rate of flow

Cannula	Rate of flow (ml/min)
14 gauge short	175–200
14 gauge long	150
16 gauge short	100–150
16 gauge long	50–100

If a peripheral site is not available in adults, central venous access is advocated. This procedure should **only** be done by experienced staff because of the potential for damaging the vein and neighbouring structures.

By the end of this assessment, the answers to the following questions should have been ascertained:

- is shock present?
- if present, what is its likely cause?

Further information from a well "phrased" history will help in deciding the answers to these questions.

Hypovolaemic shock

In hypovolaemic shock the primary aim of treatment is to prevent further bleeding if at all possible. Examples of this include the use of a Sengstaken tube for a variceal bleed. Often, however, there is no definite source for blood or fluid loss. In these cases, the clinician should move on to the next stage of management which is assessing the degree of intravascular volume loss.

Estimating volume loss and grading shock
The compensatory mechanisms evoked by "shock" are related to the decline in function of various organs. Thus by monitoring these changes it is possible to grade the degree of shock. Respiratory rate, capillary refill (see later), heart rate, blood pressure, urine output and conscious level can be readily measured and so are important indicators of both the grade of shock and the response to treatment. These physiological changes can be used to divide hypovolaemic shock into four categories depending on the percentage blood loss (Table 9.2). The important features are:

- A tachycardia often occurs early due to the sympathetic response.
- In grade II shock the diastolic blood pressure rises, without any fall in the systolic component, leading to a narrowed pulse pressure. This is due to the compensatory sympathetic nervous system mediated vasoconstriction. Consequently, a narrow pulse pressure with a normal systolic blood pressure is an early sign of shock.
- Tachypnoea can indicate shock as well as underlying respiratory or metabolic pathology.
- Hypotension indicates a loss of approximately 30% of the circulating volume.

Table 9.2 Categories of hypovolaemic shock

| | Category | | | |
	I	II	III	IV
Blood loss (litres)	<0·75	0·75–1.5	1·5–2·0	>2·0
Blood loss (%BV)*	<15%	15–30%	30–40%	>40%
Heart rate	<100	>100	>120	140 or low
Systolic BP	Normal	Normal	Decreased	Decreased ++
Diastolic BP	Normal	Raised	Decreased	Decreased ++
Pulse pressure	Normal	Decreased	Decreased	Decreased
Capillary refill	Normal	Delayed	Delayed	Delayed
Skin	Normal	Pale	Pale	Pale/cold
Respiratory rate	14–20	20–30	30–40	>35 or low
Urine output (ml/hour)	>30	20–30	5–15	Negligible
Mental state	Normal	Anxious	Anxious/confused	Confused/drowsy

*% B/V = % of blood volume

Limitations to estimations of hypovolaemia

For some patients, blindly following the signs in Table 9.2 could lead to a gross over- or underestimation of the blood loss (see box). It is therefore important that management is based on the overall condition of the patient and not isolated physiological parameters.

> **Pitfalls in assessing blood loss**
>
> - Elderly
> - Drugs
> - Pacemaker
> - Athlete
> - Pregnancy
> - Hypothermia
> - Compensation
> - Tissue damage

The **elderly patient** is less able to compensate for acute hypovolaemia as their sympathetic drive is reduced. Consequently the loss of smaller volumes can produce a fall in blood pressure. Reliance only on the blood pressure could therefore lead to an overestimation of blood loss.

A variety of **drugs** that are commonly taken can alter the physiological response to blood loss. For example, β blockers will prevent tachycardia and also inhibit the normal sympathetic positive inotropic response. Therefore, after a 15% circulating volume loss compensatory tachycardia is unlikely to occur in a β blocked patient. This could lead to an underestimation of the blood loss. It is also important to remember that the blood pressure falls at lower volumes of blood loss in these patients by the same mechanisms.

An increasing number of patients have **pacemakers** fitted each year. These devices may only allow the heart to beat at a particular rate irrespective of the volume loss. Therefore they will give rise to the same errors in estimation as β blockers.

The physiological response to training will mean that the **athlete** will have a larger blood volume and a resting bradycardia (about 50 beats per minute). The blood volume can increase by 15–20%; thus it is possible to underestimate blood loss, especially as a compensatory increase in heart rate can mean that the pulse is less than 100 beats per minute.

During **pregnancy** the heart rate progressively increases so that by the third trimester it is 15–20 beats faster than normal. Blood pressure falls by 5–15 mm Hg in the second trimester and returns to normal during the third as the blood volume has increased by 40–50%. Supine hypotension due to compression of the inferior vena cava has been discussed earlier.

Hypothermia will reduce the blood pressure, pulse and respiratory rate irrespective of any other cause of shock. Depending on the temperature, hypothermic patients are often resistant to cardiovascular drugs, cardioversion or fluid replacement. The estimation of the fluid requirements of these patients can therefore be very difficult and often invasive monitoring is required.

Prolonging the time without resuscitation (especially in the young) increases the action of the normal **compensatory mechanisms**. This can lead to improvements in blood pressure, respiratory rate, and heart rate. Thus, an underestimation of the blood loss could occur.

The degree of **tissue damage** can have a profound effect on the patient's physiological response. The initial tachycardia can convert into a bradycardia when there is a significant haemorrhage with little tissue damage (e.g. a gastrointestinal bleed). At this stage the blood pressure also begins to fall. Conversely, when there is marked tissue damage, the blood pressure and tachycardia are maintained for larger haemorrhages. Consequently the degree of blood loss can be over- or underestimated depending upon the absence or presence of significant tissue damage.

Once the degree of blood loss has been estimated, the clinician needs to consider the possible causes so that appropriate management can be introduced.

Management

General   In grade I shock, a litre of crystalloid is infused and the response monitored. If hypovolaemia is estimated to be grade II or higher, 500 ml intravenous colloid challenge is required. The aim should be to maintain the haematocrit (packed cell volume) at 30–35% so that oxygen delivery is optimised. Red cell replacement is secondary, becoming more important with progressively larger blood losses.

> **Tip**
> Remember the advantageous effect of a reduced haematocrit on blood flow

All fluids need to be warmed before they are given to patients to prevent iatrogenically induced hypothermia. A simple way of achieving this is to store a supply of colloids and crystalloids in a warming cupboard. This eliminates the need for warming coils, which increase resistance to flow and thereby slow the rate of fluid administration.

The above management should be modified in hypotensive patients where there is a definite bleeding source that has not been controlled. In these cases vigorous fluid resuscitation will lead to further bleeding and a worse prognosis. These patients require the origin of the bleeding to be controlled urgently. In the meantime fluid needs to be administered so that the blood pressure is maintained at 20 mm Hg below the baseline. This is known as **hypotensive resuscitation**.

Specific   The source of bleeding in the acutely ill medical patient is often the upper gastrointestinal tract and, as a group, accounts for 1–2% of medical admissions. The specific causes are listed in the box.

Upper gastrointestinal haemorrrhage: causes and frequency

34%	duodenal ulcer
19%	gastric ulcer
15%	no lesion identified
11%	oesophagitis
8%	gastroduodenitis
5%	malignancy (upper gastrointestinal tract)
4%	varices
4%	others

In addition to the general management principles described earlier, the clinician should also consider **early** liaison with surgical colleagues. Immediately after resuscitation has started, inform the surgical gastroenterology team of the clinical problem and request a review. Combined medical and surgical management is the ideal. The decision to operate is usually based on continuing haemorrhage and the patient's tranfusion needs.

Need for surgery with upper gastrointestinal tract bleed

- **Six units** of blood in patients aged less than 65 years, unless there is a history of non-steroidal anti-inflammatory drugs (NSAID) use or comorbid pathology
- **Four units** of blood in patients greater than 65 years of age or those less than 65 years with a history of NSAID use or comorbid pathology

---

If oesophageal varices are suspected, based on the presence of chronic liver disease stigmata or from the history, octreotide (a synthetic somatostatin analogue) should be given intravenously. The loading dose is 50 micrograms followed by an infusion of 25 micrograms/hour increasing to 50 micrograms if required to control haemorrhage. Early liaison with a gastroenterologist is important for endoscopic intervention. Tamponade devices are rarely required and should only be introduced by an appropriately trained individual.

Key point
Bleeding from varices is rare when compared with gastroduodenal inflammation/ulceration, **even** in alcohol users

---

Cardiac tamponade

The symptoms associated with cardiac tamponade (Chapter 9) can be transiently improved by administering a fluid challange to assist ventricular filling pressures. If, however, this presents as a pulseless electrical activity (PEA) or electromechanical dissociation arrest, then resuscitation according to the UK and European protocol is required augmented by pericardiocentesis. In the conscious patient echocardiography should be used to facilitate needle pericardiocentesis. If this equipment is unavailable or the patient is deteriorating, then drainage of the pericardium should be done using ECG control.

Tension pneumothorax

The clinical features and the management of this condition are described in detail in Chapter 8.

Massive pulmonary emboli (PE)

For a comprehensive description of this condition, see Chapter 8.

With greater than 25% obstruction in pulmonary flow there is an acute rise in the right ventricular afterload. Though the right ventricular pressure continues to rise with further obstruction, its maximum mean is 30 mm Hg. With a massive pulmonary embolus there is inadequate filling of the left side of the heart, impaired cardiac output and elevated right atrial pressure (Chapter 8). Acute mortality correlates with the presence of systemic hypotension, implying that early survival is dependent upon the right ventricular function. In contrast, long term survival has been shown to be largely dependent upon coexisting cardiovascular disease.

These patients present in a shocked state with marked dyspnoea and may have a preceding history of a deep venous thrombosis (DVT). In addition there can be chest pain, syncope and occasionally haemoptysis. In view of the right outflow obstruction, right heart strain is usually evident on the ECG. Due to the ventilatory–perfusion mismatch, the PaO_2 is invariably low. In addition neurohumoral factors are released which cause pulmonary vasoconstriction and occasional wheezing. Some alveoli become overventilated compared to the perfusion. As a result the dead space increases and the expired PCO_2 falls. If a pulmonary artery occlusion pressure catheter is inserted, a high right ventricular pressure will be recorded along with a low cardiac output.

Diagnosis is difficult and depends on thinking about the possibility and excluding other possible causes. Depending upon the clinical state of the patient, several investigations can be carried out (see next box). However, when dealing with a moribund patient the clinician may have to base the immediate management solely on their clinical suspicion. In such situations carry out a 12 lead ECG and a chest X-ray will help to quickly exclude other causes of cardiovascular collapse.

Investigations for diagnosing a pulmonary embolus

- Ventilation:perfusion (V:Q) scan
- Colour flow doppler of the lower limbs
- Arteriography
- D-dimer
- Spiral computed tomography (CT)
- Transoesophageal echocardiography
- Thoracic impedance

Management

As with all shocked patients, the airway needs to be cleared and high flow oxygen provided. After obtaining intravenous access, give a fluid challenge of 1000 ml of crystalloid to attempt to increase the perfusion pressure. Should this fail consider using vasopressors to maintain the diastolic pressure and thereby help coronary artery perfusion. Once the diagnosis is made thrombolytics should be administered by a peripheral line provided there are no contraindications. This should then be followed by a heparin infusion. As 20% of patients with a massive pulmonary embolus reembolise during lytic therapy, some authorities advocate insertion of a temporary vena caval umbrella.

Impaired cardiac function

Shock resulting from heart failure is common. If this is suspected, it is essential to discover the past medical history and current medications. Clinically, in addition to the more usual signs of shock, there may be evidence of left and/or right ventricular failure and/or a dysrhythmia. These are described in detail in Chapter 19. See box for summary.

Signs of cardiogenic shock

- Raised JVP
- Basal crackles
- Third heart sound
- Occasionally marked breathlessness and central cyanosis from pulmonary oedema
- Occasionally murmurs, e.g. mitral valve regurgitation (due to ventricular dilatation)

Patients with heart failure are less able to compensate for hypovolaemia, should that coexist. This problem is compounded by the fact that measurement of the central venous pressure (CVP) does not provide an accurate estimate of the left ventricular end diastolic pressure (box). These patients are therefore best managed using a pulmonary artery catheter. This enables both the filling pressure of the left side of the heart and the cardiac output to be estimated and accurate fluid resuscitation provided.

Disadvantages of CVP monitoring in heart failure

- Measures right ventricular pressure
- Often raised due to lung pathology
- Affected by positive pressure ventilation
- Malposition causing false elevations

Management

The first management priority is correction of hypoxaemia, even if this requires the patient to be intubated and ventilated with supplemental oxygen. When cardiogenic shock is due to right heart failure, give a test infusion of 200 ml of colloid and assess the effect. In contrast, when filling pressures are high, these need to be reduced in a controlled fashion. Intravenous nitrates are often used as they lower the systemic vascular resistance. Dopamine and dobutamine may also be required to provide inotropic support and improve the cardiac output. Any dysrhythmia causing haemodynamic compromise must also be treated.

It is not unusual to find that a combination of mechanical ventilation, vasodilators, inotropes, and fluids is required to increase the cardiac index and the delivery of oxygen. Clearly these procedures require the facilities available in coronary care, high dependency or intensive treatment units.

Anaphylactic shock

Clinical manifestations include:

Airway   oedema of the face and tongue
                laryngeal oedema
Breathing   bronchoconstriction
                respiratory arrest
Circulation myocardial infarction
                cardiovascular collapse.

In view of the variety of chemical mediators released, cardiovascular collapse can result from one, or more, of the following reasons:

- arrhythmia
- hypovolaemia
- decreased myocardial function
- pulmonary hypertension.

Arrhythmias may result from direct mediator effects as well as hypoxaemia, hypotension, acidosis, preexisting cardiac disease and adrenaline given during resuscitation. Hypovolaemia can occur very quickly with up to 50% of the circulating plasma volume being lost within 10–15 minutes in severe cases. This is due to a combination of increased vascular permeability, vasodilatation, and decreased venous return from raised intra-thoracic pressure secondary to bronchospasm and positive pressure ventilation.

The vast majority of serious anaphylactic reactions occur unexpectedly. Over 50% of fatalities occur within the first hour. Seventy five percent of these deaths are due to asphyxia from upper airway obstruction or bronchospasm. The remaining cases die from circulatory failure and hypotension.

> **Key point**
> The diagnosis is not difficult when a patient presents with generalised urticaria, wheeze, and hypotension following a known stimulus. However, circulatory collapse can occur without preceding warning signs

Management
The management of anaphylactic shock is dependent upon a rapid ABC assessment and resuscitation, considering the diagnosis and preventing any further absorption of the suspected causative agent. Always be wary because airway obstruction, bronchospasm, and hypotension can have a delayed presentation.

Anaphylactic reactions for adults: treatment by first medical responder (Figure 9.3)   An inhaled β agonist such as salbutamol may be used as an adjunctive measure if bronchospasm is severe and does not respond rapidly to other treatment. If profound shock is judged immediately life threatening, give cardiopulmonary resuscitation/advanced life support if necessary. Consider slow intravenous (IV) adrenaline (epinephrine) 1:10000 solution. This is hazardous and is recommended only for an experienced practitioner who can also obtain IV access without delay. Note the different strength of adrenaline (epinephrine) that is required for IV use. A crystalloid may be safer than colloid.

Following resuscitation, the patient should be admitted for 8 to 12 hours of monitoring to detect those cases which develop a protracted or biphasic response. The latter is more likely following oral antigen ingestion or when symptoms started over 30 minutes after exposure.

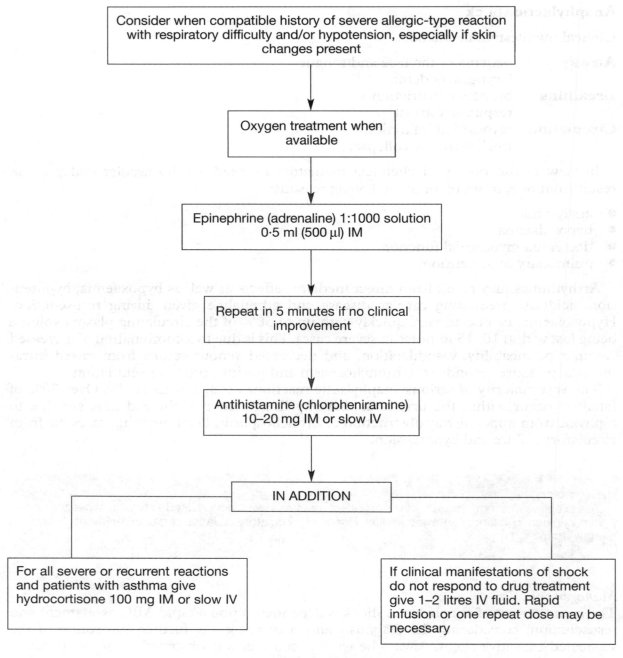

Figure 9.3 Management of anaphylactic shock

The diagnosis of septic shock can be difficult. In comparison with other causes of shock (except anaphylactic), the physiological features are usually (but not always) high cardiac output and low systemic vascular resistance (Table 9.3). The classic signs are a wide pulse pressure and warm skin due to the dilated peripheral vessels, agitation, pyrexia, and an increased respiratory rate due to hypoxaemia. Later on, the classic features of hypovolaemic shock are manifested with peripheral vasoconstriction and a low or normal core temperature. There may also be evidence of disseminated intravascular coagulation. This abnormality often manifests as blood oozing around wounds and cannula sites.

Table 9.3 Haemodynamic variables in shock (adult mean values)

	Left atrial pressure (mm Hg)	Cardiac output (l/min)	Systemic vascular resistance (dyn/s/cm²)
Normal	10	5	1200
Left ventricular failure	25	2	3000
Haemorrhage	0	3	3000
Sepsis and anaphylaxis	2	12	300

As described before, the type of septic shock known as the toxic shock syndrome has many potential causes. However, the clinical presentation remains the same:

- temperature greater than 38·9°C
- macular, blanching rash
- hypotension
- evidence of involvement of at least three systems.

The rash can be localised or general and tends to lead to desquamation after one or two weeks in survivors. Common systems which are involved are gastrointestinal (diarrhoea and vomiting); neurological (confusion, drowsy); renal (impaired function); muscle (myalgia, high creatine phosphokinase); hematological (leucocytosis, disseminated intravascular coagulation, thrombocytopenia).

Key points
- Maintain a high index of suspicion because diagnosing septic shock can be difficult
- Always check for the non-blanching purpuric rash of meningococcal septicaemia
- Consider the diagnosis in any ill patient with an altered conscious level and haemodynamic instability without any obvious cause

Management

If these patients are to survive, the source of infection needs to be removed. Repeated blood cultures are required to determine the causative organism. Antibiotic therapy should be aimed at the most likely organism. However, often a combination of a penicillin, aminoglycoside and metronidazole is used according to the hospital antibiotic policy. If meningococcal septicaemia is suspected give benzyl penicillin 2·4 g and ceftriaxone 1 g intravenously **immediately**. When there is a collection of pus, drainage will be required by either surgery or percutaneously under imaging control.

The patient will require cardiovascular and respiratory support, as well as intensive monitoring of their fluid and antibiotic regimes. The former aims to maintain a high cardiac index (over 4·5 l/min/m²), high oxygen delivery (above 600 ml/min/m²) and tissue perfusion pressure. This usually entails intubating and ventilating the patient with supplemental oxygen, correction of hypovolaemia with colloid and the use of inotropes. The response to all vasoactive drugs is unpredictable. It is therefore advisable to start with a low dose and titrate further amounts until the cardiac index is sufficient to allow acceptable tissue perfusion. In adults this is usually at a level greater than 4·5 l/min/m².

The indications for ventilation are no different from those routinely used:

- inability to maintain an airway
- inability to maintain normal PaO_2 and $PaCO_2$
- persistant tachypnoea despite adequate oxygenation and volume replacement

- persistant metabolic acidaemia
- elevated serum lactate.

Noradrenaline is frequently needed for its α agonist activity that helps counteract some of the profound vasodilatation.

Neurogenic shock

In the context of acute medical emergencies neurogenic shock is rare. Patients who are susceptible to spontaneous cervical vertebral subluxation include those with rheumatoid disease or Down's syndrome. In contrast, ankylosing spondylitis can produce an inflexible cervical spine that fractures following minimal trauma.

The effects of neurogenic shock result from the loss of sympathetic output. This gives rise to a systolic blood pressure of approximately 90 mm Hg with a heart rate of around 50 per minute. In addition the patient has warm and pink skin due to vasodilatation. However, due to an initial pressor response releasing catecholamines into the circulation, the onset of these signs can take minutes to hours to develop. This situation may persist for up to 24 hours before the levels of catecholamines fall enough to reveal the neurogenic shock.

The lack of sympathetic tone decreases the patient's response to other types of shock. It also enhances the vagal effect produced by stimulation of the pharynx, for example, during laryngoscopy. This can lead to profound bradycardia requiring treatment with glycopyrrolate. Atropine can be used but it produces dry, thick secretions which increase the lung dysfunction.

Due to the nature of the injury the patient will also present with motor and sensory loss. However, these are difficult to assess in the unconscious patient. If in doubt immobilise the cervical spine and request a neurosurgical/orthopaedic review.

Key points
- Beware of the unconscious patient who is admitted following a fall downstairs. The initial neurological features are often attributed to an underlying stroke
- Spinal stabilisation must be maintained until specialist advice is obtained if a spinal injury is suspected from either the mechanism of the injury or the physical signs

---

Management
These patients usually require intubation as the risks of regurgitation and aspiration are increased due to the presence of a paralytic ileus, a full stomach and an incompetent gastrooesophageal sphincter. As close to 100% oxygen should be given, not least because the damaged spinal cord is very sensitive to hypoxaemia. Always maintain in-line cervical spine immobilisation by an assistant holding the head or by the use of commercially available apparatus.

Key point
Intubation is not contraindicated in the presence of cervical spine instability

---

Persistent signs or symptoms of shock must not be attributed to the presence of spinal cord injury particularly if there is evidence of haemorrage or trauma. Correction of any bleeding source is still relevant in cases of spinal injury because of the risks of hypoperfusion of the spinal cord. In the presence of an isolated spinal cord injury, a systolic blood pressure of 80–90 mm Hg is initially acceptable and usually achieved with a fluid challenge of 0·5–1 litre. Patients with an enduring bradycardia of less than 50 beats per minute should be given atropine 0·5–1 mg intravenously, and repeated if necessary until the heart rate is acceptable. If this fails, inotropes may be required but this will involve the use of invasive haemodynamic monitoring to ensure that the patient does not develop pulmonary complications due to inappropriate fluid management.

Early insertion of an arterial line is necessary in these patients. This provides continuous, accurate blood pressure recordings as well as facilitating repeated arterial blood gas sampling. It is important that these patients are neither under- nor overtransfused. The former leads to further spinal injury, the latter leads to pulmonary oedema. As central venous pressure recording is unreliable a pulmonary artery occlusion pressure catheter should be inserted as soon as possible.

The loss of vascular tone in patients with high spinal injuries causes them to be prone to postural hypotension. This can occur in tipping or lifting the patient suddenly, as well as turning the trolleys at speed. As a result there can be underperfusion of areas of the body and episodes of ventilatory–perfusion mismatch. It is therefore essential that these potential problems are prevented by the careful and coordinated movement of these patients.

During the initial neurological assessment using the AVPU scale or Glasgow Coma Scale, an asymmetrical weakness may become apparent or a lack of response to peripheral stimulation. These should be noted and a definitive neurological examination performed in the secondary assessment (see Chapter 7). Finally, remember to keep the patient covered by warm sheets and blankets. This not only avoids embarrassment but also prevents heat loss from vasodilatation that occurs after high spinal injuries.

Following the primary assessment and resuscitation, specialist advice should be sought regarding investigations and further management. Following plain X-rays, CT scanning has become the mainstay for spinal cord injuries. Its axial slices and reconstructive capabilities give CT scanning the ability to visualise vertebral fractures. In addition, the degree of canal compromise can be accurately determined to within 1 mm or less. Plain CT, however, does not demonstrate the intraspinal contents other than bone fragments; for this reason contrast enhancement is required. This has been superseded by magnetic resonance (MR) scanning which is now the investigation of choice where visualisation of the contents of the spinal canal is required and for detecting ligamentous and intervertebral disc damage. However, resuscitation equipment must be magnetic resonance imaging compatible.

Published work has shown the advantage of giving high doses of methyl prednisolone in the first 24 hours after blunt spinal injury (see box). The reason for this improvement is not known but workers have postulated that it could be due to a decrease in lipid peroxidation, protein degradation, catabolic activity or an increase in impulse conduction by activation of ion pumps.

The early use of methyl prednisolone following blunt spinal injury

- 30 mg/kg IV over 15 minutes immediately
- Then 5·4 mg/kg/hour for 23 hours

Following evaluation of the spinal cord injury by plain radiography, CT and MR scanning, a decision as to the need for surgical stabilisation can be more accurately made. In the early hours of management following cervical spine injury, sufficient protection to the nervous system can be afforded by inline immobilisation and log-rolling with the patient's neck fixed in a hard collar. With radiological control, skull traction can be applied using increasing weights as necessary to maintain alignment without over-distraction.

MONITORING AND ON-GOING CARE

The shocked patient's vital signs should be continuously monitored.

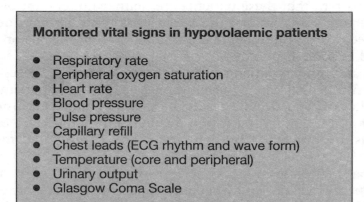

Monitored vital signs in hypovolaemic patients

- Respiratory rate
- Peripheral oxygen saturation
- Heart rate
- Blood pressure
- Pulse pressure
- Capillary refill
- Chest leads (ECG rhythm and wave form)
- Temperature (core and peripheral)
- Urinary output
- Glasgow Coma Scale

In the shocked patient coexistent pathology can be present and for those with ischaemic heart disease, the increase in cardiac work and oxygen demand may be critical. Therefore the need for high inspired levels of oxygen and accurate monitoring is extremely important. An arterial blood sample must also be sent and the result analysed. Acidosis should be initially treated with increased ventilation and fluid administration. Sodium bicarbonate is reserved for cases where the pH is less than 7.1.

Accurate measurement of urinary volume will obviously require the insertion of a urinary catheter. This should be connected to a system permitting accurate volume measurement that can be recorded whenever the other vital signs are measured.

In cases of hypovolaemia, hypotension indicates that at least 30% of the intravascular volume has been lost, therefore a blood transfusion will be required. The decision to transfuse the patient may also be made if there is a poor or transient response to the initial fluid challenge (Table 9.4).

Table 9.4 Response to a fluid challenge

Type of response	Reason
Responder	Volume loss less than 1000 ml
Transient responder	Volume loss greater than 1000 and less than 2000 ml
Non-responder	Volume loss greater than 2000 ml
	Consider another cause for shock

In the "responder" the vital signs will return to normal after the fluid challenge. However, such individuals may need an elective transfusion of fully crossmatched blood. In contrast, transiently normal vital signs that deteriorate suggest continued haemorrhage and the need for more fluid. Ideally this should be typed blood and therefore only checked for ABO and Rhesus compatibility. Most laboratories can provide this within 15 minutes. If there is no recordable blood pressure uncross matched blood (O negative) is required urgently due to the loss of over 40% of the intravascular volume. Once the uncross matched blood has been given, the typed blood should be available.

Coagulation abnormalities can occur after massive blood loss because of:

- dilution of clotting factors by administered fluids
- release of tissue factors which inhibit clotting
- low concentration of clotting factors in stored blood.

Treatment of any type of coagulation disorder has to be guided by the results of the clotting studies and liaison with the haematologist. Do not treat any bleeding problem blindly with platelets, fresh frozen plasma and vitamin K .

LATE DEVELOPMENT OF SHOCK

Shock should be identified and dealt with during the primary assessment. However, it can develop, or recur, at any stage in the patient's care. Consequently you must remain vigilant and continue to monitor and assess the patient. Should shock develop you need to repeat the primary assessment and manage the patient in the manner described earlier. However, you will usually be helped in this situation because there will be more information available regarding the patient's medical history. Consequently likely causes can be checked for first.

TIME OUT 9.3

Take a moment to write down how you would manage a 60 year old man who presents after a haematemesis. Initial vital signs recorded by the nurse are:

Respiratory rate	28/minute
SaO$_2$	92% (air)
Pulse rate	120/minute
Blood pressure	90/60
Pale, sweating and anxious.	

SUMMARY

There are many causes of shock but all lead to inadequate delivery, or utilisation, of oxygen and glucose by vital tissues. This chapter has concentrated on the oxygenation issues. In these cases the management goal is to treat hypoxaemia and hypovolaemia whilst excluding the immediately life threatening conditions. It is also important to realise that resuscitation, though crucial, only plays a preliminary part in the patient's long term management. It is therefore best that shocked patients receive multi-specialty input from the beginning.

CHAPTER

10

The patient with chest pain

OBJECTIVES

After reading this chapter you will be able to:

- resuscitate a patient with chest pain
- identify and instigate emergency treatment for the immediate life threatening causes of chest pain
- formulate a differential diagnosis for non immediately life threatening causes of chest pain
- discuss the investigation and management of the other causes of chest pain.

INTRODUCTION

Chest pain has many underlying causes and these range from the life threatening to the trivial. The nature of the pain (site, severity, radiation, and associations) varies with the actual cause, but in clinical practice immediately life threatening causes (next box) can be difficult to identify rapidly. Therefore a structured approach to care is advocated starting with a primary assessment and resuscitation followed by secondary assessment and emergency treatments.

> **Life threatening causes of chest pain**
>
> - Myocardial infarction
> - Pulmonary emboli
> - Tension pneumothorax
> - Dissecting thoracic aneurysm

PRIMARY ASSESSMENT AND RESUSCITATION

This concentrates on the evaluation and maintainance of the ABCs. If the patient is conscious it is usually also possible to gain key information about their chest pain at the same time.

137

Airway

Airway patency must be assessed and secured where necessary. If the patient's conscious level is fluctuating then simple airway adjuncts may be needed. If the airway cannot be maintained despite these measures then either endotracheal intubation or surgical airway management may be needed.

Breathing

All patients will require high flow oxygen at 12–15 litres per minute via a non-rebreathing mask with reservoir.

The rate, symmetry, and effort of respiration should be noted. Palpation in the sternal notch will determine whether there is either tracheal deviation or tug. After percussing the anterior chest wall for areas of hyperresonance or dullness, breath sounds should be auscultated and any additional sounds, such as a pleural rub, identified.

Inadequate breathing should be supported – initially by bag–valve – mask ventilation and then by intubation and mechanical ventilation. Pulmonary emboli producing pleuritic chest pain are, in themselves, rarely life threatening. However, such a symptom should raise the clinician's suspicion of a potential, larger embolus that may have a significant haemodynamic effect including pulseless electrical activity (PEA, or previously electromechanical dissociation (EMD)).

Tension pneumothoraces are a rare cause of chest pain but are rapidly fatal if ignored. The clinician must be alert to this problem, in particular in patients with preexisting lung disease. Once the diagnosis has been made, time should not be wasted getting X-rays. An immediate needle thoracocentesis is required. This converts the tension into a simple pneumothorax and allows time for chest drain insertion.

Circulation

The clinician must check for the presence of an arterial pulse and assess the rate. The carotid artery is first choice but radial, carotid, and femoral arteries should be palpated to determine their pressure, volume, and radio-carotid or radio-femoral delay. Check the precordium for the position and character of the apex beat plus any thrills or heaves. Listen for the presence of normal, altered, and added heart sounds, as well as murmurs.

Ideally, all patients should have IV access – the antecubital fossa is usually the easiest site. A central line may be used provided that the clinician has appropriate experience.

Monitoring should include SpO_2, pulse, blood pressure, and ECG.

Immediate investigations

Once access has been secured, blood should be taken for full blood count, cardiac enzymes, electrolytes, and blood glucose. If a dissecting aneurysm is suspected, blood transfusion will be required and therefore a sample should be taken for cross match. Arterial blood gas measurement is also ideally required to exclude any underlying acid–base disturbance, ventilation–perfusion mismatch and inadequate ventilation.

All patients with non-traumatic chest pain will require an early 12 lead ECG as it can help in differentiating the causes of chest pain (next box).

Key point
A normal ECG does not exclude a myocardial infarct

ECG features of immediately life threatening causes of chest pain

Myocardial infarction (ACEP)	Normal 1 mm (0·1 mV) ST elevation in two of the inferior leads 1 mm (0·1 mV) ST elevation in leads 1 and aVL 2 mm (0·2 mV) ST elevation in two contiguous leads New bundle branch block True posterior infarct
Pulmonary emboli	Normal Sinus tachycardia Atrial fibrillation Right axis deviation P pulmonale Right ventricular strain Right bundle branch block
Thoracic aorta dissection	Normal Signs of left ventricular hypertrophy and strain due to hypertension Acute ischaemic changes when coronary ostia are involved (rare) Heart block if the haematoma extends into the atrioventricular node (very rare)

A diagnosis made on ECG should lead to rapid emergency treatment. A 12 lead ECG may be normal during the evolution of myocardial infarct. If pericarditis is present then the classic concave ST elevation occurs in the leads that lie over the affected area.

SECONDARY ASSESSMENT

Immediately life threatening conditions are rare, but it is important that they have been excluded or treated. Attention can then be directed to the secondary assessment where the crucial exclusions are myocardial infarction, pulmonary embolus, pneumonia, and pneumothorax. These latter two conditions are easily diagnosed radiologically; therefore, the essential management plan is to rule out myocardial infarction (ROMI) and pulmonary embolus (ROPE). Other, minor conditions can be investigated often as an outpatient.

History

Clinical diagnoses are frequently made on the basis of a medical history. The features of a chest pain should be, as usual, assessed in a regular and orderly sequence paying particular attention to the site, character, radiation, precipitation, and relieving factors as well as any other associated symptoms.

A pertinent history can provide invaluable clues as to the differential diagnosis of conditions giving rise to chest pain.

Acute myocardial infarction patients with ECG changes should have been spotted straight away and treated appropriately. Those patients who remain will range from those with unstable angina to those with musculoskeletal pain. While the particular diagnosis in individual patients may take some time to establish, the risks of either myocardial infarction or of later complications can be rapidly assessed by further consideration of the ECG, by taking a focused history and by carrying out a brief examination. This will allow appropriate decisions about further care to be made.

The ECG findings are considered first – ischaemic changes not known to be old predict both a high risk of myocardial infarction and also a high risk of complications. If the ECG is normal then clinical risk factors are sought – these include any history consistent with unstable ischaemic heart disease (worsening of previously stable angina, new onset of post infarction or post coronary revascularisation angina, or pain the same as a previous myocardial infarction) and findings of either hypotension (systolic blood pressure less than 120 mm Hg) or significant heart failure (crepitations not just including the bases). If more than two are present then the patient is at high risk. If one risk factor is present or there are none at all then the history should be reconsidered to see whether one of two particular scenarios that go along with a moderate risk of myocardial infarction is present. These are shown below.

> **Scenario 1:** Typical cardiac pain in a patient over 40 years old where the pain is not reproduced by palpation, is not stabbing in nature and does not radiate atypically.
> **Scenario 2:** A history of anginal pain lasting longer than one hour that was either worse than usual angina pain or as bad as the pain of a previous acute myocardial infarction.

The whole approach to clinical risk assessment is shown in Figure 10.1. This assessment tool is derived from the multicentre chest pain study and provides an objective, evidence based tool. It ensures that acute myocardial infarction patients are identified rapidly and provides a framework for subsequent care of all those remaining.

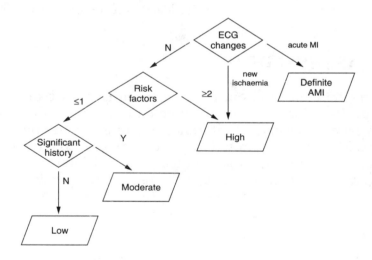

Figure 10.1   Clinical risk assessment in patients with chest pain

Tension pneumothorax can present with progressive dyspnoea, occasionally pleuritic pain, and in extreme cases, a cardiorespiratory arrest (see later). A similar range of presentations may be encountered in patients with pulmonary emboli. It is therefore important to enquire about the history of breathlessness and haemoptysis, as this may help in establishing the correct diagnosis.

The pain from a dissecting thoracic aortic aneurysm usually starts in the centre of the chest and radiates through between the scapulae and may involve the upper limbs. It is often described as tearing but the nature of the pain may change as the dissection progresses. With most of these conditions, there are no identifiable precipitating causes.

Risk factors need to be sought, in particular a family history of ischaemic heart disease, hyperlipidaemia, hypertension, diabetes mellitus, Marfan's syndrome, homocystinuria, procoagulant disorder and a history of cigarette smoking. Oral contraceptive pill use or pregnancy may influence the differential diagnosis, as may the patient's occupation.

The clinician should ascertain additional information so that a well "phrased" history has been obtained by the end of the secondary assessment.

Examination

The secondary assessment ensures that the physical examination started in the primary assessment is completed in a comprehensive fashion. The blood pressure, pulse pressure, and the height and character of the jugular venous pulse should also be recorded. Assessment of the site and character of the apex beat as well as the presence of normal and additional heart sounds can then be done. Occasionally an immediate blowing diastolic murmur may be heard when a dissecting thoracic aortic aneurysm has involved the aortic valve.

The clinician should then consider and integrate the facts from the history with the examination findings to pin point the cause of the chest pain. The commonest causes of chest pain are listed in Tables 10.1–10.5. For clarity these are divided into body systems

Table 10.1   Clinical features of cardiac chest pain

	Ischaemia	Pericarditis
Site	Retrosternal Deep Arms (infrequently)	Surface – according to site of pericarditis
Character	Constricting, band like Heavy, heavy weight	Sharp
Radiation	Left arm > right arm Throat/jaw/teeth Rare but pathognomic	Left arm >> right arm Very rare – throat
Precipitation	Exertion Cold winds Anxiety Heavy meals	Deep inspiration Coughing Postural variation (depending on site of inflammation)
Relief	Rest Nitrates (within 1–2 minutes)	Postural variation
Associated symptoms	Strangling sensation in the throat	Occasionally pleuritic
Clinical examination	Limited value Occasionally signs of hyperlipidaemia/atherosclerosis	Pericardial rub

Table 10.2 Clinical features of chest pain caused by respiratory disease

	Pleuritic	Spontaneous pneumothorax	Spontaneous pneumomediastinum
Site	Anterior/lateral/ posterior	Anterior/lateral/ posterior or none	Mid-line Retrosternal
Character	Sharp Stabbing, catching	Sharp Stabbing, catching	Stabbing
Radiation	Shoulder tip if basal pleuritis	–	Neck Back
Precipitation	Coughing Deep inspiration	Coughing Deep inspiration	Coughing Deep inspiration Postural variation
Relief	Shallow breathing Postural variation	Shallow breathing	Postural variation
Associated symptoms	(a) *Infective* Cough Purulent sputum Prodromal symptoms (b) *Embolic* Cough Breathless Haemoptysis (see earlier)	Breathless Cough (see earlier re tension pneumothorax)	Cough Neck/facial subcutaneous emphysema
Clinical examination	Pleural rub ± signs of consolidation	Hyperresonant percussion note Reduced breath sounds	Subcutaneous emphysema

Table 10.3 Clinical features of chest pain caused by gastrointestinal disease

	Peptic ulcer disease	Gastrooesophageal reflux disease	Diffuse oesophageal spasm
Site	Epigastric Right hypochondrium	Retrosternal Epigastric	Retrosternal Deep
Character	Postprandial constant/ gnawing	Burning	Squeezing Constricting
Radiation	Posteriorly (posterior duodenal ulcer)	Retrosternal Throat	Throat Arms (rare)
Precipitation	Eating Alcohol	Drinking Eating Lying/bending	–
Relief	Acid suppressants Antacids	Standing Antacids Acid suppressants	Antispasmodics Nitrates
Associated symptoms	Nausea Vomiting Waterbrash	Nausea Waterbrash Bronchospasm	Dysphagia
Clinical examination	Epigastric tenderness	–	–

Table 10.4 Clinical features of chest wall pain

	Muscular	Cervical spondylosis	Costochondritis	Herpes zoster (shingles)
Site	Intercostal Periscapular	Upper chest, arms (corresponding to nerve root involved)	Costochondral junctions	Chest wall dermatomes
Character	Sharp, stabbing ache	Ache Constant	Ache Sharp	Severe lancing
Radiation	Shoulder	Arms Inframammary	–	Affected nerve root(s)
Precipitation	Coughing Deep inspiration Physical effort	Movement Physical effort	Deep inspiration Lying on anterior chest wall	Previous varicella zoster
Relief	Rest Analgesia (NSAID) Heat	Rest Analgesia (NSAID) Immobilisation	Anti-inflammatory drugs (NSAID)	Analgesia Aciclovir Carbamazepine
Associated symptoms	Focal tenderness over muscle mimicked by compression of thoracic cage, movement of muscle/group	Paraesthesia (nerve root distribution)	Focal erythema/ swelling Tenderness over joint	Erythematous vesicular rash (pain precedes rash)
Clinical examination	Focal tenderness	Restricted neck movement Nerve root signs	Focal erythema/ tenderness	Rash

Table 10.5 Clinical features of functional chest pain

Site	Anywhere Usually left inframammary
Character	Sharp, stabbing Unrelenting
Radiation	None, usually Arms, infrequently
Precipitation	Anxiety Tension
Relief	Reassurance Treat underlying cause
Associated symptoms	Palpitations Breathless Headaches Other somatic symptoms
Clinical examination	Unremarkable

EMERGENCY TREATMENT

Myocardial infarction

In the presence of myocardial infarction, aspirin and vasodilators, i.e. sublingual or intravenous nitrates, will be required. If this combination fails to relieve pain, then opiates should be used. Irrespective of the patient's age, thrombolysis must be started as soon as possible provided there are no contraindications (next box). Clinical trials have shown that the beneficial effect of thrombolysis is significantly reduced with time, particularly if it is started over 12 hours after the onset of chest pain.

Contraindications to thrombolysis

- History of bleeding, gastrointestinal or genitourinary, in the previous two months
- Aortic dissection
- History of spinal cord or intracranial haemorrhage, aneurysm or neoplasm
- Transient ischaemic attack or stroke within the previous six months
- Reduced level of consciousness
- History of bleeding disorder
- Pregnancy
- Recent major surgery, trauma, biopsy or head injury
- Prolonged cardiopulmonary resuscitation within the previous 10 days
- Non-compressible diagnostic intraarterial procedure within previous 14 days
- Systolic blood pressure greater than 200 mm Hg or diastolic greater than 110 mm Hg

---

Unstable angina

In common with all patients with possible cardiac chest pain patients with unstable angina should receive aspirin and appropriate analgesia. Antithrombotic therapy should be given to all patients with unstable angina or non-Q wave myocardial infarction. Low molecular weight heparin is more effective than unfractionated heparin at reducing the incidence of ischaemic events and the need for revascularisation procedures. The incidence of major bleeding complications is the same for both forms of heparin. Thus all patients who fall into the high risk chest pain group who are not eligible for fibrinolytic drugs should receive low molecular weight heparin.

Pulmonary embolus

If the diagnosis is suspected, start treatment with heparin (either unfractionated or low molecular weight) immediately, after which embolic, pleuritic pain often melts away within 2–6 hours. Thrombolysis is a useful therapeutic adjunct but is best given via a transvenous pulmonary catheter (for large emboli).

Dissecting aneurysm

This condition is rare; however, when a dissecting aortic aneurysm is suspected, the optimum systolic blood pressure is considered to be 100 mm Hg. This may be achieved by either pharmacological reduction of hypertension or titrated fluid replacement with hypotension. Cardiothoracic advice must be sought.

DEFINITIVE CARE

After taking a history and examining the patient, the clinician will have either established a diagnosis or postulated a differential diagnosis. The patient with a suspected myocardial infarction will be transferred to coronary care, whilst patients with other causes of chest pain will be managed on a medical ward. Appropriate investigations will then be required to confirm or refute these conclusions. The choice will depend upon which body system(s) is involved.

INVESTIGATIONS

ECG

All patients with chest pain should have continuous electrocardiograph monitoring, at least during their initial assessment. An exercise ECG is a useful test after a myocardial infarction and is often used to identify potential candidates for coronary angiography. In addition, it is particularly useful in detecting ischaemic chest pain when the exercise provokes chest pain identical to that experienced by the patient in association with ST depression.

Chest X-ray

A chest X-ray is of limited diagnostic use in patients with angina and myocardial infarction unless the latter is complicated by heart failure and/or aneurysm of the left ventricle. Similarly, it is usually unremarkable in patients with pericarditis unless there is a co-existing pericardial effusion. A plain chest radiograph may be normal in uncomplicated pleuritis and even with pulmonary emboli. It may, however, show evidence of pulmonary parenchymal infection or a wedge shaped peripheral defect associated with pulmonary embolus. A chest X-ray is essential for diagnosing spontaneous, simple pneumothorax, especially when the film is taken in expiration.

In the case of dissecting aneurysm, a chest X-ray may show widening of the mediastinum, deviation of trachea to the right, elevation of right main bronchus and depression of left main bronchus, a pleural cap, the obliteration of the aorticopulmonary window, and, more obviously, the aortic knuckle.

Echocardiogram

An echocardiogram is helpful in the diagnosis of pericardial effusion and dissecting aneurysm. However, in the latter, angiography is the investigation of choice.

Cardiac enzymes

Cardiac enzymes should be requested in all patients with chest pain.

Cardiac enzymes
The traditional markers of creatine kinase (CK), aspartate transaminase (AST) and lactate dehydrogenase (LDH) are being superseded by newer tests. Entirely new markers such as the cardiac troponins have been developed, and new approaches to traditional enzymes have become available.

VQ scans

Ventilation perfusion (VQ) scans, if immediately available, may be useful in the diagnosis of pulmonary embolic disease, but pulmonary angiography remains the gold standard. Spiral CT scans show promise.

Endoscopy

Endoscopy is essential for investigating peptic ulcer as well as gastrooesophageal reflux disease. A normal endoscopy, however, does not exclude this disease and formal pH, manometry and a semisolid phase barium swallow may be required to confirm the diagnosis – similarly for diffuse spasm.

DIAGNOSTIC PITFALLS

- Patients with chest pain, irrespective of the cause, will manifest clinical features of anxiety.
- Always reassess every episode of chest pain as though it were the first even in frequent attenders.
- The absence of deep vein thrombosis does not rule out a diagnosis of pulmonary embolus.
- If the patient's history suggests a pneumothorax but there is no radiological evidence, reevaluate the X-ray for evidence of pneumomediastinum.
- A normal chest X-ray and white cell count does not exclude the diagnosis of pulmonary infection.
- Rapid pain relief with nitrates does not point to a diagnosis of angina – diffuse oesophageal spasm responds in an identical fashion.
- Gastrooesophageal reflux is a common problem and does not indicate that chest pain is due to this cause.

SUMMARY

- Chest pain is a common presentation requiring acute medical admission.
- Most causes of chest pain are not immediately life threatening.
- Rule out myocardial infarction (ROMI) and pulmonary embolus (ROPE) in patients with a compatible history.

CHAPTER

11

The patient with altered conscious level

OBJECTIVES

After reading this chapter you should be able to:

- understand the physiology of the conscious state and how this may be disturbed
- understand how the structured approach can be applied to the unconscious patient
- discuss the initial management of such a patient
- discuss how clinical signs detected in the secondary assessment will influence your diagnosis and subsequent management.

INTRODUCTION

The care of the unconscious patient is a common medical emergency. To understand why patients become unconscious it is necessary to review briefly the physiology of consciousness by considering:

- neurophysiology
- metabolic needs of the brain
- cerebral perfusion
- intracranial pressure.

Neurophysiology

Consciousness is a function of the integrated process of the brain. There are, however, two interlinked areas that are of paramount importance in maintaining the conscious state. These are the reticular formation and the cerebral cortex.

The reticular formation arises in the brain stem in the midst of a host of neural pathways communicating between the brain and spinal cord and vice versa. The reticular formation contains the primary centres for cardiovascular and respiratory control as well as a distinct area called the reticular activating system. This is crucial for maintaining the conscious state. Neurones in the reticular activating system pass via the thalamus to synapse in the cortex. There is no specific individual area in the cortex that is responsible for the conscious state, but the coordinated interaction of many cortical areas is required.

147

Cerebral metabolism

Glucose and oxygen are the essential fuels for cerebral metabolism. The brain only has a small store of glucose. This supply is maintained by adequate cerebral blood flow. In practice, the brain can only function for approximately 2–3 minutes in the absence of glucose. In contrast, if the brain is deprived of both glucose and oxygen, as in cardiorespiratory arrest, then normal energy metabolism can only continue for about 15 seconds.

Cerebral perfusion

Adequate ventilation and cerebral perfusion are necessary to ensure that the brain is provided with oxygen and glucose. Under normal resting conditions the brain receives approximately 15–20% of the resting cardiac output. Cerebral blood flow is autoregulated to ensure a constant supply of blood with a mean arterial pressure of 60–160 mm Hg. Within this range a rise in blood pressure is balanced by intracranial vasoconstriction and conversely, a fall by vasodilatation. Cerebral blood flow depends not only on the mean arterial pressure, but also the resistance to blood flow due to intracranial pressure and to a lesser extent the central venous pressure.

Cerebral perfusion pressure (CPP) = mean arterial pressure – intracranial pressure

Autoregulation is impaired in conditions like infection and trauma, and, in particular, chronic hypertension. However, under normal circumstances if cerebral blood flow falls (mean arterial pressure below 60 mm Hg) then cerebral ischaemia occurs. In contrast, cerebral oedema and hypertensive encephalopathy may ensue if the mean arterial pressure exceeds 160 mm Hg.

Intracranial pressure

The volume of the intracranial contents, comprising the brain, cerebrospinal fluid, blood, and blood vessels, is fixed by the surrounding rigid skull. These contents produce an intracranial pressure of 6–13 mm Hg. To maintain this normal range any increase in volume of one of the contents must be balanced by a corresponding decrease in one or more of the others. The brain is a compliant organ that will mould to accommodate any increase in pressures. Furthermore, cerebrospinal fluid can be displaced into the spinal system and the volume of cerebral venous fluid, in particular within the dural sinuses, can be displaced into the systemic venous circulation. These two mechanisms will initially offset any rise in intracranial pressure. Once these normal compensatory measures are exhausted, any further small increase in intracranial volume will cause large increases in intracranial pressure, which in turn will reduce cerebral perfusion pressure.

Therefore disruption of one or more of these four mechanisms will result in loss of consciousness.

PRIMARY ASSESSMENT AND RESUSCITATION

In the primary assessment, airway, breathing, and circulation are assessed and managed appropriately. Irrespective of the underlying pathology every effort should be made to prevent secondary brain damage by identifying and treating hypoxaemia, hypercapnia, hypotension, hypoglycaemia, and raised intracranial pressure.

The structured approach to the unconscious patient includes:

• primary assessment

- resuscitation
- secondary assessment
- emergency treatment
- definitive care.

Senior help and an anaesthetist should be called immediately for all comatose patients, who should be managed in the resuscitation area.

A – airway and cervical spine

In the patient with altered consciousness, the potential for airway obstruction is high.

Clear and control the airway using the techniques described in Chapter 4. If a patient is comatosed (a Glasgow Coma Score of eight or less) or the gag reflex is absent, then the airway is unprotected. In such cases the use of a cuffed endotracheal tube should be considered. All patients require high flow oxygen using an appropriate delivery system.

Cervical spine problems are rare in acute medicine, but be wary of the patient found unconscious/confused at the bottom of the stairs. Therefore consider a "potential neurological injury" if there is no clear history, and especially if there are external signs of trauma above the clavicle. Seek specialist help to immobilise the cervical spine.

B – breathing

Unconscious patients usually have low respiratory rates and if less than 10 per minute, may need assisted ventilation.

Patients in respiratory distress (i.e. respiratory rate greater than 30) may have a life threatening chest problem. Examination of the chest during the primary assessment is designed specifically to pick up any such chest problems.

The patient should be connected to the pulse oximeter.

Give naloxone to any patient if any of the following are present:

- intubation is necessary or the respiratory rate is less than 10 per minute.

C – circulation

Intravenous access has to be established and blood should be taken for immediate glucose estimation using a glucometer. Hypoglycaemia (< 4 mmol/l) should be treated with intravenous dextrose or glucagon 1 mg intravenously. Shock should be treated appropriately to prevent secondary brain injury.

In addition to the routine blood tests, a serum sample for toxicology and arterial blood gases must be measured.

Patients should be connected to the cardiac monitor, and urinary catheterisation is necessary for all unconscious patients.

D – disability

The initial neurological assessment should be a rapid evaluation of the Glasgow Coma Score and pupil size, equality, and reaction to light. Check for meningeal irritation – if there are no contra-indications. Remember, at this stage, you are looking for conditions which are immediately life threatening! Consider:

- Hypoglyceamia
- Antedotes e.g. naloxone if pinpoint pupils/needle track marks
- Antibiotics
- Acyclevir
- Antiepileptic drugs

E – exposure

The patient must be fully exposed to allow complete assessment. The temperature must be taken with a low reading rectal thermometer if necessary. Do not forget that hypothermia is an important cause of coma and should not be missed. Be wary of inducing hypothermia by fully exposing the patient.

The patients' clothes should be searched for useful information such as medical cards, drugs, next of kin, etc.

SECONDARY ASSESSMENT

The secondary assessment should only be done once the immediately life threatening conditions have been treated. A well "phrased" history should be sought followed by a complete examination. Further appropriate investigations can be requested.

History

The history is particularly important in this context and must be sought from attending relatives, friends, paramedics and other witnesses. Additional and useful information may be obtained from the hospital notes or the general practitioner.

Examination

A thorough head to toe examination of the patient should then take place, looking for evidence of precipitating factors such as head injury, infection, drug use, and vascular pathology. In the unconscious patient, particular attention should be paid to the following:

- level of consciousness
- assessment of brain stem function
- focal neurological signs.

Level of consciousness
The Glasgow Coma Scale (GCS) gives a qualitative measurement of the patient's conscious level. The GCS is the sum of scores in three areas of assessment and each modality is graded separately.

E – best eye opening
V – best verbal response
M – best motor response

If the patient does not respond to commands, then a painful stimulus is applied by pressure on the supraorbital ridge.

Eye opening response

Response	Score
Spontaneous	4
To speech	3
To painful stimuli	2
Nil	1

Verbal response

Response	Score
Orientated	5
Confused	4
Inappropriate words	3
Incomprehensible sounds	2
Nil	1

If assessment of a verbal response is not possible, for example, due to an *in situ* endotracheal tube, then this fact should be documented in the patient's notes.

Motor response

Response	Score
Obeys commands	6
Localises pain	5
Withdraws from pain	4
Abnormal flexion (decorticate)	3
Abnormal extension (decerebrate)	2
Nil	1

The best response of any limb is recorded. If there are differences between limbs this may suggest a potential neurological lesion.

Patients who have a GCS of eight or less are by definition comatose. It is important to recheck the GCS every 15 minutes.

Metabolic causes of coma

Drug overdose	Daily
Ischaemia/hypoxia	Daily
Hypoglycaemia	Daily
Cardiac failure	Daily
Respiratory failure	Daily
Alcohol	Daily
Renal failure	Weekly
Diabetic ketoacidosis	Weekly
Hepatic failure	Monthly
Hyponatraemia	Monthly
Septicaemia	Monthly
Wernicke's encephalopathy	Monthly
Carbon monoxide poisoning	Annually
Hypernatraemia	Annually

Assessment of brain stem function
The brain stem assessment focuses initially on the following:

- pupillary response
- eye movements
- corneal response
- respiratory pattern.

Pupillary response   The size, shape and response to light of the pupils should be assessed. An understanding of the common changes in pupillary reflexes is important as this will localise lesions; for example, with lesions that directly affect the brain stem (pontine haemorrhage) the pupillary responses are abnormal from the outset. Common pupillary changes are shown in Table 11.1.

Table 11.1   Pupillary abnormalities

	Pupillary response	Cause
Equal pupils	– small + reactive	– metabolic encephalopathy – midbrain herniation
	– pin point + fixed	– pontine lesion – opioids, organophosphates
	– dilated + reactive	– metabolic cause – midbrain lesion – ecstacy, amphetamines
	– dilated + fixed	– peri ictar – hypoxaemia – hypothermia – anticholinergics
Unequal pupils	– small + reactive	– Horner's syndrome
	– dilated + fixed	– Uncal herniation – IIIrd nerve palsy

Eye movements   Many comatose patients have roving or dysconjugate eye movements; these are common and are of no particular significance.

The oculocephalic response (doll's head/eye movement) provides useful information about the oculomotor and vestibular components of brain stem function. The response is elicited by quickly turning the head to the right, while holding the eye lids open and observing eye movements. Repeat the movement, but turn the head to the left.

- Eyes move to opposite direction – normal
- Eyes move to one side but not the other – unilateral brain stem lesion – lateral gaze palsy
- Eyes fail to move in any direction – bilateral brain stem lesions

Key point
Do not attempt to elicit the oculocephalic response if cervical spine pathology is suspected

The oculovestibular (caloric) test is a much more potent stimulus to the brain stem function than the oculocephalic reflex. It is more time consuming to perform and often unsuitable for emergency assessments. It is useful, however, in one instance, that of psychogenic unresponsiveness. Having first ensured that the ear drums are intact, the head is inclined at 30° to the trunk, and the external auditory canal of one ear is irrigated with ice cold water while the eyes are held open. In those comatose patients with an intact vestibular component there is a tonic deviation of the eyes to the irrigated ear, while in patients not in coma it produces nystagmus and vomiting. (The quick phase is away from the irrigated side.) There is no movement of the eyes when brain stem function is lost.

Corneal reflexes are usually preserved in coma. In the absence of drugs, the loss of this reflex is a very poor sign.

Respiratory pattern Alterations in brain stem function produce a variety of respiratory patterns, which may help to localise the lesion. In practice, however, they are of limited value.

- Eupnoeic – normal, e.g. postictal, metabolic coma
- Periodic breathing (Cheyne–Stokes) e.g. lesions in the thalamus and hypothalamus, though there are many non-cerebral causes including heart failure
- Central neurogenic hyperventilation, e.g. lesions in the midbrain or upper pons
- Apneustic breathing (slow and irregular) lesions in the medulla
- Deep sighing respiration (Kussmaul) associated with a metabolic acidosis

Focal neurological signs

When assessing motor response to pain, tone, and deep tendon reflexes you are looking for asymmetry. Such signs with intact brain stem reflexes occur with a focal hemispheric lesion whereas focal signs with absent brain stem reflexes are signs of a lesion in the posterior fossa. Assessment of the brain stem reflexes can be very valuable in localizing the lesion and help select patients needing immediate further investigation, e.g. CT scanning.

The fundi must always be examined. The presence of papilloedema indicates raised intracranial pressure.

Key point
The absence of papilloedema does not exclude raised intracranial pressure.

Subhyloid haemorrhage should be sought as this may indicate subarachnoid haemorrhage or basal skull fracture. Furthermore, changes associated with diabetes mellitus and hypertension should also be noted.

It cannot be overemphasised that the initial neurological examination is only the beginning. The initial findings are only a "baseline" for comparison with repeated neurological examinations.

Do not forget that specific evidence should also be sought of meningeal irritation (usually neck stiffness and Kernig's sign, Brudzinski's sign). This test should not be elicited if cervical spine instability is suspected. It is important to realise that neck stiffness is often absent if the patient's conscious level is depressed.

Coma can be caused by the broad pathophysiological insults listed in the box on p. 154.

Investigations

Neuroradiology

Computerised tomography (CT) is the primary investigation in coma. It is relatively quick to perform and will identify 99% of supratentorial masses, especially when combined with intravenous contrast. It is important to maintain adequate resuscitation during the scan. Restless or uncooperative patients will need to be electively intubated to get good quality images by avoiding movement artefacts. It is dangerous to sedate agitated or restless patients in this situation as optimum management of the airway can not be guaranteed when the patient is being scanned.

In comparison with CT scanning, cranial magnetic resonance imaging (MRI) is a more sensitive imaging modality. It will not only demonstrate most cerebral disease processes, but is also the ideal method for imaging posterior fossa lesions. These cannot be seen on CT imaging because of obtrusive artefacts. MRI is highly sensitive for infective/inflammatory changes to cerebral tissue, enabling identification of encephalitic disorders at an early stage when, for example, the CT scan will be normal. A further advantage is that magnetic resonance angiography can be performed as a non-invasive, radiation free technique for the investigation of intra- and extracerebral vascular structures. Unfortunately MRI is a very lengthy process when compared with CT scanning. Furthermore, it is extremely difficult to continue resuscitation in the MRI scanning area as metal components are not allowed within the area of the "magnet". For practical reasons CT is still the modality of choice. It is important to realise that the scan must not delay the diagnosis of conditions like meningitis and encephalitis. These should be treated early with appropriate antibiotics or antiviral agents based on clinical diagnosis before scanning.

Lumbar puncture
A lumbar puncture should not be done in the unconscious patient until a CT scan has excluded a mass lesion. Failure to do this may precipitate central/uncal herniation as cerebrospinal fluid is drained via the lumbar puncture needle. Furthermore, a diagnosis of subarachnoid haemorrhage on CT will negate the need for lumbar puncture, especially as this is now believed to further destabilise patients with this condition. However, a lumbar puncture must be done in patients who have a clinical history of subarachnoid haemorrhage and a negative CT scan. Other conditions which may cause coma and neck stiffness are shown in the box.

Causes of coma and neck stiffness

Bacterial meningitis
Encephalitis
Subarachnoid haemorrhage
Cerebral or cerebellar haemorrhage with extension to the subarachnoid space
Cerebral malaria

It is important to remember that meningeal irritation may be absent when conscious levels are depressed. The unconscious victim without evidence of mass lesion but who is pyrexial will warrant a lumbar puncture. However, the prognosis is extremely poor for patients with meningitis who are unconscious before treatment is started.

Emergency management

The aims of emergency management are to maintain adequate cerebral metabolism, and prevent and or treat intracranial hypertension, whilst a specific diagnosis is made and specific treatment is commenced.

Maintain cerebral metabolism
The principal metabolic requirements of the brain are oxygen and glucose. Delivery of adequate levels of these substrates must be ensured. The oxygen content of the blood depends on arterial haemoglobin and oxygen concentration. The arterial oxygen concentration can be assessed using blood gas analysis and pulse oximetry. Supplementary oxygen must be given to maintain arterial PO_2 greater than 10·5 kPa (80 mmHg).

The concentration of glucose in the blood must be considered early and the brain must be protected from hypo- or hyperglycaemia. Close control of blood sugar concentrations between 4 and 8 mmol per litre offers better preservation of cerebral function in hypoxia and traumatic damage.

Maintain cerebral blood flow

The cerebral blood flow depends on the difference between systemic arterial pressure and intracranial pressure.

Systemic arterial pressure   The aim is to maintain a normal blood pressure, considering the nature of the intracranial pathology and preexisting medical conditions, e.g. hypertension. Although autoregulation will endeavour to preserve cerebral perfusion, causes of hypotension, for example hypovolaemia and sepsis, must be identified and treated immediately. Conversely, hypertension is often a compensatory response to maintain cerebral perfusion in patients with raised intracranial pressure. Therefore treat the underlying condition and **not** the hypertension. Any reduction in blood pressure will reduce cerebral perfusion pressure resulting in global cerebral infarction.

Intracranial pressure   Several steps can be taken to keep pressure to acceptable levels.

1. $PaCO_2$ should be kept within the normal range. Elevations in $PaCO_2$ will be associated with cerebral vasodilatation and exacerbate the raised intracranial pressure. In contrast, hyperventilation will not only reduce the arterial carbon dioxide tension and hence reduce cerebral oedema but also cerebral blood flow resulting in ischaemia. The ideal, therefore, is to seek an early liaison with an intensivist/neurosurgeon, maintain a normal $PaCO_2$ and monitor the $PaCO_2$ and intracranial pressure.
2. Overhydration must be avoided as this may increase cerebral oedema.
3. Hyperosmolar fluids must be avoided.
4. Diuretics, either loop or osmotic, can be used in certain situations. Oedema formation is reduced as right atrial pressure is lowered. As the diuresis will produce a negative fluid balance it is important to avoid jeopardising the circulation. Therefore, they should only be used in consultation with a neurosurgeon, physician, intensivist or neurologist. Diuretics are usually the immediate management of raised intracranial pressure associated with a tumour mass and surrounding oedema.
5. Corticosteroids. These are commonly used in less urgent situations. Dexamethasone 4 mg six hourly may produce symptomatic relief by reducing tumour associated oedema. They have not been shown to be of benefit in any other situations.
6. Seizures. Prolonged seizures are associated with brain damage. Therefore, they should be controlled rapidly. Diazemuls 2 mg per minute up to a maximum of 20 mg may be given intravenously. (Lorazepam is a useful alternative as it has a longer anti-seizure effect.) If this is unsuccessful, then phenytoin, 15 mg per kg diluted in 0.9% saline, should be infused over 30 minutes. Fosphenytoin is a new water soluble predrug that is converted into phenytoin by non-specific phosphatases. In comparison with phenytoin, it can be infused faster, causes phlebitis and is soluble in dextrose. The patient should have ECG monitoring as too rapid an infusion of phenytoin can cause hypotension, bradycardia, and asystole. If this fails an anaesthetic induction agent should be used and the patient anaesthetised and ventilated as necessary.
7. Temperature control. Hyperthermia is detrimental to patients with intracerebral pathology. An elevated temperature increases metabolism and therefore substrate requirements, i.e. oxygen and glucose.

TIME OUT 11.1

Take a 15 minute break from reading.

a. List the mechanisms that maintain consciousness.
b. Describe briefly how you would assess brain stem function.

SPECIFIC CONDITIONS

Subarachnoid haemorrhage

Pathophysiology
The causes of subarachnoid haemorrhage are shown in the box.

Causes of subarachnoid haemorrhage

Intracranial saccular aneurysm
Arteriovenous malformation
Others   extension from intracranial haemorrhage
            intracranial venous thrombosis
            haemostatic failure
            vascular tumour
            drug use

The commonest cause is rupture of an intracranial saccular aneurysm. In contrast, only about 5% of patients bleed from an arteriovenous malformation.

Intracranial saccular aneurysms develop on medium sized arteries at the base of the brain. The commonest sites are the distal internal carotid/posterior communicating artery and the anterior communicating artery complex. Multiple aneurysms are present in approximately 25% of patients. Aneurysms vary in size from a few millimetres to several centimetres in diameter. Whilst some are undoubtedly congenital, others develop during adult life possibly as a consequence of atherosclerosis and hypertension. Conditions associated with intracranial saccular aneurysms are shown in the box.

Conditions associated with intracranial saccular aneurysms

Polycystic kidney disease
Aortic stenosis
Infective endocarditis
Coarctation of the aorta
Thyromuscular dysplasia
Others   Marfan's syndrome
            Ehlers–Danlos syndrome
            Pseudoxanthoma elasticum

Many aneurysms remain asymptomatic and are only detected at post mortem.

Assessment

Clinical features   The clinical picture is usually, but not always, dominated by an acute severe occipital headache. Often there is a preceeding history (usually over 1–2 weeks) of an acute transient severe headache, indicating a sentinel bleed. This can radiate over the head and down into the neck, some times as far as the back or legs – as blood tracks down the spinal canal. If the haemorrhage is extensive then the patient may become comatosed. If not, consciousness may be either lost transiently or impaired. Vomiting is common. Chemical meningitis (induced by bleed) may take several hours to develop and focal signs are rare unless blood has extended into, or emanated from, the cerebral parenchyma. Occasionally there is an oculomotor nerve palsy from posterior communicating artery aneurysm. Arteriovenous malformations may be diagnosed from the history because of recurrent unilateral migrainous headaches or very rarely on examination when an intracranial bruit is heard.

The patients are often irritable, confused and drowsy for several days. Headache may persist for weeks. Fundoscopy may reveal subhyloid haemorrhages which are believed to follow a rapid rise in intracranial pressure at the onset of intracranial haemorrhage.

Diagnosis

The diagnosis of subarachnoid haemorrhage is usually made on CT and lumbar puncture. However, a negative head CT does not exclude a subarachnoid haemorrhage. Therefore a lumbar puncture is still required. Remember to collect cerebrospinal fluid in at least three tubes to differentiate between a traumatic spinal puncture and preexisting subarachnoid haemorrhage. Furthermore, the white blood cell count will be significantly higher in the peripheral blood in the initial phases of a subarachnoid haemorrhage. If the haemorrhage is more than 4 hours old then the cerebrospinal fluid becomes xanthochromic due to altered blood pigments. The CT scan and cerebrospinal fluid features will resolve two to three weeks after the haemorrhage, provided that no intracerebral complications occur.

The complications of subarachnoid haemorrhage are shown in the box.

Complications of subarachnoid haemorrhage

Local recurrent haemorrhage
Cerebral oedema
Haemorrhage into brain substance
Hydrocephalus
Secondary cerebral infarction due to vasospasm
Epileptic seizures
Hyponatraemia (inappropriate antidiuretic hormone production)
Central/uncal herniation
General hypoxia
Pulmonary embolus
Hypertension
Dehydration
Pneumonia/septicaemia
Hyperglycaemia

Occasionally organised blood clot within the subarachnoid space may obstruct cerebrospinal fluid flow, causing acute hydrocephalus. This may lead to a deterioration in the patient's conscious level within days or weeks after the haemorrhage. Other causes of neurological deterioration correspond to the complications of subarachnoid haemorrhage shown in the earlier box. Any change in neurological status is likely to warrant a CT scan to assess the presence of any treatable complication, e.g. hydrocephalus.

Management

The aim is to prevent secondary brain injury by following the structured approach. In addition severe vasospasm may occur and this can be reduced by nimodipine. Other conditions that can arise include hypertension, cardiac dysrhythmias and neurogenic pulmonary oedema. Treatment should be initiated following discussions with an intensivist and neurosurgeon.

Do not forget that haemorrhage into the 4th ventricle can cause a *transient* rise in blood sugar. This is believed to be due to rapid autonomic nervous system discharge. The blood sugar will rapidly return to normal. Treatment with insulin could be fatal in precipitating hypoglycaemia.

Definitive treatment is neurosurgical for both aneurysms and arteriovenous malformations. However, embolisation and stereotactic radiotherapy are occasionally used when surgery is not technically feasible.

Outcome

Approximately 25% of patients die within 24 hours of their subarachnoid haemorrhage. A further 25% die within the first month as a consequence of either recurrent haemorrhage or vasospasm induced infarction. The remainder survive for longer but with an increased risk of rebleeding of approximately 2% per year.

Bacterial meningitis

Bacterial meningitis can occur in a number of clinical settings. Causative organisms will influence the clinical presentation, management, and outcome. Bacterial meningitis may be classified as:

- spontaneous
- posttraumatic
- postsurgical.

Spontaneous

Spontaneous meningitis is usually community acquired. The majority of cases are caused by *Streptococcus pneumoniae* or meningitides. Of the remainder (approximately 20%) *Listeria monocytogenes*, anaerobic Gram negative bacilli (e.g. *Eschericia coli*), *Haemophilus influenzae* and *Staphylococcus aureus* are responsible. Risk factors for *Streptococcus pneumoniae* meningitis are shown in the box.

Risk factors for *Streptococcus pneumoniae* meningitis

Hypogammaglobulinaemia (primary or secondary, e.g. chronic lymphatic leukaemia)
Sickle cell disease
Previous skull trauma

Listeria tends to affect people at the extremes of age as well as pregnant women and those patients who have prolonged immunosuppression from steroids or alkalating agents, for example, azathioprine. Contaminated foods, in particular unpasteurised soft cheeses, pâté and poorly refrigerated precooked chicken, have been implicated.

Posttraumatic

Posttraumatic meningitis can follow trauma to the skull or spine. It often occurs early in the post traumatic period due to a breach in the meninges; however, it may occur years later. If the infective organism is acquired in the community, then *Streptococcus pneumoniae* or *Haemophilus influenzae* are the likely responsible organisms. In contrast, hospital acquired infections are usually caused by the anaerobic Gram negative bacilli (*E. coli*, *Klebsiella*, *Enterobacter* and *Pseudomonas* species).

Postsurgical

Postsurgical meningitis may follow an operation on the head, neck and spine or insertion of cerebrospinal fluid drains and shunts. The majority of the postsurgical meningitides are caused by anaerobic Gram negative bacilli (as described earlier). Most infections affecting cerebrospinal fluid drains and shunts are hospital acquired, predominantly caused by coagulase negative staphylococci and *Staphylococcus aureus*.

> **Key point**
> It is important to remember that:
>
> - approximately 2% of meningitides will be culture negative
> - with recurrent meningitis, cerebrospinal fluid leak, hypogammaglobulinaemia and complement deficiencies should be excluded

Whilst it is easy to understand how organisms may contaminate the cerebrospinal fluid as a result of trauma or surgery, the precise mode of invasion in spontaneous meningitis is currently unknown.

All organisms induce inflammatory injury to the meninges. This increases permeability of the blood–brain barrier and raises intracranial pressure due to cerebral oedema. This is due to a combination of:

- interstitial fluid accumulation
- communicating hydrocephalus due to decreased cerebrospinal fluid reabsorption
- cellular swelling
- vasculitis affecting the large vessels traversing the subarachnoid space.

A major consequence of increased intracranial pressure and vascular inflammation is decreased cerebral perfusion and therefore impaired delivery of oxygen and substrates. As the acute inflammatory response affects the pia and arachnoid mater, the cerebrospinal fluid contains numerous neutrophils and fibrin. Therefore pus accumulates over the surface of the brain, in particular around its base, and can extend over the associated cranial nerves and spinal cord.

The early diagnosis of meningitis is difficult as many of the symptoms are non-specific and include malaise, fever, headache, myalgia, and vomiting. As the disease progresses, the picture is dominated by irritability, severe headache and vomiting with the exception of meningococcal infection where diarrhoea is common. The classic non-blanching purpuric rash is common to people with meningococcal septicaemia but occurs in only approximately 50% of those with meningococcal meningitis. The precise reason why some patients will develop meningococcal septicaemia rather than meningitis or vice versa is unknown.

Assessment

Clinical signs Patients with bacterial meningitis are usually ill and distressed. Limitation of neck movement is obvious but meningitis is unlikely if the patient can shake their head or place their chin on their chest. Meningism is best elicited by passive flexion of the neck when the patient is supine. Confirmatory evidence may be obtained from Kernig's test where the lower limb is flexed at the hip and the knee gradually extended. Resistance to this manoeuvre by contraction of the hamstrings is indicative of meningeal irritation. In contrast, Brudzinski's test is performed with the patient seated with their legs straight. Flexion of the neck in the presence of meningeal irritation will be associated with flexion of the hips and knees. Marked meningeal irritation can manifest as opisthotonos, i.e. the neck and back fully extended. **Meningism may be absent in patients who are either immunosuppressed or deeply comatosed.**

Herpes labialis is commonly seen in **all** forms of bacterial meningitis.

Physical examination must exclude primary sites of infection, in particular otitis media, sinusitis, mastoiditis, and pneumonia. Watery rhinorrhoea or otorrhoea should be collected and tested for glucose. Under these circumstances a basal skull fracture must be excluded. The other clinical signs in the box are not always present.

Clinical signs of a basal skull fracture

Bruising over mastoid process – Battle's sign
Otorrhoea – CSF ± blood
Rhinorrhoea – CSF ± blood
Periorbital bruising (panda or racoon eyes)
Subhyloid haemorrhage

As the disease progresses cranial nerves may become involved as they cross the inflamed basal meninges – commonly II, III, VI, VII, and VIII. Papilloedema suggests that either cerebral oedema, hydrocephalus, a subdural effusion or empyema is contributing to the development of intracranial hypertension. Headache, vomiting, fever, and decreasing level of consciousness usually dominate the clinical picture. Patients with infected shunts may present as described earlier. These devises can become infected in the cranium, the venous circulation or the peritoneal cavity, where they may produce symptoms akin to meningitis, right sided infective endocarditis, and peritonitis, respectively.

Diagnosis
The diagnosis is made clinically and often confirmed by lumbar puncture, provided there are no contraindications. The cerebrospinal fluid features of bacterial meningitis, in the majority of patients, are as follows:

- raised white cell count (> 100 wbc/ml) the majority of which are neutrophils
- cerebrospinal fluid glucose less than 40 mg/dl or lower
- cerebrospinal fluid protein elevated
- Gram staining of the cerebrospinal fluid will reveal organisms in over 50% of cases (see box).

Gram staining of cerebrospinal fluid in pyogenic bacterial meningitis

Appearance	Probable organism
Gram positive cocci	*Strep. pneumoniae, Staph. aureus*
Gram negative cocci	*N. meningitides*
Gram positive rods	*L. monocytogenes*
Gram negative rods	*H. influenzae, enterobacter*

The causes of a predominant lymphocyte count are listed in the box.

Meningitis with high cerebrospinal fluid lymphocyte count

Early or partially treated cryogenic bacterial infection
Tuberculosis, leptospirosis, brucellosis, syphilis, *Listeria*
Viral infection
Fungal infection, e.g. *Cryptococcus*
Parameningeal infection – intracerebral abscess or subdural empyema
Neoplastic infiltration

Specific treatment
Antibiotic therapy must be started immediately as bacterial meningitis progresses rapidly and has a high mortality.

Suspected meningococcal meningitis/septicaemia The patient should be given an immediate dose of benzyl penicillin 2·4 g either IV or IM, combined with 1 g of either ceftriaxone or chloramphenicol.

Suspected meningitis In adults spontaneous meningitis is usually caused by *Streptococcus pneumoniae* or *Neisseria meningitidis*. There is an increased risk of *Listeria monocytogenes* and infections caused by anaerobic Gram negative bacilli, e.g. *E. coli*. The first line management would be 2 g of ampicillin (IV every four hours) or 1 g ceftriaxone (IV every 12 hours). **This regime will also be suitable for community acquired posttraumatic meningitis.**

Postsurgical meningitis is usually caused by hospital acquired, multiresistant organisms. Often specific hospital antibiotic policies exist; if not, an initial choice is ceftazidine 2 g every eight hours as this will also provide antipseudomonal cover. Ceftazidine or ceftriaxone is also a good first line antibiotic for patients who have acute infections of either shunts or drains, before they are removed.

Outcome
Mortality rates vary considerably depend on the study and type of organism. The overall mortality ranges from approximately 10% for *Neisseria meningitidis* and *Haemophilus influenzae* to in excess of 20% either for *Listeria monocytogenes* or *Streptococcus pneumoniae* meningitis. Mortality is much greater in the very young and elderly, and patients with debilitating illnesses. Furthermore, progression from consciousness through to confusion and then coma is associated with an increased mortality. Complications are not uncommon and are listed in the box.

Complications of meningitis

Raised intracranial pressure
Seizures
Hyponatraemia
Venous sinus thrombosis
Cranial nerve deficit
Hydrocephalus

Tuberculous meningitis

There has been an increased incidence of tuberculosis in many parts of the world, related to the human immunodeficiency viral infection. These patients have a high risk of meningeal involvement. Other high risk groups include immigrants from Pakistan, India, Africa, and the West Indies, as well as alcoholics, intravenous drug users, immunocompromised patients, and those with previous pulmonary tuberculosis.

Pathophysiology

Infection spreads from the primary lesion, or site of chronic infection, through the blood stream to the brain and meninges where microtubercles are formed. These rupture and discharge tubercular protein and mycobacteria into the subarachnoid space, inciting an inflammatory response. Many patients develop miliary tuberculosis at this stage because of haematogenous spread. As with bacterial meningitis, the base of brain and associated cranial nerves can be affected. Tuberculous meningitis is also associated with endarteritis. This can produce ischaemia/infarction of superficial cortical areas, internal capsule, basal ganglia, and brain stem.

Assessment

Symptoms   The onset is usually subacute with two to eight weeks of non-specific prodromal symptoms including malaise, irritability, lethargy, headache, and vomiting.

Clinical signs   Meningeal irritation and cranial nerve damage are common, as is papilloedema. Raised intracranial pressure usually occurs because of obstruction of cerebrospinal fluid circulation, in particular, through the basal cisterns. The neurological features associated with raised intracranial pressure and/or hydrocephalus have been described earlier. The development of focal neurological signs, however, does not always imply raised intracranial pressure as these patients are prone to arteritis and hence cerebral infarction. Inappropriate antidiuretic hormone secretion is also common and may precipitate or exacerbate unconsciousness.

Diagnosis

The cerebrospinal fluid is clear or slightly turbid with a white cell count less than 500 cells per millilitre. This is composed of both lymphocytes and neutrophils in varying proportions. The cerebrospinal fluid glucose is low and the protein concentration is elevated. Tubercle bacilli are rarely seen on cerebrospinal fluid microscopy; however, centrifugation of the sample can increase the diagnostic yield. The most sensitive and specific test uses the polymerase chain reaction (PCR) to detect the *Mycobacterium tuberculosis* genome.

Treatment

This comprises combination chemotherapy with isoniazid (300 mg), rifampicin (600 mg) and pyrazinamide (1500 mg) for 12 months. Streptomycin can also be added for the first two months. Para-aminosalicylic acid should not be used because it does not enter the cerebrospinal fluid. In view of the numerous complications and morbidity and mortality, specialist advise should be sought early.

Outcome

Mortality is still high, at approximately 25%, irrespective of whether patients have co-existant human immunodeficiency virus. Unfortunately permanent sequelae occur in approximately 25% of survivors, ranging from cranial nerve deficit (including blindness) to hemiparesis or intellectual impairment.

Encephalitis

There is considerable variation in geography and type of virus causing distribution of encephalitis. In the UK, however, the commonest diagnosed cause of encephalitis is mumps. Other causes are shown in the box.

Causes of viral encephalitis

Mumps
Echo virus
Coxsackie virus
Herpes simplex
Herpes zoster
Epstein–Barr virus
Adenovirus
Enterovirus

Many of these infections occur in seasonal peaks or epidemics; for example, mumps encephalitis is common in the late winter or early spring whilst enterovirus infections occur in summer and early autumn. Other viral infections, in particular herpes simplex encephalitis, are sporadic. Although viral infections affect all age groups they are most frequent and severe in children, the elderly or those who have decreased T cell immunity, for example Hodgkin's disease. It is interesting to note that whilst herpes simplex encephalitis affects all age groups it shows distinct peaks in those patients aged either between five and 30 years or greater than 50 years.

Pathophysiology

Most viral infections reach the central nervous system via the blood stream from the primary site of infection. Nervous system damage is a consequence of direct invasion and immunological reaction. These processes culminate in:

- destruction and phagocytosis of neurones
- inflammatory oedema
- vascular lesions
- demyelination.

Characteristically viral encephalitides cause lymphocytic infiltration of the meninges. Other features include perivascular cuffing of lymphocytes, plasma cells, and histiocytes within the cortex and white matter as well as proliferation of microglia. Neuronal degeneration and demyelination are invariable.

Herpes simplex encephalitis has characteristic features, in particular gross oedema, severe haemorrhage, and necrotising encephalitis. These features are often asymmetrical and localised to the temporal lobe, and to a lesser extent the frontal lobe. Demyelination is rare. The unique localisation of herpes simplex encephalitis has not, as yet, been satisfactorily explained.

Assessment

Clinical features   The symptom profile is similar to that of meningitis, dominated by headache, vomiting, fever, and malaise.

Clinical signs   A wide spectrum of clinical signs is seen including confusion, convulsions, coma, focal neurological signs, features of raised intracranial pressure, and psychiatric manifestations.

163

However, specific symptoms may arise as herpes simplex encephalitis involves primarily the temporal and frontal cortex. These include gustatory and olfactory hallucinations, amnesia, expressive dysphasia, temporal lobe seizures, anosmia, and behavioural abnormalities. Cerebral oedema is common with herpes simplex encephalitis and untreated patients usually lapse into coma towards the end of the first week.

Diagnosis

The aim is to demonstrate a specific viral agent, especially herpes simplex, or exclude potentially non-treatable causes. Providing there are no contraindications, as described earlier, a lumbar puncture is needed. The cerebrospinal fluid pressure is usually increased, especially in herpes simplex encephalitis (related to the intense cerebral oedema) unless it is early in the evolution of the illness. There is often a marked increase in white cells, with lymphocytes and other mononuclear cells predominating. Furthermore, the cerebrospinal fluid may contain erythrocytes or be xanthochromic if there is a haemorrhagic element to the encephalitis as with herpes simplex. Protein concentration is usually increased in excess of 50 mg per decilitre with an increase in the proportion of immunoglobulin G (IgG). A prominent monoclonal IgG band will be seen in the cerebrospinal fluid due to *de novo* synthesis of IgG combined with leakage of IgG from the serum. The cerebrospinal fluid glucose is usually normal.

A specific virus can be found in the majority of patients from either a throat swab or samples of stool, cerebrospinal fluid and blood. Unfortunately this is not the case for herpes simplex encephalitis. **This is important as it is the only viral condition for which specific therapy is currently available.** The viral genome of herpes simplex can be identified early after the onset of symptoms by the polymerase chain reaction. Hopefully this technique will become widely available in the near future.

Magnetic resonance imaging has provided greater detail about the structural damage in patients who have encephalitis. Further supporting evidence may be provided by an EEG that shows irregular activity over the affected area.

Specific treatment

Aciclovir (Zovirax), a nucleoside analogue, is an effective treatment for herpes simplex encephalitis. It has the advantage that it is only taken up by infected cells and is therefore non-toxic to normal uninfected cells. If the diagnosis is suspected clinically, then treatment should be started immediately as the virus is extremely toxic. Corticosteroids can be used in an attempt to combat cerebral oedema but there is no convincing evidence that this drug is beneficial.

Outcome

Neurological sequelae are common in patients following herpes simplex encephalitis and include mental retardation, amnesia, expressive aphasia, hemiparesis, ataxia, and recurrent seizures, along with various behavioural and personality disturbances.

Cerebral malaria

Malaria remains the most important human parasitic disease globally. Of the four species of malarial parasite (Plasmodium) that have man as their natural vertebral host, only *Plasmodium falciparum* causes cerebral pathology. This is the predominant species in the highly endemic areas of Africa, New Guinea, and Haiti.

Infection in man is acquired from either the female anopheles mosquito, which inoculates parasites into the human blood stream, or by transfusion of blood containing the parasite. The parasite, at this stage referred to as a sporozoite, enters hepatic parenchymal cells. *Plasmodium falciparum* does not have a dormant phase within the liver so relapses do not occur. However, this infection can persist for years in a chronic state if left untreated. After a period of 6–8 days mature forms (merozoites) are liberated into the blood stream. Here they attach to and invade circulating erythrocytes. Parasites undergo many morphological changes in the erythrocytes to eventually produce shizonts containing daughter erythrocytic merozoites. These are liberated by red cell lysis and immediately invade uninfected erythrocytes, resulting in a cycle of invasion and multiplication. The intraerythrocytic division is relatively regular, as is red cell lysis and merozoite release. These processes and the inflammatory components they provoke (e.g. cytokines) are responsible for the regular attacks of fever that occur at approximately the same time of day for the duration of the infection.

In contrast, some of the extraerythrocytic merozoites undergo maturation into gametocytes. These may be ingested by a mosquito during a blood meal. The gametocytes develop in the mosquito's midgut to form sporozoites which migrate into the salivary glands to complete the life cycle.

Pathophysiology

Plasmodium falciparum, in contrast to the other three forms of human malaria (*P. ovale, P. malariae, P. vivax*), affects the brain as well as other tissues. This unique difference is attributed to the fact that the mature intraerythrocytic form of the parasite adheres to specific endothelial receptors, in particular on the venule. As a consequence, partial occlusion of small vessels occurs which reduces perfusion. The resulting tissue anoxia and damage is exacerbated by red cells impacting on the parasites adhering to the vascular endothelium. Consequently areas of the brain will be deprived of oxygen and appropriate substrates, in particular glucose.

Assessment

Clinical features   Prodromal symptoms often predominate and include malaise, headache, myalgia, anorexia, and mild fever. These are present for several days before the first rigor. This typically starts with the patient feeling cold and apprehensive. Shivering rapidly evolves into a rigor lasting for one hour associated with vomiting, throbbing headache, palpitations, breathlessness, and fainting. This culminates in a drenching sweat. The whole episode lasts for approximately 8–12 hours, after which the exhausted patient sleeps. A high irregular continuous fever is not uncommon in a patient with falciparum malaria. In addition, generalised seizures, confusion, delirium, irritability or loss of conscious may occur. Mild meningism can be present but neck stiffness, photophobia and papilloedema are rare. A conjugate gaze palsy is common, but pupillary, corneal, and oculocephalic reflexes are normal. Muscle tone is increased symmetrically, knee reflexes are generally brisk and both plantar responses are extensor. Furthermore, extensor posturing is not uncommon and can be associated with sustained gaze. Other clinical features are shown in the box.

Non-neurological features associated with cerebral malaria

Anaemia
Spontaneous bleeding from the gastrointestinal tract
Jaundice
Hypoglycaemia
Shock
Oliguria
Acute renal failure
Pulmonary oedema

Diagnosis

Malaria should be considered in the differential diagnosis of any acute febrile illness until it can be excluded by definite lack of exposure, repeated examination of blood smears or following a therapeutic trial of antimalarial chemotherapy. Examination of several thick and thin blood films is required to exclude the diagnosis. **Do not dismiss the possibility of malaria in patients who have taken prophylactic drugs, as protection is never complete.** Absence of parasites in peripheral blood smears may indicate partial antimalarial treatment or sequestration in deep vascular beds. Treatment must be started and the diagnosis may be made on bone marrow aspirate.

If there are no contraindications, lumbar puncture must be done because it is important to exclude other treatable encephalopathies. The cerebrospinal fluid will show approximately 15 lymphocytes per millilitre with increased protein and normal glucose, unless the patient is hypoglycaemic.

Specific therapy

Quinine is the drug of choice. This should be given by an intravenous infusion to patients who are seriously ill or unable to swallow tablets.

- Loading dose 20 mg/kg of quinine salt diluted in 5% dextrose over four hours.
- Maintenance dose 10 mg/kg of quinine salt given over four hours by intravenous infusion every 8 to 12 hours until the patient can swallow tablets to complete a seven day course. If patients require more than 48 hours of parenteral therapy, the maintenance dose should be halved to 5 mg/kg.

Note that quinine can induce hypoglycaemia as a result of islet cell stimulation. This may be combined with hypoglycaemia due to extensive hyperparasitaemia. Thus, regular monitoring of blood glucose is necessary. Contraindications to quinine therapy are shown in the box.

Contraindications to quinine therapy

Hypersensitivity to quinine
Concurrent use of cimetidine, amiodarone or digoxin
Therapeutic administration of mefloquine within the previous 14 days
Resistant *Plasmodium falciparum*

Side effects from quinine are rare and usually follow rapid intravenous injection (see next box). Thus, careful monitoring of the infusion speed is required.

Side effects following quinine administration

Cardiovascular	sinus arrest, junctional rhythms, arteriovenous block, ventricular tachycardia/fibrillation, sudden death, prolongation of QT interval
Neurological	visual disturbances, partial deafness, headache, tinnitus, myopathy
Haematological	thrombocytopenia, haemolytic anaemia
Endocrine	hypoglycaemia

Any of the following regimes are appropriate for patients who are not seriously ill and can swallow tablets:

- quinine 600 mg three times a day for seven days. If quinine resistance is known or suspected this should be followed by either

- panzidol three tablets (sulfadoxine 500 mg plus pyrimethamine 25 mg per tablet)
- tetracycline 200 mg four times each day for seven days (provided renal function is normal)
- methalquine 20 mg/kg (maximum 1·1 g given as two doses, 6–8 hours apart)
- halothantrine (three doses of 500 mg given orally every six hours). This course should be repeated after one week.

Key point
Tetracyclines, sulfadoxine and pyrimethamine are contraindicated in pregnancy

Outcome

Mortality is approximately 10%, but varies according to the medical facilities available. Severe falciparum malaria can occur with the following conditions:

- impaired acquired immunity
- post splenectomy
- pregnancy
- immunosuppression.

Complications such as retinal haemorrhage, renal failure, hypoglycaemia, haemoglobinuria, metabolic acidaemia, and pulmonary oedema carry a poor prognosis.

Intracranial abscess

These can be extradural, subdural or intracerebral. Occasionally subdural and intracerebral abscesses may rupture into the subarachnoid space, resulting in meningitis.

Pathophysiology

Extradural abscess   As the dura mater is tightly adherent to the periosteum of the skull, epidural collections of pus are usually localised. They are related to either infections within the mastoid and nasal sinuses or focal osteomyelitis of the skull. Occasionally infection may spread intracranially to involve all layers of the meninges and even result in focal cerebritis. This is more likely to occur in penetrating trauma to the skull or rarely following craniotomy. Common organisms include *Haemophilus influenzae*, *Streptococcus pneumoniae*, *Staphylococcus aureus*, and many anaerobic species.

Subdural abscess   This is often a sequel to an infection in the paranasal sinuses or middle ear. Other causes include meningitis and septicaemia related to cyanotic congenital heart disease and lung abscesses. Penetrating trauma and intracranial surgery, as described earlier, can also be implicated. Subdural abscesses may be extensive with pus extending over the surface of the brain. The most common organisms include *Streptococcus pneumoniae*, *Streptococcus milleri*, *Streptococcus pyogenes*, *Staphylococcus aureus* and *Bacteroides* species along with *Haemophilus influenzae*.

Intracerebral abscess   These occur as a consequence of middle ear infection, frontal sinusitis and penetrating trauma to the head. Other causes include septicaemia related to infective endocarditis, lung abscess and bronchiectasis. As most abscesses are related to disease affecting either the middle ear or sinuses, they tend to be found in the temporal lobes, cerebellum or frontal lobes. Not surprisingly septicaemia can be associated with multiple intracerebral abscesses.

Large intracerebral abscesses may rupture into the ventricular system producing ventriculitis. Some of the organisms involved are described earlier under subdural abscess/empyema.

Assessment

Clinical features   The clinical features will depend upon the number, site, and extent of the lesions, as well as the impact on surrounding structures.

Extradural abscess is often difficult to diagnose clinically, but may present with a localised headache in association with mastoiditis and sinusitis.

Subdural abscess is often associated with severe headache, pyrexia, confusion, seizures and coma. A contralateral hemiparesis can be present. There may be evidence of mastoiditis, frontal sinusitis or a scalp infection.

Intracerebral abscess can present as headache, vomiting, impaired consciousness, hemiparesis, and seizures. There may also be features to suggest either a pulmonary or cardiac primary focus of infection.

Diagnosis

This is usually made on either a CT scan or magnetic resonance imaging.

Specific management

Neurosurgical opinion is necessary. Most supratentorial abscesses can be sterilised by aspirating via a burr hole. Subdural collections tend to be evacuated through a craniotomy. Small abscesses are usually treated with antibiotics. The prognosis is usually poor.

Outcome

The mortality is 10–20%. However, one third of survivors will have persistent epilepsy, in particular, as a sequel to temporal lobe or subdural abscesses.

Intracranial haematoma

Classification is identical to "intracranial abscess", i.e. extradural, subdural, and intracerebral.

Extradural haematoma

This classically follows a tear to the middle meningeal artery following a fracture in the temporoparietal region. The sequence of events is diagnostic. The patient initially suffers a head injury, becomes unconscious for a short time then recovers (the lucid interval, where confusion is common) only to become comatosed once more, minutes or hours later. The increasing volume of blood within the extradural space raises the intracranial pressure.

Subdural haematoma

This may be acute in patients who are overanticoagulated or chronic in the elderly, epileptic or alcoholic. A chronic subdural haematoma is usually associated with a trivial injury that may go unnoticed by the patient. Haemorrhage is due to rupture of the small veins crossing the subdural space with blood forming a localised collection between the dura and arachnoid mater. Absorption of fluid from the adjacent arachnoid space causes expansion of the blood clot. The onset of symptoms is insidious with headache, often mental changes, drowsiness, and vomiting. There may be mild hemiplegia, but raised intracranial pressure is not initially prominent.

Intracerebral haematoma
Occasionally spontaneous haemorrhage can produce a haematoma within the substance of the brain. The site and extent of the lesion will determine the clinical findings. One such condition which deserves mention is a cerebellar haematoma because surgical treatment can be life saving. The patient presents with acute occipital headache, dizziness, truncal ataxia, and rapid reduction in consciousness.

Diagnosis
In all cases the diagnosis is confirmed by either a CT scan or magnetic resonance imaging.

Specific management
For all of these conditions urgent neurosurgical consultation is required. It is important to realise that patients with such lesions can deteriorate very quickly. Regular monitoring is mandatory, as is prevention of secondary brain injury.

Intracranial tumours

These may be benign or malignant, primary or secondary. The clinical effects are related to the site and extent of the lesion(s) as well as the impact on neighbouring structures. An in-depth discussion on the different types of tumour is beyond the scope of this text. Furthermore this will not influence the initial management.

Pathophysiology
The effect of any intracranial neoplastic lesion depends upon the following:

- type of tumour
- growth rate
- site
- extent
- capacity to incite oedema formation in the adjacent brain tissue
- effect on neighbouring structures
- potential to obstruct flow of cerebrospinal fluid and blood.

The precise effects that these will have on intracranial pressure have been explained earlier.

Assessment

Clinical features Patients with intracerebral tumours tend to present with either epilepsy, or focal neurological signs, or raised intracranial pressure or a combination of these.

Late onset epilepsy (patients over 25 years) should always raise the suspicion of an intracranial tumour. Focal neurological deficits will obviously be related to the site and extent of the tumour, as well as its effect on adjacent structures. The effects of raised intracranial pressure have been discussed earlier.

The progressive development of clinical signs is the most significant factor in the diagnosis of intracerebral tumours.

Investigations
Imaging, either CT scan or magnetic resonance (imaging), is the investigation of choice.

Specific management

Dexamethasone (4 mg tds) can reduce oedema surrounding the tumour(s). Neuro-surgical consultation is required.

TIME OUT 11.2

Check your knowledge acquisition by answering the following questions.

a. What is the commonest site for a saccular aneurysm?
b. List the two common causes of subarachnoid haemorrhage.
c. How long does it take for xanthochromia to develop?
d. What is the mortality in the first 24 hours after a subarachnoid haemorrhage?
e. List the two common bacteria that cause spontaneous meningitis.
f. Which categories of patients are "high risk" for TB meningitis (a clue – six major groups)?
g. List the characteristic features of herpes simplex encephalitis.
h. In which patients would you consider a diagnosis of cerebral malaria?
i. List the non-neurological features of *Plasmodium falciparum* infection.
j. List any differences between abscess in the extradural, subdural, and intra-cerebral locations
k. List any differences between haematoma in the extradural, subdural, and intra-cerebral locations.

SUMMARY

- The patient with altered conscious level is a common medical problem.
- Prevent secondary brain injury by ensuring appropriate provision of supplemental oxygen and glucose.
- It is important that CT scanning is the critical first investigation providing all immediately life threatening problems have been treated and hypoglycaemia excluded. If meningitis encephalitis is suspected treatment should be given before investigations are done.
- Late onset epilepsy may indicate an intracranial tumour.
- Early liaison with specialist colleagues in microbiology, neurology or neurosurgery is important.

CHAPTER
12

The collapsed patient

OBJECTIVES

After reading this chapter you will be able to:

- describe the structured approach to the collapsed patient
- understand the pathophysiology of collapse
- describe the causes and investigation of transient loss of consciousness.

INTRODUCTION

Patients with stroke may present in a variety of ways but will commonly be referred to hospital having been found "collapsed". This chapter will cover the acute management of these patients. It will also cover the large number of patients who present with transient loss of consciousness.

STROKE

Introduction

Stroke is a syndrome characterised by an acute onset of focal (at times global) loss of function lasting more than 24 hours (or causing earlier death) due to cerebrovascular disease. Therefore, it is a clinical diagnosis.

Acute stroke affects about two per 1000 population per annum. This incidence increases steeply with increasing age (20 per 1000 in the over 85s). Stroke is more common in men.

Mortality is high (20% within 30 days after a first stroke). It causes a high prevalence of disability in survivors (about one third are dependent on others at one year).

Pathophysiology

The pathology underlying stroke is listed in the box.

171

Pathology of stroke

- Cerebral infarction   80%
    (large vessel disease 50%)
    (small vessel disease [lacunar] 25%)
    (cardiogenic embolism 20%)
- Primary intracerebral haemorrhage   10%
    (hypertension 50%)
- Subarachnoid haemorrhage   5%
- Unknown   5%

Atherosclerosis of the major vessels supplying the brain can precipitate a stroke by causing either embolisation from atherosclerotic plaques or major vessel occlusion. Small vessel disease, with occlusion of small penetrating arterioles, leads to small infarcts in the subcortical white matter, internal capsule, and basal ganglia (lacunar infarcts). Atrial fibrillation, valvular heart disease, recent myocardial infarction, and ventricular aneurysm can cause embolic strokes.

Intracerebral haemorrhage usually follows the sudden rupture of microaneurysms caused by hypertensive vascular disease, characteristically in the basal ganglia, brain stem and cerebellum.

Subarachnoid haemorrhage is commonly caused by rupture of an aneurysm arising on one of the arteries at the base of the brain, but it may arise from an arteriovenous malformation. (See Chapters 11 and 14 for further details.)

The distinction between strokes in the internal carotid territory and those in the vertebrobasilar territory is not always easy on clinical grounds. Dysphasia or visual spatial apraxia indicates definite carotid distribution. In contrast, simultaneous bilateral weakness or sensory loss, cortical blindness, diplopia, vertigo, ataxia and dysphagia suggests vertebrobasilar distribution.

Lacunar strokes tend not to affect conscious level or cognitive function. They may cause pure motor stroke, pure sensory stroke, sensorimotor stroke, ataxic hemiparesis and rarely, movement disorders such as hemiballismus or hemichorea.

Primary assessment and immediate treatment

In a patient presenting with stroke, it is essential to follow the structured approach previously described to optimise oxygenation and cerebral perfusion, and to limit secondary cerebral damage. Specific problems in the stroke patient include:

A – Airway may not be maintained. Clear and secure if necessary.

B – Respiratory drive may be depressed.

C – Cardiovascular compromise may have precipitated the stroke. Treat hypotension and tachycardias/bradycardias appropriately.

D – Check glucose. Hypoglycaemia may present with focal signs or depressed conscious level.

E – Check temperature. Hypothermia may complicate stroke.

Secondary assessment

History

An account of the onset of symptoms must be obtained from the patient or relative. A rapid onset of a focal neurological deficit is characteristic of a stroke (minutes or hours).

A history of sudden onset of a severe headache associated with neck stiffness suggests subarachnoid haemorrhage. In contrast a slower onset of symptoms suggests other diagnoses, for example, intracranial tumour or chronic subdural haematoma.

Note any vascular risk factors including history of transient ischaemic attacks, hypertension, atrial fibrillation, ischaemic heart disease, cigarette smoking, diabetes mellitus, and hyperlipidaemia.

Examination

A full neurological assessment will help localise the lesion and record the degree of disability.

Examination of the fundi may reveal changes of raised intracranial pressure or show evidence of previously undiagnosed hypertension or diabetes mellitus.

Cardiovascular examination includes:

- assessment of heart rhythm (atrial fibrillation?)
- blood pressure, taken in both arms (subclavian steal, aortic dissection)
- evidence of valvular heart disease
- listen for carotid bruit
- examination of peripheral pulses.

Listen carefully at the lung bases. Patients with swallowing difficulty are at risk of aspiration.

Investigations

CT scan

This is essential to exclude possible cerebral tumour or subdural haematoma and to establish whether the underlying pathology is infarction or haemorrhage.

> **Key point**
> It is not possible to distinguish cerebral infarction from cerebral haemorrhage on clinical grounds

CT scanning has several advantages over magnetic resonance imaging (MRI) in the acute stage and is the current method of choice due to the following:

- more widely available
- cheaper
- more sensitive at identifying haemorrhage in the early stages
- monitoring the patient during a CT scan is easier.

However, there are disadvantages to CT scanning.

- It will not identify an infarction in the first few hours after the onset of symptoms.
- It has limited ability to show vascular lesions in the brain stem and cerebellum and small ischaemic infarcts deep in the cerebral hemispheres.

Other investigations

- ECG is essential, examining rhythm disturbance and evidence of ischaemic, hypertensive or valvular heart disease.

- Chest X-ray may reveal features consistent with a potential cardiogenic source of emboli.
- Full blood count and clotting will exclude polycythaemia, thrombocytosis and clotting disorders.
- Plasma viscosity, as a screen for infection, vasculitis.
- Blood glucose, to exclude hypoglycaemia and thrombocytopaenia diabetes mellitus.
- Urea and electrolytes, to identify:
  (a) electrolyte disturbances in patients on diuretics
  (b) evidence of renal impairment in patients with hypertension
  (c) hyponatraemia as a rare case of focal neurological deficit.
- Fasting lipids, in all but the very elderly (although levels in acute phase of a stroke may not reflect premorbid profile).
- Syphilis serology, to identify meningovascular syphilis as a treatable, but rare, cause of cerebral ischaemia.

Management
The immediately life threatening problems will have been identified and treated as part of the primary assessment. Other important considerations at this stage would include the following.

Cardiovascular   Hypotension must be corrected (hypovolaemic hypotension may occur due to inadequate oral fluid intake). Hypertension must be managed cautiously. Some elevation in blood pressure is often seen with an acute stroke. Too drastic a reduction in blood pressure may reduce cerebral blood flow in the area around the infarct, causing extension of the stroke. Mild to moderate elevations in blood pressure do not require treatment unless they are maintained for several days after the acute event. If the diastolic blood pressure is persistently above 120 mm Hg the blood pressure must be lowered cautiously, using oral agents e.g. sublingual nefedipine. Avoid intramuscular preparations which may cause precipitous falls in blood pressure.

Respiratory   Patients with swallowing difficulty are at risk of bronchopulmonary aspiration. Monitor carefully for evidence of aspiration in the early stages and treat accordingly. An early review by the SALT (speech and language therapy) team is beneficial.

Metabolic   Blood sugar must be maintained within normal limits. Hyperglycaemia is harmful. Also take care with fluid and electrolyte balance, with the likelihood of an inadequate oral intake in the early stages.

Antiplatelet therapy   In acute stroke, aspirin should be started as soon as the diagnosis of cerebral infarction has been made. A starting dose of 150–300 mg daily should be given and continued until decisions have been made about secondary prevention.

Anticoagulant therapy   There is no evidence at present to support the use of anticoagulants in **acute** stroke, even for patients in atrial fibrillation. However, all patients who are in atrial fibrillation will require anticoagulation, providing there are no contraindications.

Thrombolysis Intravenous thrombolytic therapy is potentially an effective treatment of acute stroke, offering the possibility of early reperfusion of ischaemic cerebral tissue and limitation of infarct size. However, all thrombolytic drugs need to be given early after the onset of symptoms (probably within six hours) and involve a risk of cerebral haemorrhage. Results of trials so far suggest an increase in the proportion of patients making a good recovery by six months, but a substantial increase in cerebral haemorrhage within the first two weeks. In view of the potential risks and service implications, a consensus statement on the medical management of stroke produced by the Royal College of Physicians of Edinburgh (June 1998) stated that thrombolysis should not be used at present, except in the context of a randomised controlled trial. However, it is likely that the recommendations on the use of thrombolysis in acute stroke will change in the near future.

Surgery Neurosurgery may need to be considered for some cases of intracerebral haemorrhage. Evacuation of a cerebellar haematoma may be life saving and result in good long term recovery. Evacuation of supratentorial haematomas may also be life saving but the survivors usually have greater disability.

Other investigations and treatments will need to be considered later with regard to reducing the risk of recurrent stroke, but these will not be considered further here.

Summary

- Stroke is common.
- Mortality is high.
- Prevalence of dependency in survivors is high.
- The history and clinical assessment provide the diagnosis in the majority of patients, but a CT brain scan is necessary to exclude other pathology and to distinguish between thrombosis and haemorrhage.
- In the acute phase, the main aim is to optimise cerebral oxygen supply and ensure normal glucose, fluid and electrolyte balance.
- Aspirin is of benefit and should be started once cerebral thrombosis has been confirmed.
- It is likely that thrombolysis will have a significant role in the future but routine use is not at present recommended.

TRANSIENT COLLAPSE

Collapse is common. It accounts for about 3% of visits to the Emergency Department and between 1 and 6% of general medical admissions.

Recurrent collapse is important because:

- it is common
- it is disabling
- it may cause serious injury
- it can indicate life threatening underlying pathology.

Cerebral function can be disturbed by interruption of blood supply, epilepsy or metabolic factors. Some causes are listed in the box.

Causes of transient disturbances of consciousness

- Reduction in cerebral blood flow
  - (a) Generalised cerebral hypoperfusion (syncope)
    - (i) Cardiac:
      - reduced cardiac output
        - severe myocardial ischaemia – daily
        - aortic stenosis – monthly
        - hypertrophic obstructive cardiomyopathy (HOCM) – annually
        - (pulmonary hypertension) – only in exams
      - reduced ventricular filling
        - pulmonary embolism – weekly
        - atrial myxoma – only in exams
      - Arrhythmias – daily
    - (ii) Reflex mediated:
      - Vasovagal – weekly
      - Situational (micturition, cough) – weekly
      - Carotid sinus hypersensitivity – weekly
    - (iii) Postural hypotension – daily
  - (b) Localised vascular disease
    - Vertebrobasilar transient ischaemic attack – weekly
    - Basilar artery migraine – annually
- Epilepsy – daily
- Metabolic disturbances/drugs
  - Hypoxaemia
  - Hypoglycaemia – daily
  - Hyperventilation – only in exams
  - Phaeochromocytoma – daily

The prevalence of the various causes will depend on the population studied. Some recently published pooled data are summarised in the box. However, carotid sinus hypersensitivity may cause up to 47% of syncope in the elderly.

Causes of recurrent collapse – prevalence	
Vasovagal syncope	18%
Arrhythmias	14%
Epilepsy	10%
Postural hypotension	8%
Situational syncope	5%
Organic heart disease	4%
Medications	3%
Psychiatric	2%
Carotid sinus hypersensitivity	1%
Unknown	35%

Pathophysiology

Syncope

Syncope is defined as a transient loss of consciousness associated with an acute reduction in cerebral blood flow; although cerebral autoregulation compensates for minor changes in blood pressure more severe reductions will cause a fall in cerebral perfusion pressure. This will cause loss of consciousness.

Syncope is the most common cause of recurrent loss of consciousness. The other main differential diagnosis to consider is epilepsy. The distinction is usually clear from the history. However, seizures can sometimes be precipitated by cerebral hypoperfusion due to a primary cardiac problem.

Mean arterial blood pressure is affected by:

- **Heart rate**
  - bradycardia
  - tachycardia
- **Reduced stroke volume** due to
  - reduced preload
    - reduced circulatory volume
    - pulmonary embolism
    - atrial myxoma
  - cardiac
    - cardiomyopathy
    - tamponade
  - outflow obstruction
    - aortic stenosis
    - HOCM
- **Inappropriate vasodilatation**
  - postural hypotension
  - vasovagal syncope
  - autonomic neuropathy
  - drugs

Postural hypotension is common in the elderly, due to a combination of reduced baroreceptor sensitivity, excessive venous pooling and autonomic dysfunction. It is often exacerbated by drugs and dehydration.

With vasovagal syncope, venous pooling in the upright posture reduces venous return, resulting in increased sympathetic activity. In response to the vigorous contraction of the underfilled ventricles stimulation of ventricular mechanoreceptors initiates a brain stem reflex. This causes profound hypotension due to a combination of vagal stimulation (causing bradycardia) and withdrawal of sympathetic stimulation (causing vasodilatation) – the Bezold–Jarisch reflex.

Situational syncope occurs when the parasympathetic nervous system is activated by a trigger such as micturition or coughing.

Localised vascular disease
Any disorder of the cerebral blood vessels can result in reduced cerebral perfusion. Syncope in isolation is not typically a feature of transient ischaemic episodes. Loss of consciousness would not usually occur with a stroke in the carotid artery territory. A brain stem vascular episode may result in impaired consciousness but other symptoms usually occur, for example, vertigo, diplopia and ataxia.

Metabolic causes
Metabolic causes of transient loss of consciousness are uncommon. Hypoglycaemia must not be forgotten. It is usually due to overtreatment of diabetes mellitus but may occur in other situations, for example, Addison's disease, postgastrectomy and insulinoma.

Hyperventilation can cause a respiratory alkalosis which can predispose to syncope.

Chronic catecholamine oversecretion with phaeochromocytoma can be associated with postural hypotension.

Drugs
Drugs can cause collapse by:

- interfering with cardiac conduction (digoxin, β blockers, calcium channel blockers, amiodarone, etc.)

- causing postural hypotension (e.g. diuretics, antihypertensives, antidepressants, levodopa preparations, etc.).

Assessment

The paroxysmal nature of the problem means that you are likely to see the patient between episodes of collapse, when primary assessment is likely to reveal no major problems. Secondary assessment with a careful history and physical examination will provide the diagnosis in the majority of patients.

History

It is important to obtain a history from a witness, in addition to the patient, where possible. The circumstances of the collapse may be relevant, e.g. cough or micturition syncope. Vasovagal syncope is usually associated with a hot environment or stressful, emotional situations. Collapse associated with head turning may indicate carotid sinus hypersensitivity. Episodes associated with exertion suggest mechanical limitation of cardiac output (aortic stenosis, HOCM) or an exercise induced arrhythmia. Symptoms on prolonged standing suggest postural hypotension or vasovagal syncope.

Ask specifically about cardiovascular symptoms (palpitations, chest pain, breathlessness) and neurological symptoms (headache, weakness/parasthesiae, autonomic dysfunction). **The importance of an accurate drug history cannot be overemphasised.** A family history of syncope or sudden death may be relevant.

The distinction between epilepsy and syncope can be difficult. A witnessed tonic–clonic convulsion associated with tongue biting and incontinence is obviously helpful in making a diagnosis, but the story may not always be so clear.

- A patient with syncope will usually report symptoms of light headedness, nausea, sweating or blurring of vision before consciousness is lost. In contrast, a generalised tonic–clonic seizure will usually have minimal prodromal symptoms.
- With syncope the duration of unconsciousness will be shorter than epilepsy (seconds versus minutes) and the recovery will be more rapid, without the usual drowsy, confused postictal period.
- Brief twitching may be seen with an episode of syncope but this will usually be very transient.
- Pallor may be seen before the collapse. This is common with syncope, although it may be seen with epilepsy.

> **Key point**
> The distinction between epilepsy and syncope is important. A careful history from the patient and witnesses will clarify the situation in the majority of cases

Examination

Assess the pulse rate, rhythm, and character. Measure the lying and standing blood pressure. A fall in systolic blood pressure of 20 mm Hg after two minutes standing is significant. Examine the precordium for evidence of structural heart disease, especially aortic stenosis or other causes of outflow obstruction. Listen for carotid bruits.

A thorough neurological assessment is essential. Look for patterns of signs including upper motor neurone lesions, extrapyramidal pathology, cerebellar features, brain stem signs or evidence of peripheral neuropathy.

Investigations

Further investigations will be guided by the history and clinical findings.

(a) Cardiological
- 12 lead ECG. All patients with recurrent collapse need an ECG. It may reveal evidence of ischaemia, left ventricular hypertrophy or conduction abnormalities.
- 24-hour ECG monitoring may be useful if there is a suspicion of paroxysmal rhythm disturbances, even though 12 lead ECG may be normal.
- Echocardiography is invaluable if either left ventricular outflow obstruction is suspected or left ventricular function is impaired.
- Exercise testing may be useful when collapse is associated with exertion (providing left ventricular outflow obstruction has been excluded). It may reveal ischaemia, hypotension or an arrhythmia.

(b) Neurological
- Electroencephalogram (EEG) is of little value in the assessment of patients with recurrent collapse. It may be helpful in confirming a diagnosis of epilepsy, when this is suspected clinically, but it is not indicated routinely in the assessment of syncope.
- CT/MRI scanning is not required unless there are focal neurological signs or there has been a witnessed seizure.
- Carotid or transcranial doppler ultrasonography is rarely helpful. It should only be considered in the presence of bruits, a palpaple discrepancy between carotid pulses or when the history suggests either carotid or vertebrobasilar insufficiency.

(c) Laboratory tests
- Laboratory tests have a poor yield unless there is clinical suspicion of an abnormality. However, it is worth checking glucose, urea and electrolytes and haemoglobin.
- Rarely the clinical features may indicate either Addison's disease (adrenocortical failure) or phaeochromocytoma; therefore a short Synacthen® test or 24-hour urine collection for dopamine degradation products (adrenocortical) may be needed.

(d) Other investigations
- Carotid sinus massage. This is contra-indicated:
  (i) in the presence of carotid bruits or cerebrovascular disease
  (ii) if there is a history of ventricular arrhythmias or recent myocardial infarction.

Providing there are no contraindications, place the patient in the supine position and monitor ECG and blood pressure. The right carotid artery is massaged longitudinally, with the neck slightly extended, for a maximum of five seconds. If the response is negative there should be a 30 second interval before the left carotid artery is massaged (maximum five seconds).

> **Key point**
> Bilateral carotid massage must never be attempted

A positive cardioinhibitory response is defined as a sinus pause of three seconds or more. A positive vasodepressor response is defined as a fall in systolic blood pressure of more than 50 mm Hg.

- Tilt testing

Tilt testing is useful in the further assessment of unexplained recurrent syncope after conclusion of other cardiac causes including arrhythmias. Briefly:

(i) Baseline pulse and blood pressure recordings are measured with the patient lying supine for 30 minutes.

(ii) The patient is tilted to 60–75° for up to 45 minutes and asked to report any symptoms.

(iii) A positive result is a cardioinhibitory response and/or a vasodepressor response in association with symptoms.

(iv) If a positive response occurs, the patient is immediately returned to the horizontal position.

Other measures may be used to increase the sensitivity of the test.

> **Key point**
> With both carotid sinus massage and tilt testing full resuscitation facilities must be available immediately

SPECIFIC CONDITIONS

Status epilepticus

Status epilepticus is defined as either a single seizure lasting for 30 minutes or repeated seizures between which there is incomplete recovery of consciousness. However, seizures lasting more than 5 minutes can indicate impending status epilepticus. This may be prevented by immediate treatment. A working definition is therefore: continuous seizures lasting at least 5 minutes, or, two or more discrete seizures betwen which there is incomplete recovery of conciousness.

> **Key point**
> Generalised convulsive status epilepticus is a common and serious medical emergency. There is a significant risk of permanent brain damage and death from cardiorespiratory failure (5–10% mortality in those admitted to an intensive care unit)

Primary assessment and resuscitation – specific summary for epilepsy management.

A – Maintain patency/initially with nasopharyngeal airway
Give oxygen ($FiO_2 = 0.85$)
Do not attempt to insert oral airway/intubate while jaw is clenched
Early liaison with anaesthetist

B – Pulse oximeter

C – Establish IV access
Monitor ECG

D – IV diazepam 10 mg over 2–5 minutes
Check glucose
IV thiamine (250 mg over 10 minutes) if history of chronic alcohol abuse
Look for head trauma

E – Check temperature
Look for purpura (meningococcal septicaemia)

Respiratory depression and hypotension may occur after IV diazemuls. Give 2 mg up to a maximum of 20 mg per minute. If control is not achieved, phenytoin 15 mg/kg IV should be given with ECG monitoring (reduce dose if patient previously on phenytoin). The infusion rate should not exceed 50 mg/min because of the risk of cardiac arrhythmias. Further doses up to a total of 30 mg/kg may be given if seizures persist. Then maintenance doses of 100 mg IV should be given every 6–8 hours. Phenytoin has the advantage of suppressing seizures without causing cortical or respiratory depression. See Chapter 11 for alternative drugs e.g. lorazepam and fosphenytoin. If seizures continue, the patient should be anaesthetised and ventilated. Cerebral function monitoring is very useful in this situation. Anaesthesia and ventilation should continue until 12–24 hours after the last seizure.

Secondary assessment

A history from a relative is important. Are there any symptoms to suggest tumour, meningitis, head injury? Ask about alcohol consumption. If the patient is a known epileptic, ask about current drug regime, compliance or any recent changes in drug therapy.

Physical examination will include a careful neurological assessment, looking particularly for evidence of meningeal irritation, raised intracranial pressure and focal neurological deficits.

Arrhythmia

Bradycardia

Bradycardia may be diagnosed on 24-hour ECG monitoring but it is important to document associated symptoms. Review the patient's medications and stop those which may cause bradycardia.

In the presence of sino-atrial node disease, pacing may be considered if pauses greater than three seconds are documented.

With atrioventicular node dysfunction, pacing should be considered for second degree or third degree heart block, in the absence of a reversible cause (drugs or ischaemia).

Tachycardia

Supraventricular tachycardia including atrial fibrillation, for example, often cause palpitations and dizziness but rarely present with syncope. Ventricular tachycardia is more likely to cause syncope. The Wolff–Parkinson–White syndrome and the prolonged QT syndrome should be considered in patients with recurrent syncope. The type of tachycardia will determine the treatment. This comprises antiarrhythmic drug therapy, occasionally an antitachycardia pacemaker/defibrillator or radio-ablation. Transient rhythm abnormalities are increasingly common with increasing age, for example, short runs of atrial fibrillation and sinus bradycardia occur at night. Do not treat unless there is clear evidence that these arrhythmias are associated with symptoms or predispose to further pathology, for example, paroxysmal atrial fibrillation and stroke.

Vasovagal syncope

The mechanism of collapse in vasovagal syncope and the assessment of patients by tilt testing has been described. Treatment is not always satisfactory. β blockers may be used to inhibit the initial sympathetic activation in vasovagal syncope. With a positive cardio-inhibitory response to tilt testing, disopyramide may be useful (to block the vagal outflow) or dual chamber pacing may be necessary. With a predominant vasodepressor response, ephedrine, dihydroergotamine or fludrocortisone have been tried with variable success.

Carotid sinus hypersensitivity

Hypersensitivity of the carotid artery baroreceptors can cause bradycardia and/or vasodilatation due to vagal activation. The patient complains of dizziness or syncope associated with head turning or the wearing of a tight collar. Diagnosis is by carotid sinus massage as described previously. A positive cardioinhibitory response to this technique responds well to cardiac pacing. As with vasovagal syncope, a vasodepressor response is more difficult to treat.

Postural hypotension

Postural hypotension is associated with:

- hypovolaemia (dehydration, haemorrhage, diuretics)
- drugs
- autonomic failure (diabetes mellitus, Parkinson's disease, old age).

It is difficult to treat patients who have postural hypotension offering correct intravascular volume and rationalising the drug therapy as much as possible. They should be advised to stand up slowly and to avoid prolonged standing. Graduated elastic stockings may reduce venous pooling. Fludrocortisone increases salt and water retention and is occasionally helpful.

Left ventricular outflow obstruction

Advanced aortic stenosis may cause exertional dizziness and syncope because cardiac output is reduced. Such symptoms indicate urgent assessment with a view to aortic valve replacement.

Hypertrophic obstructive cardiomyopathy (HOCM) is associated with restricted cardiac output during stress. Treatment is with negatively inotropic drugs (β blockers, verapamil) to reduce the outflow tract gradient. Dual chamber pacing or surgery may be needed in more advanced cases.

SUMMARY

Recurrent collapse is common.
- It can be associated with life threatening underlying pathology and can cause serious injury.
- History and physical examination provide a likely diagnosis in the majority of patients.
- Further investigation will be guided by clinical judgement and by the frequency and severity of the symptoms.

Following stroke:
- patients in atrial fibrillation should be immediately anticoagulated;
- hypertension must be aggressively treated if diastolic blood pressure is greater than 90 mm Hg;
- a normal CT brain scan excludes cerebral thrombosis.

In transient collapse:
  loss of consciousness is an uncommon feature of transient ischaemic attack;
- prodromal symptoms of light headedness, nausea, and sweating suggest syncope rather than epilepsy as a cause of collapse;
- a sinus pause of three seconds or more with carotid sinus massage is significant.

TIME OUT 12.1

a. Define "stroke".
b. Describe your immediate management of a patient with a suspected transient ischaemic attack.

CHAPTER

13

The overdose patient

OBJECTIVES

After reading this chapter you will be able to:
- describe how the structured approach can be applied to patients who have taken an overdose
- discuss the diagnostic clues that are available in the primary assessment
- understand the use of various measures that can be used to eliminate drugs from the body
- describe some specific treatments for overdose.

INTRODUCTION

The management of overdose is one of the most challenging aspects of emergency medical care. In the absence of a clear history (for example, in the unconscious patient) the diagnosis can be difficult. Furthermore, many patients are reluctant to cooperate during their initial assessment. The pharmacological effects of the substances taken in overdose may be significant, necessitating emergency intervention to limit morbidity and mortality.

The majority of cases are as a result of deliberate self harm; however, accidental overdose is also common, especially in the paediatric population. More alarmingly, a minority of patients may present with non-accidental overdose (both deliberate poisoning and Munchausen by proxy). Care should also be taken to recognise iatrogenic overdose, which is more common in the elderly, those on multiple medications and in patients with long-standing health problems such as chronic renal failure. The presentation is generally variable; some patients may self refer with a full history whilst others may attend with symptoms such as unusual behaviour, decreased conscious level, fits and those related to an arrhythmia.

Whatever the presentation, medical care should follow the structured approach discussed in Chapter 3 – with primary assessment and resuscitation preceding a secondary assessment, emergency treatment, and definitive care. Psychiatric assessment is often necessary in this group of patients but should only take place once the above medical assessment is complete.

185

PRIMARY ASSESSMENT AND RESUSCITATION

Airway

The simple question, "Are you all right?" will allow the examining doctor to establish whether the patient is conscious, has good laryngeal function, and an adequate vital capacity. As discussed in Chapter 3, a failure to answer this question should lead to the use of a simple airway opening manoeuvre and an assessment of breathing.

Endotracheal intubation is required in the unconscious patient, to provide airway protection and facilitate gastric lavage (if appropriate).

Breathing

Since a number of agents taken in overdose (particularly narcotics) can produce respiratory depression it is very important to look for adequate breathing. The rate, depth, and work of breathing should be assessed. If there are any signs of inadequacy, breathing should be supported using a bag–valve–mask device with added oxygen. Even in the patient who appears to be breathing adequately, oxygen should be given until it is deemed unnecessary.

Circulation

Pulse rate, cardiac rhythm, blood pressure, and adequacy of peripheral perfusion should be assessed. Inadequate circulation is generally caused by hypotension or arrhythmia. Hypotension is commonly caused by a relative hypovolaemia secondary to peripheral vasodilatation and will respond to fluid resuscitation. The cause of cardiac dysrhythmias differs from those seen in ischaemic heart disease, and requires a different approach to management. Dysrhythmias are often surprisingly well tolerated. If treatment becomes necessary cardioversion is preferable to antiarrhythmic drugs, as potential drug interactions can be avoided. Intravenous access should be established at this stage, providing an opportunity to take blood samples for relevant investigations.

Diagnostic clues from the primary assessment may provide a pointer towards the specific drug or drugs ingested. These are listed in Table 13.1.

Disability

Assess disability in the standard manner using either the AVPU or Glasgow Coma Scale (see Chapter 3) and measure the pupillary size and responses. These latter observations can be helpful in establishing a diagnosis if the agent that has been taken is unknown. Many drugs, e.g. paracetamol, can cause rapid hypoglycaemia. As this has **protean manifestations** always check a serum glucose concentration.

Exposure

Full exposure is necessary, looking for both marking and rashes. It is very important to assess temperature at this stage since a number of drugs can alter thermoregulatory mechanisms, e.g. **phenothiazines**. Once patients have been fully exposed and the required examination has been completed, cover immediately; as many will lose heat rapidly in this situation.

Table 13.1 Diagnostic clues from the primary assessment

	Sign	Drug
B	Tachypnoea	Aspirin
	Bradypnoea	Opiates
		CNS depressants
C	Tachycardia	Antidepressants
		sympathomimetics
		amphetamines
		cocaine
	Bradycardia	β Blockers
		digoxin
		clonidine
	Hypertension	Amphetamines
		cocaine
D	Small pupils	Opioids
		cholinesterase inhibitors
	Large pupils	Tricyclic antidepressants
		anticholinergics
		antihistamines
		ephedrine
		amphetamines
		cocaine
	Coma	barbiturates
		tricyclic antidepressants
		opiates
		benzodiazepines
		ethanol
E	Hypothermia	tricyclic antidepressants
		barbiturates
		phenothiazines
	Hyperthermia	amphetamines
		cocaine

By the end of the primary assessment, the minimum essential monitoring should include pulse oximetry and continuous ECG trace. The respiratory rate, pulse, blood pressure, Glasgow Coma Score, temperature and glucose concentration should have been documented. These observations need to be repeated on a regular basis in order to monitor the patient's condition and response to treatment.

LETHALITY ASSESSMENT

At the end of the primary assessment it is important to assess the potential lethality of the overdose. This requires knowledge of the substance, the time it was taken and the dose. Corraborative evidence may need to be sought from other sources, such as family members or paramedic staff, to establish this information. Regional poisons centres will provide advice on specific treatment. If the nature of the overdose is unknown then a high potential lethality should be assumed.

IMMEDIATE MANAGEMENT

Drug elimination

If the drug overdose is assessed as having a potentially high lethality or if the exact nature of the overdose is unknown, use measures designed to reduce drug levels.

Reducing absorption

Methods to stop or decrease absorption of drugs have been used liberally in the past. Recent evidence shows such techniques are of limited effect and probably only have a role in a minority of patients. It should be noted that they should never be used as a punishment and that their use does not act as a deterrent to further episodes of overdose.

Gastric lavage

The use of lavage should be limited to patients who have taken life threatening overdoses and present within the first hour after ingestion. This time period may be increased for certain drugs which prolong gastric emptying, most commonly aspirin and tricyclic antidepressants (Table 13.2). Gastric lavage use may also be considered for those drugs which are not absorbed by charcoal, such as iron and lithium. It is contraindicated after ingestion of caustic agents and when the airway is compromised. Therefore a cuffed endotracheal tube will protect the airway.

Table 13.2   Indications and timing for gastric lavage

Drug	Minimum dose	Maximum time since ingestion
Paracetamol	10 g	4 hours
Theophyllines	>2.5 g	4 hours
Barbiturates	>1000 mg	8 hours
Unknown		8 hours
Tricyclic antidepressants	>750 mg	8 hours
Aspirin	15 g	12 hours
Benzodiazepines	Lavage not indicated	

Contraindications to gastric lavage	
Corrosive agents, e.g.	acid
	alkali
	bleach
	kettle descaler
Petroleum derivatives, e.g.	petrol
	paraffin
	white spirits
	turpentine substitute
	kerosene

Therapeutic emesis

A centrally acting emetic (usually ipecacuanha) is used to promote active vomiting. The symptoms it produces can often cloud an already complicated clinical picture. There is no evidence that it decreases absorption and its use in emergency practice is now obsolete.

Activated charcoal

Charcoal works by absorbing ingested drugs on to its large surface area. It is now the treatment of choice for decreasing absorption in the overdose patient, but its use should be limited to those patients with life threatening overdose presenting within one hour of ingestion. Charcoal will only absorb 10% of its own weight of a drug (i.e. 50 g will absorb 5 g of drug). Thus it is relatively ineffective in overdoses where the total concentration of toxin ingested is large (> 5 g). The initial use of gastric lavage may be justified in these circumstances, but should be followed by charcoal.

Compliance with taking charcoal is generally low, due to its appearance and taste. The use of a nasogastric tube will help those patients who are unwilling to drink charcoal.

Increasing elimination

Attention to cardiovascular problems elicited in the primary assessment will ensure that the body's natural elimination routes via the liver or kidneys are maximised. Other measures to increase elimination include therapeutic diuresis, alkalinisation, chelation, haemoperfusion, and haemodialysis. Such treatment should be done **only** on the advice of, or under the supervision of, specialists.

SECONDARY ASSESSMENT

As in all other emergency presentations the secondary assessment involves taking as full a history as possible. A full examination is also necessary. Appropriate investigations based on this assessment should be ordered. A 12 lead ECG should be recorded in all patients with predicted cardiac sequelae from their overdose or if continuous cardiac monitoring shows any rhythm disturbance. A chest radiograph is necessary in a patient who is unconscious or shows evidence of aspiration. Blood may be taken for renal and liver function, clotting studies, and osmolality. Arterial blood gases will help with quantifying any respiratory compromise and also indicate an acid–base disturbance. Toxicology screening is generally limited by local resources to paracetamol and salicylate estimation, but blood and urine may be saved for further testing, depending on the services available.

Some symptoms and signs elicited in the secondary assessment may provide clues to specific types of overdose. These are listed in the box.

Clues from secondary assessment

Pulmonary oedema	salicylate
	ethylene glycol
	opiate
	organophosphates
	paraquat
Hypoglycaemia	insulin
	oral hypoglycaemic
	ethanol
	paracetamol
	salicylate
Hyperglycaemia	salbutamol
	theophylline
Hypokalaemia	salbutamol
	theophylline
	salicylates
Metabolic acidosis	salicylates
	paracetamol
	ethanol
	ethylene glycol
	tricyclics
Raised osmolality	ethanol
	methanol
	ethylene glycol
Prolonged prothrombin time	salicylates
	paracetamol

EMERGENCY TREATMENT

In addition to the general management described previously, some poisons require specific antedotes (Table 13.3).

Table 13.3 Specific measures in overdose

Drug	Treatment
β Blockers	Glucagon, dobutamine
Cyanide	100% oxygen, amyl nitrite, sodium thiosulphate, high dose vitamin B12
Digoxin	Specific Fab antibodies
Ethylene glycol	Ethanol
Iron	Desferrioxamine
Methanol	Ethanol
Opiates	Naloxone
Organophosphates	Atropine, pralidoxine
Paracetamol	N-acetyl cysteine
Tricyclic antidepressants	Alkalinisation
Aspirin	Dose dependent: diuresis, alkaline diuresis, haemodialysis

Fab, fragment of immunoglobulin G involved in antigen binding.

DEFINITIVE CARE

Some patients may require admission to the medical wards because of their physical condition. A large number, however, will be fit for discharge after immediate treatment and a short period of observation. However, it is important to realise that many sequelae to overdose are **not** instantly apparent, e.g. nephrotoxic renal failure due to either paracetamol or aspirin. Thus you have to be proactive and treat to prevent such conditions. This may not always be possible, for example, due to the prolonged time between ingestion and presentation. Therefore, actively seek/monitor for complications. It is absolutely essential that patients who are to be discharged (whether immediately or after medical care) are adequately assessed from a psychiatric point of view and in particular that their level of intent is considered. A number of issues can be investigated to try and define the intent and these are summarised in the box below.

> **Factors defining intent in deliberate self harm**
>
> Patient's perception of lethality
> Evidence of premeditation
> Measures to prevent discovery
> Social circumstances
> Evidence of depression
> Evidence of psychosis

SUMMARY

- The structured approach to the seriously ill patient should be used when dealing with patients who have taken overdoses.

- The potential lethality of the overdose must be assessed at the end of the primary assessment.
- If indicated, measures should be taken to stop absorption and increase excretion of the ingested compound.
- Specific treatment may be indicated once the substance has been identified.
- An assessment of intent must be made to determine the nature of further care.

CHAPTER

14

The patient with a headache

OBJECTIVES

After reading this chapter you should be able to:

- understand the causes of headache
- describe a classification of headache that will be useful in clinical practice
- discuss the initial management of a patient with headache
- describe how clinical signs detected in the secondary assessment influence diagnosis and subsequent management.

INTRODUCTION

Patients presenting with a headache of acute onset account for less than 2.5% of new emergency attendances. Of these only 15% will have a serious cause for their headache. Therefore, the aim is to identify the relatively small group of high risk patients.

PATHOPHYSIOLOGY

Pain sensitive structures in the head include:

- dura
- arteries
- venous sinuses
- paranasal sinuses
- eyes
- tympanic membranes
- cervical spine.

These are innervated by somatic afferents from the V, VII, IX, and X cranial nerves (linked via the spinal tract of the trigeminal nerve) and the upper three cervical nerve roots. Pain will occur if there is traction, inflammation or distension of these structures, in particular, the dura, blood vessels, and nerves. A throbbing headache is non-specific because it is common to many intracranial conditions. Similarly the site of pain is non-specific, but it can provide clues to underlying pathology as outlined below.

- Frontal — **ipsilateral forehead and eye pain**, referred via the trigeminal nerve, can indicate a lesion in the anterior or middle cranial fossa.
  - **bifrontal** headache can be a presenting feature of acute hydrocephalus secondary, for example, to either a supra- or infratentorial lesion. The pain is attributed to vascular distortion following dilatation of the lateral ventricles.
- Frontotemporal — **unilateral** pain is common with sinusitis and dental problems. In addition, orbital cellulitis, glaucoma, and cavernous sinus thrombosis have a similar presentation.
- Occipital — posterior fossa or upper cervical spine pathology (referred via the upper three cervical nerve roots) can present with occipital pain.

In contrast, the distribution of pain can be more specific.

- Trigeminal — neuralgia is restricted to the distribution of the trigeminal nerve. The searing paroxysms of intense pain are usually unilateral and confined to one division. Occasionally, two or all three divisions are involved. This specific distribution of pain is attributed to distortion of the blood vessels supplying the trigeminal nerve.
- Somatic afferent — postherpetic neuralgia is secondary to inflammation and will occur in the distribution of the affected nerve, i.e. the V, VII, IX, and X cranial nerves.

CLINICAL ASSESSMENT

A useful way to categorise patients presenting with a headache is shown in the box.

Clinical classification of headache

- Headache with **altered Glasgow Coma Score** and/or **focal neurological signs**
- Headache with **papilloedema** but **no** focal neurological signs
- Headache with **fever** but **no** focal neurological signs
- Headache with **extracranial** signs
- Headache with **no** abnormal signs

This classification will form the framework of the remaining sections in this chapter. It is important to note that some conditions occur in more than one category – reflecting the diverse manifestations. The structure of the initial assessment and the earlier classification is designed to ensure early detection and management of an immediately life threatening problem, i.e. headache with **altered Glasgow Coma Score** and/or **focal neurological signs**. The remaining, non-immediately life threatening causes will be identified in the secondary assessment.

HEADACHE WITH ALTERED GLASGOW COMA SCORE AND/OR FOCAL NEUROLOGICAL SIGNS

After assessing "D" the following will have been identified:

- a reduction in the Glasgow Coma Score
- the presence of lateralising signs

- pupillary abnormalities
- meningeal irritation.

Although the specific diagnosis is often unknown at this stage, the patient should receive optimum oxygenation and appropriate control of both blood pressure and serum glucose.

An immediately life threatening event either causing or following a headache will be identified in the **primary assessment**. Such conditions are listed in the box below.

Causes of headache with altered Glasgow Coma Score and/or focal neurological signs

● Vascular	Stroke	Daily
	Subarachnoid haemorrhage	Weekly
	Chronic subdural haematoma	Monthly
● Infective	Meningitis	Daily
	Encephalitis	Monthly
	Cerebral abscess	Monthly
	Subdural empyema	Annually
	Cerebral malaria	Annually
● Neoplastic	Secondary intracerebral tumour	Weekly
	Primary intracerebral tumour	Monthly

Key point
Remember that the goal of initial management is to prevent secondary brain injury

---

Key management issues

- The mode of onset of symptoms will help distinguish different conditions, e.g.
  acute onset   = vascular/meningeal irritation
  subacute onset   = infective
  chronic onset   = neoplastic
- If the patient is febrile take blood cultures and start appropriate antibiotic therapy to cover bacterial meningitis. If there is a history of foreign travel to relevant areas request thick and thin films to exclude malaria. Subsequent investigations will include imaging, either CT or MR, and this should precede lumbar puncture.
- Further management should be discussed with appropriate clinicians, i.e. neurologist, microbiologist, neurosurgeon or infectious disease physician.

Specific management of the conditions shown in the earlier box is considered in the unconscious patient (Chapter 11).

Key point
Emphasis should be placed on seeking meningeal irritation, fever, reduced conscious level, focal neurological features, and skin rash

---

The primary assessment will detect any changes in the Glasgow Coma Score, pupillary response, and lateralising signs. However, physical signs can change. Thus, the secondary assessment facilitates reevaluation combined with obtaining further information and a more comprehensive examination. The relevant secondary assessment features are summarised in the box.

Most patients presenting with a headache will have a non-immediately life threatening condition. Thus, in the **secondary assessment** the doctor has time to take a full history. A new headache, or one different from normal, can indicate intracranial pathology.

> **Key point**
> Over one third of patients will have a minor (sentinel) bleed hours or days before a major sub-arachnoid haemorrhage

It is important to ellicit the frequency of headache and what the patient was doing at the onset of the pain, for example, a headache that wakes a patient from sleep suggests significant pathology. Furthermore, headaches that become progressively more severe or chronic ones that are different from usual may be caused by raised intracranial pressure.

An important part of this assessment is to exclude raised intracranial pressure. Features that would indicate this diagnosis are listed in the box.

> **Headache with features suggestive of raised intracranial pressure**
>
> Worse on waking
> Aggravated by coughing, vomiting, straining, standing, and sitting
> Relieved by lying down
> Eventually associated with papilloedema and neurological signs

> **Key point**
> It is important to realise that the classic early morning headache of raised intracranial pressure is uncommon

Headache exacerbated by changes in posture or associated with nausea, vomiting or ataxia requires further investigation, especially cranial imaging, when neurological signs are detected.

Specific information should also be sought regarding photophobia, neck stiffness, altered mental function, neurological dysfunction as well as the presence of a fever or skin rash. These features may be transient.

> **Key features of the assessment of a patient with a headache**
>
> - Characteristics
>   - New onset
>   - Acute onset
>   - Progressive
>   - Wakens from sleep
>   - Worst ever
> - Associated symptoms
>   - Photophobia
>   - Neck stiffness
>   - Fever
>   - Altered mental state
>   - Neurological dysfunction
> - Examination findings
>   - Temperature
>   - Meningeal irritation
>   - Abnormal neurological signs
>   - Rash

HEADACHE WITH PAPILLOEDEMA BUT NO FOCAL NEUROLOGICAL SIGNS

The pathophysiology of cerebrospinal fluid production and the relationship to intracranial pressure is discussed in Chapter 11.

The dynamic components that influence intracranial pressure are shown in Figure 14.1. This diagram is a useful *aide-mémoire* for the pathophysiology of raised intracranial pressure. The brain is contained within a rigid skull with little room for expansion. There are four ways to disturb the normal cerebral homeostasis:

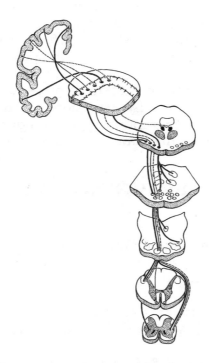

Figure 14.1   The components responsible for intracranial pressure

- increasing the pressure in the arteries, e.g. vasodilatation
- adding to the intracranial contents, e.g. tumour or oedema
- obstructing cerebrospinal fluid drainage
- preventing venous drainage, e.g. congestion.

In the context of headache, the relevant causes are listed in the box below.

Causes of headache and papilloedema, but with no focal or neurological signs	
• Arterial	Accelerated hypertension/arterial dilatation
• Intracranial	Mass lesions, e.g. tumour, haematoma
	Cerebrospinal fluid accumulation
	Cerebral oedema
	Benign intracranial hypertension
• Venous	Obstruction to outflow, i.e. sinus thrombosis
	Congestion

Key point

Papilloedema is:
- usually bilateral and causes minimal interference with vision
- associated with hypertension; it is due to optic nerve vascular damage and cerebral oedema

Key management issues

- Antihypertensive therapy is required if the diastolic blood pressure is greater than 120 mm Hg and retinal haemorrhages are present.
- CT is warranted especially if the blood pressure is normal.
- The CT scan result will guide further management; for example, dexamethasone for tumour associated oedema and neurosurgical referral for evacuation of haematoma.
- Further management will follow discussion with appropriate clinicians, especially a neurologist or neurosurgeon.
- Although neurological signs may be absent at presentation they can develop as the condition progresses. For example, hypertension can lead to a stroke; a host of focal features can be associated with an intracerebral tumour (depending on the site and extent) and sinus thrombosis. In addition they can all present as epilepsy.

HEADACHE WITH FEVER BUT NO FOCAL NEUROLOGICAL SIGNS

This is a common mode of presentation and the major conditions are listed in the box below. However, headaches and fever are common to many infectious diseases. One particularly useful differentiating feature is the presence of neck stiffness.

Causes of headache with fever but no focal neurological signs

Intracranial		Meningitis	Daily
		Subarachnoid haemorrhage	Weekly
		Encephalitis	Monthly
Extracranial	– focal	Acute sinusitis	Daily
	– systemic	Viral illness	Daily
		Malaria	Annually
		Typhoid	Annually

Key point

Do **not** assess neck stiffness in patients with potential cervical spine instability, e.g. rheumatoid disease, ankylosing spondylitis, Down's syndrome and trauma

---

Neck stiffness is a non-specific sign that should be assessed with the patient flat, your hands supporting the occipital region and by feeling for increased tone while:

1. gently rotating the head (as if the patient is saying no)
2. slowly lifting the head off the bed. During this manoeuvre also watch for hip and knee flexion. This response, referred to as Brudzinski's sign, indicates meningeal irritation. The latter will also produce a positive Kernig's sign, i.e. whilst the patient is

lying flat with one leg flexed at both the hip and knee, resistance is experienced when trying to extend the knee. Repeat on the other limb. A bilateral response indicates meningeal irritation. In addition, a positive Kernig's sign can occur with a radiculopathy where other signs of nerve root irritation will be found.

Neck stiffness can be elicited in the following conditions.

- Meningeal irritation – meningitis   infective – commonly bacterial or viral
                                        chemical – subarachnoid haemorrhage
- Cervical spondylosis
- Parkinsonism
- Myalgia, e.g. as a prodromal feature of a viral illness
- Pharyngitis
- Cervical lymphadenopathy

Other features from the history and examination will provide clues to the underlying diagnosis.

> **Key point**
> In a patient with neck stiffness:
> - Kernig's sign usually indicates meningeal irritation
> - discomfort only on forward flexion suggests pharyngitis and/or cervical lymphadenopathy

If meningeal irritation is present a lumbar puncture is necessary after a C.T. scan, to exclude either meningitis or subarachnoid haemorrhage. Similarly cerebrospinal fluid is required to establish a diagnosis of encephalitis. In contrast, if there is a history of foreign travel further details and investigations are required to exclude relevant infectious diseases, especially malaria and typhoid.

TIME OUT 14.1

During your five minute break answer the following questions.

a. List the conditions that can present as "headache with fever but no focal signs".
b. List the diagnostic signs of a radiculopathy.

HEADACHE WITH EXTRACRANIAL SIGNS

Many conditions can present with headache and extracranial signs; some examples are listed in the box.

Causes of headache with pericranial signs	
Acute sinusitis	Daily
Cervical spondylosis	Daily
Giant cell arteritis	Monthly
Acute glaucoma	Annually

Acute sinusitis

This acute infection commonly causes frontal and/or maxillary sinusitis. However, it may extend to involve the ethmoid and sphenoid sinuses. In contrast, isolated infection in these areas is rare. Sinusitis is usually secondary to either the common cold or influenza and both streptococci and staphylococci are involved. On occasions anaerobes can be present when maxillary sinusitis is associated with a dental apical abscess.

Patients usually relate an initial history of an upper respiratory tract infection. This can be followed by headache and facial pain which is often supraorbital (frontal sinusitis) and infraorbital (maxillary sinusitis). The pain is often worse in the morning and exacerbated by head movements or stooping. Nasal obstruction is invariably present. The clinical signs are listed in the box.

Clinical signs of sinusitis

Pyrexia
Tenderness over the affected sinus
Oedema of the upper eye lid

Key point
Swelling of the cheek:

- is very rare in maxillary sinusitis
- is commonly of dental origin
- from antral pathology usually implies a carcinoma

The treatment comprises:

- analgesia
- antibiotics
- nasal decongestants.

Most patients with acute sinusitis will recover completely. However, liaison with an ear, nose, and throat (ENT) specialist is required when either chronic infection or complications may occur.

Further investigations are often needed and the results will dictate referral to the relevant specialist colleague.

Indications for ENT referral

Potential for chronic infection	Poor drainage
	Virulent infection
	Dental infection
	Immunocompromised patient
Complications	Laryngitis
	Pneumonia
	Orbital cellulitis/abscess
	Meningitis
	Cerebral abscess
	Osteomyelitis
	Cavernous sinus thrombosis

Cervical spondylosis

This is a common condition caused by intervertebral disc degeneration that produces two main effects.

- Annulus bulging   which elevates the periosteum from adjacent vertebral bodies, resulting in osteophyte formation.
- Disc space narrowing   causes malalignment of posterior facet joints, which develop hypertrophic osteoarthritic changes, and ligament folding and disruption as the vertebral bodies become closer.

These chronic degenerative changes are referred to as spondylosis and in the cervical spine occur commonly at the C4/5, C5/6, and C6/7 interspaces. The combination of disc space narrowing, posterior facet joint malalignment and ligament folding results in either anterior or posterior displacement of one vertebral body on another. Any of these effects, either individually or combined, can cause compression of the spinal cord (producing a myelopathy) or adjacent nerve roots (radiculopathy).

Another feature of this degenerative condition is headache. This is thought to arise not only from posterior facet joints and the associated ligaments, but also osteophytes which may irritate the C2 nerve root and branches of the greater occipital nerve. The pain classically involves one or both sides of the neck, extending to the occiput or even the temporal and frontal areas. It is often aggravated by movement and worse in the morning after the neck has been inappropriately positioned on, or inadequately supported by, pillows.

Clinical examination usually reveals restriction of neck movements, especially lateral flexion and rotation.

> **Key point**
> Always check for signs of a myelopathy or radiculopathy

The headache will usually respond to antiinflammatory drugs, but local infiltration with lignocaine and hydrocortisone may be required. It is best to leave this type of treatment to the "pain specialist".

Despite the extensive degenerative changes and associated neurology, the cervical spine is usually stable and acute cord compression is rare (the exception is an acute disc prolapse). Assessment for spinal surgery is advocated, as it may be possible to prevent further neurological compromise.

Giant cell arteritis (cranial arteritis, temporal arteritis, and granulomatous arteritis)

This condition predominantly affects large/medium sized arteries. It is rare before the age of 50 and commonly affects those aged between 65–75 years.

Giant cell arteritis classically involves the branches of the arteries originating from the aortic arch in a patchy distribution. Microscopically, the affected vessels show infiltration with lymphocytes, macrophages, histiocytes, and multinucleate giant cells. These changes frequently occur around the internal elastic lamina. In contrast, a panarteritis can develop that causes disruption of the whole vessel wall. Both types of infiltrate have a final common pathway of intimal fibrous thickening producing narrowing or occlusion of the vessel lumen.

The onset of the arteritis may be acute, but the symptoms are present for many months before the diagnosis is made. Thus, a high degree of suspicion is needed. Most patients have clinical features related to the arteries involved, i.e. mainly those originating from the aortic arch. Therefore, symptoms and signs related to the head and neck are common. Headache is a frequent presentation, localised to the superficial temporal or occipital arteries, and described as throbbing and worse at night. On examination these vessels can be tender, red, firm and pulseless. In addition, increased scalp sensitivity may predominate with complaints like, "It is painful to comb my hair". Visual problems (see next box) are associated with involvement of the following:

- ciliary artery producing an ischaemic optic neuropathy
- posterior cerebral artery leading to hemianopia
- vessels supplying the III, IV, and VI cranial nerves resulting in ophthalmoplegia.

Visual problems associated with giant cell arteritis

Blurred vision
Visual hallucinations
Amaurosis fugax
Loss of vision   – transient
                   – permanent
Hemianopia
Ophthalmoplegia

Although the head and neck vessels are commonly affected, arteritis can be widespread (see next box). However, these features are rare. In contrast, constitutional symptoms are common and include weight loss, fever, malaise, and a low-grade anaemia (often a normocytic hypochromic picture). Furthermore, polymyalgia rheumatica is present in approximately 50% of patients who have giant cell arteritis.

Other manifestations of giant cell arteritis

Intermittent claudication
Peripheral neuropathy
Myocardial ischaemia/infarction
Gut ischaemia/infarction
Stroke
Aortic arch syndrome

The diagnosis is confirmed, in approximately 75% of cases, by biopsy of an affected vessel, usually the temporal artery. Other laboratory investigations yield non-specific results, which reflect the inflammatory response, for example, elevated ESR and CRP.

Key point
A normal ESR and CRP does not exclude the diagnosis of giant cell arteritis

The lack of readily available supportive laboratory data means that the diagnosis relies on the clinician's skills. Despite the many potential modes of presentation, treatment should be started as soon as the condition is suspected because of the profound morbidity and mortality. Do not wait for a biopsy to confirm the diagnosis. This can be done at a later stage, if required, as the histological changes persist for approximately 14 days.

Prednisolone 60 mg daily, in divided doses, is an effective treatment. This is reduced slowly according to the patient's response to achieve a maintenance dose of 10 mg after one year. On occasion "pulse" intravenous methylprednisolone is used to treat ocular involvement. Early liaison with specialist colleagues is necessary when patients present with clinical signs or when giant cell arteritis has entered into the differential diagnosis. This is very important as correct diagnosis and treatment will reduce morbidity and prevent inappropriate chronic therapy with corticosteroids (and their related side effects).

Acute glaucoma

Acute closed angle glaucoma results from raised intraocular pressure. It commonly occurs in patients who are over 50 years old. Under normal circumstances aqueous humour circulates from the capillaries of the iris and ciliary muscle in the posterior chamber (between the iris and the lens) to reach the anterior chamber (between the iris and the cornea) (Figure 14.2).

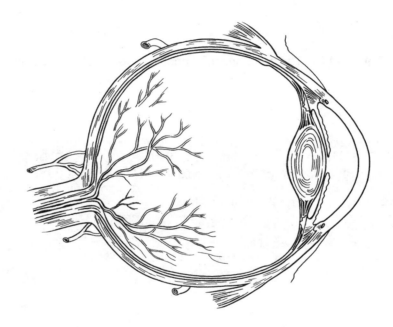

Figure 14.2   The anterior chambers of the eye

   With raised intraocular pressure the iris root protrudes into the back of the cornea and closes the canal of Schlemm, preventing drainage of aqueous (Figure 14.3). The precise cause of glaucoma is unknown but patients who have diabetes mellitus or an affected first-degree relative are at risk. Furthermore, it is more common in individuals who are long sighted (hypermetropia). The shorter eyeball has a shallow anterior chamber, hence a very narrow drainage angle, which is more readily obstructed. The sudden rise in intraocular pressure causes vascular insufficiency which, if untreated, can lead to ischaemia of the optic nerve and retina.

   Acute glaucoma usually presents with severe pain in, and around, the eye. Visual changes include blurring, photophobia and marked impairment to such an extent that only light can be perceived. In addition, the patient experiences either nausea or vomiting.

   The affected eye is red (ciliary congestion) with a cloudy cornea (oedema) and a dilated, oval pupil that is unreactive to light.

   Urgent referral to an ophthalmologist is required.

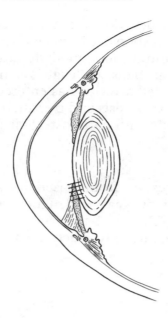

Figure 14.3   The mechanism of acute closed angle glaucoma.

Key points
Subacute glaucoma occurs with mild, transient episodes of intraocular hypertension. The patient may describe "coloured haloes around lights" especially at night. This should be regarded as a danger signal indicating an imminent acute attack

Coloured haloes around lights can also occur as:

- light diffuses through an early cataract
- a scintillating aura associated with migraine

TIME OUT 14.2

Assess your knowledge by answering the following questions.

a. What is the differential diagnosis in a patient presenting with a headache with extracranial signs?
b. List the major complications associated with each condition.

HEADACHE WITH NO ABNORMAL SIGNS

In most patients presenting with an acute headache, no abnormal signs are detected.

Causes of headache with no abnormal signs	
Tension	Daily
Migraine	Daily
Drugs	Daily
Toxins	Daily
Subarachnoid haemorrhage	Weekly
Giant cell arteritis	Monthly
Cluster headache	Annually
Coital migraine/cephalgia	Annually
Hyponatraemia	Annually

Tension type headache

This is common and also referred to as muscle contraction headache. Patients are usually aged 20–40 years, predominantly female (female:male = 3:1) and may describe either an acute or chronic history.

Acute

After an acute onset, the pain rapidly increases in severity over a few hours. The patient often appears pale and anxious with a tachycardia, photophobia and neck stiffness (attributed to muscle spasm). These clinical features mandate lumbar puncture to exclude meningitis, irrespective of the cause. The main treatment is to reassure the patient, provide adequate analgesia and help to sort the emotional problems that are invariably associated.

Chronic

This common problem is the classic, presentation of a tension type headache. The features are listed in the box below but patients can seek medical advice at any stage. Therefore, a comprehensive history is important to exclude other conditions and identify patient concerns (usually a brain tumour) and possible therapeutic avenues. Clinical examination provides some reassurance, but referral for psychological advice may be necessary as drug therapy has little to offer. The shorter the history, the better the chance for effective treatment.

Features of tension type headache	
Site	Diffuse, but commonly at the vertex
	Often starts at forehead or neck
	Frequently bilateral
Character	Pressure sensation or pain
	Tight band, vice or clamp like, squeezing
	"As if my head is going to explode"
	"On fire or stabbing from knives or needles"
	Daily, increasing throughout the day
Radiation	Forehead to occiput or neck – vice versa
	Over the vertex or around the side – band like
Precipitation	Stress, anxiety
Relief	Nothing
Associated symptoms	Nausea, tiredness
Clinical examination	Often unremarkable

Key points
Important discriminating factors in a patient with a tension headache:

- headache starts each morning and increases in severity throughout the day
- vomiting does not occur
- visual disturbances do not occur

Migraine

This common condition affects approximately 20% of women and 15% of men who usually present with paroxysmal headaches before the age of 30 years. There is often a family history but the genetic basis remains unknown. Many patients will identify specific things that will precipitate an attack of migraine.

Common migraine precipitants	
Dietary	Fasting
	Alcohol
	Specific foods
Drugs	Oral contraceptives
Affective	Anxiety/stress
	Post stress relaxation
Physiological	Exercise
	Menstruation
Visual	Bright light

Migraine appears to be of neural/cerebral origin. This primary event somehow triggers the release of substances that influence vasomotor tone and neuronal activity. The resultant distension of arteries in the scalp and dura causes pain whilst decreased neuronal activity is responsible for the aura.

Migraine is often described as common, classic, or variant. As its name suggests, most patients (75%) have the common variety and only 20% experience classic symptoms. However, all of these people will have prodromal features and paroxysmal headaches.

Prodromal features occur in the 24 hours before the headache and comprise changes in mood, ranging from excess energy to euphoria to depression and lethargy, and diet, including craving or distaste for specific foods.

Paroxysmal headaches can be either unilateral, bilateral or unilateral progressing to bilateral. They occur on wakening or during the day are described as throbbing or pounding.

In contrast, patients with classic migraine can have other presenting symptoms.

Visual aura is described as, for example, flashing lights, fragmented images and micropsia. The aura lasts for 30 minutes and is followed by headache.

Sensual disturbances can signify the onset of an attack with numbness and tingling of one or both hands or the face, lips, and tongue.

Motor disturbances include weakness, hemiparesis and dysphasia.

Most patients experience nausea, prostration and vomiting. Other somatic symptoms include shivering, pallor, diarrhoea, fainting, and fluid retention.

The attacks gradually subside after 48 hours. Some relief is gained from rest in a dark room but vomiting or sleep usually relieves the pain.

Immediate treatment

- Rest in a dark, quiet environment
- Analgesia – usually aspirin, paracetamol or a non-steroidal antiinflammatory drug, such as diclofenac or piroxicam melt.
- Antiemetics, e.g. metoclopramide or domperidone, can be given as either suppository or intravenous preparations.
- Sumatriptan, a selective $5HT_1$ antagonist, can be used if the patient has failed to respond to analgesia. A 6 mg **subcutaneous** injection provides prompt, effective relief in nearly 70% of patients. Only one dose should be given for each attack. However, if a second attack occurs a further 6 mg can be administered providing one hour has lapsed following the first dose (maximum: 12 mg in 24 hours).

> **Key point**
> Sumatriptan is contraindicated in patients with ischaemic heart disease

Prophylactic treatment

- Seek and exclude known precipitants.
- Treat precipitants appropriately, e.g. amitriptiline if anxiety/stress related; atenolol for the tense patient.
- Oral pizotifen (1·5 g at night) is useful if a specific precipitant cannot be identified.

> **Key points**
> Migraine should not be:
>
> - diagnosed in anyone presenting for the first time over the age of 40 years until other conditions have been excluded
> - confused with tension headache (non-paroxysmal, no vomiting or visual features)

Drugs

A variety of drugs can cause headache because of their effect on vascular muscle tone, e.g. nitrates and calcium channel antagonists. A medical history will establish the link and provocation tests are rarely required.

> **Key point**
> Caffeine is often added to analgesic preparations to enhance their effect. This is bad for the patient but a good marketing ploy as either the addition or withdrawal of caffeine can cause headache

Toxins

Alcohol: your own experience, either personal or professional, will have equipped you with the necessary information.

Carbon monoxide is covered in detail in Chapter 13.

Subarachnoid haemorrhage

Always consider this condition for any patient with an unexplained headache of acute onset. Please see Chapter 11 for further information.

Giant cell arteritis

The differential diagnosis of a sudden headache, in any patient over the age of 50 years, includes giant cell arteritis as described earlier in this chapter.

Cluster headache

This distinctive condition comprises:

- unilateral headache with
- ipsilateral
    corneal injection and epiphora (90%)
    nasal congestion or rhinorrhoea (90%)
    transient Horner's syndrome (25%)

It can present at any age, commonly between 20 and 50 years, and predominantly affects men (male:female = 10:1). The headache is centred around the orbit and is described as severe, boring or stabbing with radiation to the forehead, temple or cheek and jaw. Brief bouts of this unilateral pain last 30–120 minutes each day for between four and 16 weeks. Characteristically, the pain occurs shortly after the onset of sleep, although it can occur during the day. During attacks the patient is usually crying, restless, and prefers to walk. The cause remains unknown, but alcohol can precipitate an attack, as can other vasodilators.

Prophylactic ergotamine should be given approximately one hour before an attack. Suppositories are the most useful preparation and should be continued for one week. If the headache recurs, treatment should be restarted on a weekly basis until the cluster ends. Oral sumatriptan and verapamil are alternatives if the patient does not respond to ergotamine.

Coital migraine/cephalgia

This is a severe headache that begins suddenly during sexual intercourse or immediately following orgasm. It is more common in males and nearly 50% will have a previous history of migraine. Some patients require propranolol 40–80 mg before intercourse. This drug can be stopped once the patient has remained asymptomatic for one month.

> **Key point**
> Subarachnoid haemorrhage must be excluded in patients who present with coital migraine

Hyponatraemia

This can be associated with headache, nausea, vomiting, and weakness. The diagnosis and management are considered in detail in Chapter 26.

TIME OUT 14.3

a. List the features that would differentiate between tension headache, migraine, and cluster headache.
b. In a patient presenting with headache and no abnormal signs, under what circumstances would you consider doing a lumbar puncture?

SUMMARY

Headache of acute onset accounts for less than 2.5% of new emergency attendances. Of these, 15% will have an immediately life threatening condition. These need to be identified and treated in the primary assessment. Some of the remaining patients will have sinister pathology. The characteristics of headache that suggest a serious underlying cause are:

- new onset
- acute onset
- progressive
- wakens from sleep
- worst ever.

Important associated symptoms that should be sought include:

- photophobia
- meningeal irritation
- fever
- altered mental state
- neurological dysfunction.

Physical examination should be thorough, with particular emphasis on:

- meningeal irritation
- papilloedema
- pyrexia
- pericranial signs
- focal neurological features
- rash.

CHAPTER

15

The patient with abdominal pain

OBJECTIVES

After reading this chapter you should be able to describe:

- the different mechanisms of abdominal pain
- the primary assessment and resuscitation of the patient with abdominal pain
- the secondary assessment of the patient with abdominal pain
- the initial treatment and disposition of the patient with abdominal pain.

INTRODUCTION

Making an accurate diagnosis and starting appropriate treatment for the patient with abdominal pain may be difficult. This can be the presenting symptom of a wide range of conditions which have their origin both within and outside the abdomen. Although the majority do not have an immediately life threatening problem, identification of those who require urgent investigation and treatment is essential to avoid preventable mortality and morbidity. The structured approach gives priority to life threatening conditions and initial resuscitation, and a "phrased" history and examination are, therefore, particularly important in the patient with abdominal pain.

ANATOMY AND PATHOPHYSIOLOGY

Abdominal pain may arise from the peritoneal cavity, the retroperitoneum, the pelvis, and occasionally outside the abdomen itself (see next box).

The basic pathological processes in intraabdominal causes of abdominal pain are:

- inflammation (e.g. gastroenteritis, appendicitis, pancreatitis, pyelonephritis)
- perforation (e.g. peptic ulcer, carcinoma of the colon)
- obstruction (e.g. intestine, bile duct, ureter)
- haemorrhage (e.g. leaking aortic aneurysm, bleeding ulcer, ectopic pregnancy)
- infarction (e.g. bowel, spleen).

211

Major causes of abdominal pain

Intraabdominal

Non-specific abdominal pain	Daily
Gastroenteritis	Daily
Acute appendicitis	Daily
Acute cholecystitis and gall bladder disease	Weekly
Peptic ulcer disease	Weekly
Intestinal obstruction	Weekly
Pseudoobstruction	Monthly
Acute pancreatitis	Monthly
Perforated viscus	Monthly
Malignancy (carcinoma, lymphoma)	Monthly
Diverticular disease	Monthly
Vascular	Monthly
• leaking abdominal aortic aneurysm	
• infarction of bowel or spleen	
Inflammatory bowel disease	Annually
Primary infective peritonitis	Only in exams

Urological

Lower urinary tract infection/pyelonephritis	Daily
Ureteric/renal colic	Weekly
Acute urinary retention	Weekly
Testicular torsion	Monthly

Gynaecological

Miscarriage	Daily
Pelvic inflammatory disease	Daily
Accident to an ovarian cyst	Monthly
Ectopic pregnancy	Monthly
Retained products of conception	Annually

Obstetric

Labour	Monthly
Abruption	Annually
Red degeneration of a uterine fibroid	Only in exams

Extraabdominal causes

Poisoning/toxins	
• alcoholic gastritis	Daily
• food poisoning	Weekly
• aspirin, iron, lead	Variable
Psychosomatic (including Munchausen's syndrome, drug seeking behaviour)	Weekly
Chest (myocardial infarction, basal pneumonia, pulmonary embolus)	Monthly
Haematological (sickle cell crisis, haemophilia)	Annually
Metabolic (diabetic ketoacidosis, Addisonian crisis, uraemia, porphyria)	Annually
Neurological	Annually
• herpes zoster	
• radiculopathy	
• spine/disc disease	
Vasculitis (e.g. polyarteritis nodosa, systemic lupus erythematosus)	

As you will have seen, the box giving the major causes of abdominal pain is neither a comprehensive list nor user friendly. A better way to distinguish the causes of abdominal pain is to consider three mechanisms of pain in the clinical assessment of patients:

- visceral pain
- parietal or somatic pain
- referred pain.

Visceral pain

Visceral pain is characteristically caused by inflammation, ischaemia, neoplasia and distension of either the wall of a hollow viscus or the capsule of a solid intraabdominal organ. Most abdominal organs are served by afferent nerves from both sides of the spinal cord. Visceral pain is usually perceived in the midline transmitted via autonomic nerve fibres in the wall or capsule of the organ; and the site of pain is characteristically poorly demarcated and may not correspond to the site of tenderness on examination. It is often described as cramp like, colicky, dull, burning or gnawing, and associated with autonomic features such as nausea, vomiting, pallor, and sweating. The pain is usually localised to one of three regions according to the embryological origin of the organ involved. Foregut structures – stomach, liver, gall bladder, pancreas and most of the duodenum – produce pain in the epigastrium. Midgut structures – distal duodenum, small intestine, appendix and ascending and proximal part of the transverse colon – produce pain.

In hindgut structures – descending colon, kidneys, bladder, ureter and pelvic organs – pain is characteristically felt in the hypogastrium or lower back.

Parietal pain

Parietal or somatic pain is characteristically caused by inflammation (bacterial or chemical) of the parietal peritoneum. It is mediated by segmental spinal nerves associated with specific dermatomes. Consequently the pain is more precisely localised to the structure from which the pain originates. This corresponds to the site at which tenderness and guarding develop. The pain is also characteristically sharper, and is aggravated by movement, coughing, and sometimes breathing.

Referred pain

Referred pain is localised to a site distant from the organ that is the source of pain. The organ involved and the site at which the pain is felt share a common embryological origin, and associated peripheral nerves share common central pathways. A classical example is pain felt in the shoulder tip, supraclavicular area, and side of the neck due to subphrenic irritation (by blood or pus) of the diaphragm that is derived from the fourth cervical segment. Pain may be referred to the abdomen from the chest (myocardial infarction, pneumonia or pulmonary embolism), the back and external genitalia.

PRIMARY ASSESSMENT AND RESUSCITATION

Rapidly life threatening conditions presenting with abdominal pain should be recognised by the end of the primary assessment (see box). Patients with abdominal pain generally have a patent airway, although it is important to be aware of the risk of aspiration of gastric contents in patients with profuse vomiting, particularly if there is any depression of conscious level. A nasogastric tube should be passed early in patients with small bowel obstruction, to drain fluid and air and reduce the risk of aspiration.

Life threatening conditions in the patient with abdominal pain

Hypovolaemic shock
- gastrointestinal bleeding — Daily
- leaking abdominal aortic aneurysm — Monthly
- ectopic pregnancy — Monthly
- splenic rupture (usually traumatic but may be spontaneous) — Annually

Small bowel infarction (mesenteric artery occlusion) — Monthly
Acute pancreatitis — Weekly
Septicaemia (e.g. following perforation of colon) — Weekly
Acute myocardial infarction — Monthly
Diabetic ketoacidosis — Monthly

Abnormalities on the assessment of breathing, such as dyspnoea, tachypnoea, and signs of hypoxia (including low oxygen saturation), in the patient with abdominal pain may occur for a variety of reasons. Severe abdominal pain may cause splinting of chest movement. There may be symptoms and signs of pathology within the chest (causing pain localised to the upper abdomen), such as pneumonia or myocardial infarction. Abnormalities on assessment of breathing may be a manifestation of shock (due to intra-abdominal or retroperitoneal haemorrhage) or sepsis. Tachypnoea and deep inspiration (Kussmaul's respiration) suggest metabolic acidosis as in diabetic ketoacidosis or sepsis.

Initial treatment is usually with high flow oxygen via a facemask with a non-rebreathing reservoir bag. Intubation and ventilation may be required if oxygenation is inadequate (despite the administration of supplemental oxygen) in patients with severe acute pancreatitis who develop acute respiratory distress syndrome or in patients with septic shock.

Evidence of an immediately life threatening condition in the patient with abdominal pain is more commonly encountered when assessing circulation (see next box and Chapter 6).

Assessment of circulation: signs of circulatory failure

Peripheral perfusion: pallor, cool extremities, sweating, prolonged capillary refill time
Pulse: tachycardia, low volume
Blood pressure: hypotension (but remember systolic blood pressure may be normal in a patient who has lost up to 30% of circulating volume); check for pulse pressure

---

Occult bleeding can occur in the gut lumen, peritoneal cavity or retroperitoneum. Patients with septic shock are classically vasodilated and warm with hypotension and a fever, but many (particularly if presenting late) are peripherally vasoconstricted and have a normal or even low body temperature. Atrial fibrillation in the elderly patient with abdominal pain means that mesenteric artery embolism should be considered in the differential diagnosis.

Insert two large bore (14 gauge) peripheral intravenous cannulae. Take blood for baseline full blood count, biochemistry (including glucose stick test and amylase) and blood crossmatch or save serum, coagulation screen, blood cultures and when appropriate pregnancy test and sickle screen.

If hypovolaemia is suspected, start fluid resuscitation with two litres of crystalloid, followed by blood; if there is evidence of anaemia as well as circulatory failure, it may be preferable to substitute blood for crystalloid earlier.

A portable ultrasound scan (if available) may confirm the cause of hypovolaemic shock (for example, a leaking aortic aneurysm, free intraperitoneal fluid or an ectopic pregnancy). This should not delay urgent referral to a surgeon or gynaecologist when prompt surgery may be life saving (see next two boxes).

Indications for urgent referral to a surgeon

- Abdominal pain or tenderness plus a pulsatile mass and/or a history of aortic aneurysm or a leaking aortic aneurysm suspected for any other reason
- Gastrointestinal bleeding in a patient of 60 years or over or in a patient of any age with signs of shock, haemoglobin less than 10 g/dl or significant coexistent disease
- Any evidence of free intraperitoneal fluid in the patient with abdominal pain and signs of circulatory failure
- Suspected pancreatitis
- Suspected mesenteric ischaemia

Indications for urgent referral to a gynaecologist

- Suspected ectopic pregnancy
- Suspected torsion or rupture of an ovarian cyst

Key point
Urgent surgical (or gynaecological) referral of the patient with abdominal pain and shock may be life saving; do not wait for the results of investigations

---

If a diagnosis of either myocardial infarction or pulmonary embolism is considered investigate and start specific treatment (see Chapters 8 and 10). If septic shock is suspected, treat with intravenous broad spectrum antibiotics before the result of cultures is known.

If there is any depression of conscious level in the patient with abdominal pain, check that hypoxaemia and shock are being adequately treated, consider hypoglycaemia, sepsis, and diabetic ketoacidosis.

TIME OUT 15.1

a. What is the differential diagnosis of abdominal pain and shock in (i) a 75 year old man and (ii) a 25 year old woman?
b. What are the management priorities?

SECONDARY ASSESSMENT

A focused history and careful examination are important for making a diagnosis in the patient with abdominal pain. An improvement in diagnostic and decision making skills has been attributed to the use of computer assisted diagnosis based on a proforma (Figure 15.1). This ensures more effective collection of information from the patient's history and examination findings.

History

The well "phrased" history may be applied to the patient with abdominal pain.

Problem
It is important to establish the patient's main complaints, particularly as abdominal pain may be a presenting symptom of such a wide variety of conditions.

History of presenting problem
The **site**, any change in location, and **radiation** of pain are important. Distinguish pain that the patient can localise precisely from ill defined pain (which may indicate visceral pain early in the disease process, referred pain and a metabolic, toxic, or psychological cause). Migration of pain is characteristic of an inflamed viscus; for example, from the periumbilical region to the right lower quadrant in acute appendicitis or from the epigastrium to the right upper quadrant in cholecystitis.

Pain arising from the stomach or duodenum is chacteristically localised to the epigastrium in the midline. Pain from the gall bladder is also felt in the epigastrium and/or right upper quadrant, sometimes radiating to the interscapular region. Pain from pancreatitis is generally felt in the upper abdomen, with radiation through to the back. Other important conditions to consider in the patient who reports pain radiating to the back are leaking aortic aneurysm, and renal or ureteric disease. Characteristically small bowel pain is felt symmetrically, centrally, and may radiate to the back, while pain from the large bowel is felt in the hypogastrium and may radiate to the back and thighs.

Sudden **onset** of severe pain is characteristic of either a vascular problem such as a leaking abdominal aortic aneurysm, torsion of a gonad, or of a perforated viscus. The pain of acute pancreatitis may come on relatively rapidly, but over minutes rather than seconds. Pain due to an inflammatory condition such as diverticulitis or appendicitis progresses more gradually, over hours or days. Note the **duration** of pain and whether pain can be characterised as *steady* (present all the time at a similar intensity – as with bowel infarction), *intermittent* (pain resolves for periods of time – as with pain from gastroenteritis) or *colicky* (present all the time with fluctuating intensity). Determine whether the pain is improving, worsening or remaining much the same over a period of 1–2 hours or more.

Somatic pain is characteristically described as sharp whereas vague terms are used for visceral pain. Otherwise it is difficult to draw diagnostic inferences from the description of the **character** of abdominal pain by patients who may use a variety of terms in different ways. The **severity** of pain may be assessed by the patient's own account and by observation of the patient who may appear distressed, sweating or crying out. Although conditions such as a perforated viscus, bowel infarction or acute pancreatitis often cause severe pain, this does not reliably distinguish them from non-specific abdominal pain.

Ask about the main **exacerbating/relieving** factors; *movement* (particularly movements which cause the patient to tense the anterior abdominal wall muscles and movement of inflamed peritoneal surfaces), *coughing*, and *deep inspiration*. The effect on pain

Abdominal Pain Chart

NAME		REG NUMBER	
MALE FEMALE AGE		FORM FILLED BY	
PRESENTATION (999, GP. etc)	DATE		TIME

PAIN

SITE

ONSET

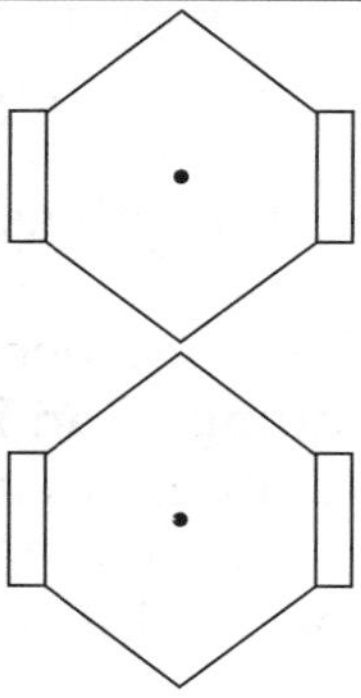

PRESENT

RADIATION

AGGRAVATING FACTORS
movement
coughing
respiration
food
other
none

RELIEVING FACTORS
lying still
vomiting
antacids
food
other
none

PROGRESS
better
same
worse
DURATION

TYPE
intermittent
steady
colicky

SEVERITY
moderate
severe

HISTORY

NAUSEA
yes   no

VOMITING
yes   no

ANOREXIA
yes   no

PREV INDIGESTION
yes   no

JAUNDICE
yes   no

BOWELS
normal
constipation
diarrhoea
blood
mucus

MICTURITION
normal
frequency
dysuria
dark
haematuria

PREV SIMILAR PAIN
yes   no

PREV ABDO SURGERY
yes   no

DRUGS FOR ABDO PAIN
yes   no

♀   LMP

pregnant

Vag. discharge

dizzy/faint

EXAMINATION

MOOD
normal
distressed
anxious

SHOCKED
yes   no

COLOUR
normal
pale
flushed
cyanosed

TEMP   PULSE

SP

ABDO MOVEMENT
normal
poor nil
peristalsis

SCAR
yes   no

DISTENSION
yes   no

TENDERNESS

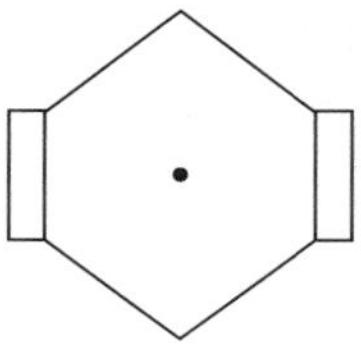

REBOUND
yes   no

GUARDING
yes   no

RIGIDITY
yes   no

MASS
yes   no

MURPHY'S
+ve   –ve

BOWEL SOUNDS
normal   absent   + + +

RECTAL – VAGINAL TENDERNESS
left
right
general
mass
none

INITIAL DIAGNOSIS & PLAN

RESULTS
amylase
blood count (WBC)
computer
urine
X-ray
other

DIAG & PLAN AFTER INVEST

(time   )

DISCHARGE DIAGNOSIS

History and examination of other systems on separate case notes

Figure 15.1   Abdominal pain chart (reproduced with permission from de Domble FT. *Diagnosis of acute abdominal pain*, 2nd edn. London: Churchill Livingstone, 1991)

of vomiting (which may provide transient relief in small intestinal obstruction, food, and antacids should also be noted.

Other gastrointestinal symptoms including anorexia, nausea and vomiting, which are common and relatively non-specific. The relationship of the onset of pain and these symptoms may be significant: pain before nausea and vomiting suggests a surgical aetiology such as peritonitis or obstruction, whereas nausea and vomiting followed by pain is more characteristic of gastroenteritis. Ask about blood or bile in vomit; faeculent vomiting indicates intestinal obstruction. Preexisting indigestion may lead to a diagnosis of a perforated or bleeding peptic ulcer and previous symptoms of cholelithiasis would indicate a cause for acute pancreatitis.

Diarrhoea and constipation may also be non-specific (either may occur in patients with appendicitis). As with vomiting, diarrhoea from the beginning of an illness is characteristic of gastroenteritis, as compared with onset after several hours that may occur in appendicitis and peritonitis. Ask about blood or mucus in diarrhoea (inflammatory bowel disease, ischaemic bowel or malignancy). Change in bowel habit over a period of time suggests possible malignancy.

Abdominal pain, vomiting, and absolute constipation are virtually pathognomonic of intestinal obstruction. Early vomiting and more frequent episodes of colicky abdominal pain are features of more proximal small bowel obstruction; on arrival at hospital the patient may not yet be aware of constipation. By contrast, constipation will be prominent in the patient with large bowel obstruction.

Relevant medical history
The past history should include details of:

- similar episodes of pain, investigation, treatment and outcome (leading to a diagnosis of inflammatory bowel disease)
- previous abdominal surgery (with possible subsequent adhesions, the leading cause of small bowel obstruction)
- other conditions, including diabetes mellitus, heart, cerebrovascular and respiratory diseases and psychiatric illness, may be relevant to the cause of abdominal pain or complicate its treatment.

Allergies
Note any previous allergy and adverse reaction to drugs, particularly antibiotics, analgesics and – if surgery is a possibility – topical antiseptic or dressing.

Systems review

- Burnua dysuria, frequency and urgency with or without haematuria are characteristic of urinary tract infection, but an inflamed appendix or diverticulum adjacent to ureter or bladder may cause urinary symptoms and pyuria. Establish whether dysuria is an exacerbation of the patient's abdominal pain or a different pain.
- A gynaecological history should be taken from women with abdominal pain, to include information about pregnancies, menstrual pattern, contraception, abnormal vaginal discharge, and – if pelvic inflammatory disease is suspected – new or multiple sexual partners.
- Ask patients with upper abdominal pain, in particular, about chest pain, shortness of breath, cough, and haemoptysis. Coexistent cardiovascular disease may be a clue to the diagnosis of intraabdominal vascular pathology.

Essential family and social history
A family history of intraabdominal conditions (such as inflammatory bowel disease or carcinoma) or inherited conditions (Marfan's, sickle cell disease, acute intermittent

porphyria, haemophilia) and ethnic origin may be relevant to diagnosis and treatment. A group of people affected by vomiting, diarrhoea, and abdominal pain suggests an infectious agent (or carbon monoxide poisoning).

Drugs
This part of the history should include inquiry about medicines taken either for the present problem or other conditions (particularly corticosteroids, non-steroidal anti-inflammatory drugs, anticoagulants and antibiotics), alcohol consumption, and drug use.

Examination

Objectives of examination include:

- assessment of the patient's general condition – the ABCDEs should be reassessed
- localisation of an intraabdominal source of pain (generally related to the area of maximum tenderness)
- detection of any extraabdominal cause of pain.

General examination
Pallor, sweating, and signs of distress in a patient with abdominal pain suggest (but are not diagnostic of) a more serious cause for abdominal pain, such as a vascular event, perforated viscus or acute pancreatitis. Classically, patients with visceral pain (e.g. ureteric colic) roll around. In contrast those with peritonitis lie immobile, showing signs of pain if the bed on which they are lying is inadvertently knocked. The lethargic patient may be septicaemic.

Mucous membrane pallor may indicate anaemia due to chronic blood loss. Look at the sclerae for jaundice. Stigmata of chronic liver disease (spider naevi, palmar erythema, Dupuytren's contracture, leuconychia and clubbing, abnormal veins around the umbilicus, loss of body hair, gynaecomastia and testicular atrophy, ascites, and signs of encephalopathy) may provide useful clues to the cause of either upper gastrointestinal bleeding or abdominal distension. Extended features of uraemia are rare. The pigmentation of Addison's disease, seen in scars, the flexor creases of the palm, over pressure areas and on the buccal mucosa opposite the molar teeth, may be missed if not actively sought. Purpura in characteristic distribution over the lower limbs will suggest the possibility of Henoch–Schönlein purpura, but abdominal pain can precede the rash. Petechiae can represent an underlying haematological abnormality. Erythema nodosum is one of the extraintestinal manifestations of inflammatory bowel disease, and photosensitivity is a feature of porphyria.

Pyrexia is significant but a normal temperature, particularly in the elderly, does not exclude conditions such as cholecystitis and appendicitis, although perforation of the appendix is usually associated with a temperatutre greater than 38°C. A temperature above 38·5°C, particularly with a history of rigors, is a common feature of bacterial infections, such as pyelonephritis, acute salpingitis or ascending cholangitis. A furred tongue and foetor are common and non-specific; the smell of acetone, if detected, may facilitate the rapid diagnosis of diabetic ketoacidosis (DKA). Signs of dehydration imply extracellular fluid loss, due to gastroenteritis, diabetic ketoacidosis or intestinal obstruction.

Rapid shallow respiration may be a feature of either peritonitis or pneumonia. In contrast look for the deep (Kussmaul's) sighing respiration of diabetic ketoacidosis or other metabolic acidoses. Signs of circulatory failure due to hypovolaemia will usually have been detected in the primary assessment; other causes of tachycardia include sepsis, untreated pain, and anxiety.

A brief systematic examination of the cardiovascular system (including peripheral pulses), the chest, and back is important to identify any extraabdominal cause of pain and to assess the patient's general condition.

Abdominal examination

Adequate exposure is vital if subtle but important signs (such as a small incarcerated femoral hernia) are not to be missed.

On **inspection** look for:

- the contour of the abdomen (particularly distension) and any gross deformity
- visible peristalsis (suggesting intestinal obstruction) or the abdominal wall held immobile in peritonitis; get the patient to move the anterior abdominal wall and ask him/her to take a deep inspiration and cough, while watching the patient's facial expression. (If there is peritonitis, coughing or any movement of the bed is likely to cause sharp pain due to the movement being transmitted to the inflamed peritoneum.)
- scars from previous surgery (which may be the clue to adhesions as the cause of small bowel obstruction)
- visible pulsation of an aneurysm
- discolouration of bruising around the umbilicus (Cullen's sign) or in the flank (Grey Turner's sign) which are rare but important features of haemorrhagic pancreatitis; retroperitoneal haemorrhage from an aortic aneurysm may also produce flank bruising.

Palpation (with a warm hand) should be gentle and start in an area of the abdomen away from the site of pain. Distinguish between the symptom of pain and tenderness on examination, and the site of each. Localised tenderness suggests the site of an inflammatory source of the patient's pain. However, it can be absent in appendicitis, either because the pain is visceral early in the inflammatory process, or because the appendix is retrocaecal. Conversely abdominal tenderness may be present in biliary colic, small bowel obstruction or gastroenteritis. A particular pitfall for the unwary is the elderly patient with bowel infarction due to mesenteric artery thrombosis or embolism: characteristically these patients present with pain of sudden onset which is steady and severe, apparently out of proportion to the limited tenderness on examination. If the diagnosis is not suspected there may be a dangerous delay in arranging surgery.

The presence of guarding (reflex contraction of the abdominal wall muscles in response to palpation) and rebound tenderness is more predictive of local peritonitis, and rigidity is a sign of generalised peritonitis.

Palpate also for any abnormal mass or organomegaly. A distended bladder may be identified on percussion or palpation.

Percussion may give information about the size of solid organs, and distinguish between gas and fluid as the cause of abdominal distension (shifting dullness in ascites). Percussion tenderness may identify signs of localised or generalised peritonitis, in which case subsequent examination should be modified to avoid unnecessary painful palpation.

On **auscultation** loud high-pitched bowel sounds – if present – suggest obstruction, and absent bowel sounds a perforated viscus with peritonitis or ileus; but neither is sensitive and normal bowel sounds do not exclude serious intraabdominal pathology. Listen for bruits over the upper quadrants of the abdomen and costovertebral angles (for renal artery stenosis or aneurysm).

Examination of the abdomen should include examination of the flanks, the external genitalia (in particular the scrotum and testes) and inguinal and femoral canals for herniae; an incarcerated hernia is the second most common cause of small bowel obstruction. **Vaginal examination** – when indicated – may provide information about gynaecological causes of abdominal pain or an inflamed appendix palpable in the pelvis.

On **rectal examination**, assess for signs of perianal disease (in inflammatory bowel disease), pelvic tenderness, abnormal masses, the prostate in men, blood or melaena, and sphincter tone.

Investigations

All patients with abdominal pain should have a glucose stick test (to exclude diabetes) and urinalysis. Microscopic haematuria can occur with either ureteric colic or urinary tract infection (but remember also the possibility of infective endocarditis, symptoms of which include abdominal pain). Pyuria (more than 5–10 white cells per microlitre) is commonly due to urinary tract infection but it may also be due to inflammation of an adjacent organ, such as in appendicitis or diverticulitis. In the presence of jaundice or suspected biliary tract disease test the urine for urobilinogen and bilirubin. A urine pregnancy test (for the β subunit of human chorionic gonadotrophin) should be done in all women of childbearing age, regardless of the history.

A raised white cell count supports the diagnosis of a significant cause for abdominal pain but is neither sensitive nor specific for a surgical condition. For example, patients with acute appendicitis may have a normal white cell count value as a raised white cell count may be due to pyelonephritis or other bacterial infection. Nevertheless, a white cell count of greater than 15×10^9/litre in a patient with acute pancreatitis is one factor associated with increased mortality (see box of adverse prognostic factors in the acute pancreatitis section). The haemoglobin concentration does not reflect acute blood loss but may indicate chronic bleeding; serial values may be useful.

A serum amylase of greater than five times the upper limit of normal suggests acute pancreatitis, but a normal amylase does not exclude pancreatitis, and a lesser rise may be seen in a variety of conditions which cause abdominal pain (incuding cholecystitis and peptic ulcer). A raised serum lipase has greater sensitivity and specificity, but is not commonly available. Estimation of electrolytes and urea does not usually contribute to the diagnosis of the patient with abdominal pain, but forms part of the assessment of the general condition of any patient who is haemodynamically unstable or dehydrated, for example, due to vomiting or diarrhoea. A liver enzyme profile and prothrombin time are required for patients who are jaundiced. Baseline coagulation studies are indicated in the patient who is bleeding, has a suspected coagulopathy or requires blood transfusion.

An arterial blood gas sample will assess oxygenation and acid–base status in the patients with hypovolaemia, pancreatitis or a suspected pulmonary problem.

An electrocardiogram is recommended in patients over the age of 40 (or younger if there is a specific indication), as can either acute myocardial infarction or pulmonary embolism that cause abdominal pain. In addition an ECG may identify coexistent cardiac disease which predisposes to an intraabdominal vascular event (e.g. atrial fibrillation leading to mesenteric artery embolism) or complicates treatment.

The role of **radiology** is primarily to confirm a diagnosis suspected on clinical assessment, and is not a substitute for an effective history and clinical examination.

Plain X-rays

The principal indications for plain X-rays in patients with abdominal pain are suspected:

- intestinal obstruction
- perforated viscus
- toxic megacolon
- foreign body
- ureteric/renal colic
- chest pathology.

The abdominal film may also yield useful information in patients with peritonitis or suspected mesenteric ischaemia, but should not be used indiscriminately in patients with abdominal pain.

Standard views are the erect chest X-ray (CXR) and the supine abdominal film. The erect CXR should be taken after the patient has been sitting upright for five to ten minutes (after which as little as 1–2 ml of free air may be shown); it may also show pneumonia or other pathology in the chest. If the patient is unable to stand or sit, the left lateral decubitus view of the abdomen is an alternative when looking for "free gas". An unsuspected abdominal aortic aneurysm may be outlined by a calcified vessel wall. The erect abdominal view does not generally add any useful information. An unprepared barium enema may be required urgently to elucidate the cause of suspected large bowel obstruction and to exclude pseudo-obstruction.

A KUB (kidney, ureter, bladder) X-ray is the initial imaging for patients with ureteric colic. Although more than 80% of ureteric calculi are radioopaque, they are often missed on plain X-ray. This film should be followed by either an intravenous urogram (IVU), ultrasound scan or computed tomography to demonstrate the size and location of a stone and the extent of obstruction to ureter and kidney.

Ultrasound
Urgent ultrasound scan is indicated in the following situations:

- suspected abdominal aortic aneurysm
- right upper quadrant pain, jaundice or suspected cholelithiasis
- suspected urinary tract colic or obstruction, particularly if any contraindication to an intravenous urogram
- lower abdominal pain in women of childbearing age
- suspected intraabdominal abscess.

Computed tomography (CT)
If available as an urgent investigation, CT may be used in the patient who is sufficiently stable to be moved to the CT suite:

- as an alternative for imaging suspected urinary tract obstruction
- to visualise retroperitoneal structures, including the pancreas and aorta.

Angiography has an occasional role in the evaluation of lower gastrointestinal haemorrhage or intestinal ischaemia. However, labelled red cell scans are more sensitive in detecting bleeding in the gut.

Potential pitfalls in the assessment of patients with abdominal pain

Elderly patients with acute abdominal pain have a higher mortality. Several factors, some of which put the elderly at risk of delayed diagnosis, may contribute to this.

- **Different spectrum of disease:** a greater proportion have malignancy or a vascular cause for pain (which may not initially be recognised).
- General peritonitis may be due to a perforated colon rather than a perforated ulcer or appendix.
- **A different presentation of intraabdominal disorders:** in comparison with younger patients, the pain is often not as marked. Fever, tachycardia and leucocytosis are uncommon with inflammatory conditions such as appendicitis. These factors can lead to a delay in diagnosis and an increased risk of perforation.
- Delayed presentation is more common.
- Coexistent illness is likely to make the elderly more vulnerable to complications.

> **Key point**
> **Glucocorticoids** can mask both clinical and laboratory responses to inflammation or perforation of a viscus in the abdomen

Similarly other immunosuppressive drugs, coexistent diabetes mellitus, and immunodeficiency can influence the patient's response to other conditions. Thus they may display minimal clinical signs and abnormal laboratory tests, despite a serious intra-abdominal disorder.

Finally, the clinical features of surgical conditions may be unexpectedly non-specific in late **pregnancy**.

EMERGENCY TREATMENT

After the primary assessment and a well "phrased" history, examine the patient; a differential diagnosis can be formulated and appropriate investigations requested. Treatment should be initiated simultaneously with assessment and investigation. Consider:

- analgesia
- review of fluid resuscitation
- antiemesis and nasogastric suction
- antibiotics.

Analgesia

Early judicious analgesia is advocated for the patient with acute abdominal pain. If opioid analgesia is given as a dilute solution by slow intravenous injection, the dose can be titrated against the patient's pain. Adequate analgesia reduces the suffering and a patient who is not distressed will give a clearer history and appropriate responses to examination.

> **Key point**
> Acute abdominal pain is **not** a contraindication to opioid analgesia

Antiemetic and nasogastric tube

An antiemetic may also be given to the patient with acute abdominal pain especially if opioid analgesia has been used. A nasogastric tube should be passed to decompress the stomach in patients with small bowel obstruction, pancreatitis, and persistent vomiting – despite administration of an antiemetic.

Fluid and electrolyte replacement

Reassess whether the patient has signs of intravascular volume depletion, and the response to fluid resuscitation.

Dehydration in patients with acute abdominal pain may be due to a combination of factors including vomiting and diarrhoea, inadequate oral intake and "third space" loss (including loss into the bowel lumen or retroperitoneum). Pathology affecting the small bowel mucosa and intestinal obstruction can produce profound electrolyte disturbances.

223

Replace fluid and electrolytes with an appropriate crystalloid solution; this may be either definitive treatment for gastroenteritis or preparation for urgent surgery in patients with intestinal obstruction.

Central venous pressure monitoring is often required in the elderly or those with cardiac disease. Careful fluid balance is necessary in any patient who is seriously ill.

Antibiotics

Antibiotics are needed for either localised infection such as pyelonephritis or where clinical sepsis is thought to have an intraabdominal source (for example, perforation of the colon in an elderly patient). Patients who are septicaemic starting a broad spectrum intravenous antibiotics must be started without waiting for the result of blood cultures.

DEFINITIVE CARE

After secondary assessment and emergency treatment some patients with abdominal pain will require referral to a surgeon (see next box). This is particularly true if the pain:

- has preceded other symptoms
- has persisted for more than six hours
- is asymmetrical and distant from the umbilicus, and accompanied by distension, bile stained or faeculent vomiting or significant abdominal tenderness.

Indications for surgical referral

Suspected generalised peritonitis
- significant diffuse tenderness, with or without a rigid silent abdomen

Suspected localised peritoneal inflammation
- significant localised tenderness with or without other signs of peritoneal irritation
- tenderness and a mass
- tenderness and a fever

Suspected bowel obstruction
- pain and bile stained or faeculent vomiting

Tenderness plus uncontrolled vomiting

Suspected pancreatitis

Suspected aortic aneurysm

Suspected bowel infarction/ischaemia

Gastrointestinal bleeding
- upper gastrointestinal bleeding in a high risk patient
- lower gastrointestinal bleeding

Age greater than 65 years

Patients with ureteric colic should be referred to the urology team or general surgeons (depending on local arrangements). Gynaecological assessment is required for women with suspected ectopic pregnancy, miscarriage, pelvic inflammatory disease or complications of an ovarian cyst. Other patients including those with gastroenteritis, gastrointestinal haemorrhage or pyelonephritis will be admitted under the medical team. Diverticulitis and acute pancreatitis can be treated "medically", but the ideal situation is combined management by physicians and surgeons on a high dependency unit.

Patients may be discharged home if they have either uncomplicated cholelithiasis, ureteric colic or gastroenteritis or where a diagnosis has not been made but the patient appears clinically well and no serious condition is suspected. Advice should be given to these patients to return to hospital without delay if their symptoms deteriorate or new symptoms develop. A proportion may have presented at an early stage of an intra-abdominal problem such as appendicitis. However, if in doubt or the patient is unable to cope at home, then admit for observation.

SPECIFIC CONDITIONS

Acute gastroenteritis

Gastrointestinal infection is one of the commonest abdominal disorders, and symptoms commonly include abdominal pain. Worldwide, intestinal infections account for significant morbidity and mortality. The elderly are particularly vulnerable to the effects of dehydration and electrolyte imbalance, and may present with life threatening cardio-vascular collapse.

Pathophysiology
There are three different pathophysiological mechanisms that will help you to understand the clinical features and the rationale of treatment.

Non-inflammatory (secretory) diarrhoea is classically due to enterotoxin of *Vibrio cholerae* in the small bowel. The toxin blocks passive absorption of sodium (and water) **and** stimulates active sodium (and water) excretion. This leads to an outpouring of iso-tonic sodium and water into the bowel lumen which exceeds the absorptive capacity of the small intestine and colon. Active sodium absorption by a glucose dependent mecha-nism is, however, generally unaffected; hence rehydration may be achieved by oral glu-cose solutions which contain both sodium **and** carbohydrate.

Characteristically the patient has profuse watery diarrhoea (and vomiting), which may lead to severe dehydration, shock, and death.

Viruses (e.g. rotavirus), *Giardia lamblia* and *Cryptosporidium*, toxins of *Staphylococcus aureus* and *Bacillus cereus* (in food poisoning) and enterotoxogenic *E. coli* (a major cause of traveller's diarrhoea) may also produce secretory diarrhoea.

Inflammatory diarrhoea (dysentery) Eschiericia can follow bacterial invasion of the mucosa of the colon and distal small intestine. This leads to both impairment of absorp-tive function and to loss of blood, protein, and mucus which contribute to diarrhoea. Bacterial infections which produce inflammatory diarrhoea include *Salmonella enteritidis*, *Shigella* and *Campylobacter jejuni*. Cytopathic toxins are produced by *Clostridium difficile* which is the commonest cause of antibiotic associated colitis and by verotoxin producing *E. coli*, one type of which (0157:H7) is associated with haemolytic uraemic syndrome. *Entamoeba histolytica* also produces dysentery of varying severity.

The patient may report blood and pus in the diarrhoea (which characteristically con-tains faecal leucocytes). Severity varies from mild self-limiting diarrhoea to severe colitis which may be complicated by toxic megacolon, perforation, and septicaemia.

Systemic infection results from infection that penetrates the mucosa of the distal small bowel, invades lymphatic structures and causes a bacteraemia. Invasive organisms include *Salmonella typhi* (typhoid or enteric fever), *Salmonella paratyphi*, and *Yersinia ente-rocolitica*.

Although about 50% of patients with typhoid may develop diarrhoea, fever and other features are prominent (including headache, cough, malaise, myalgia, abdominal tenderness and hepatosplenomegaly, relative bradycardia, 'rose spots' on the trunk). Complications include small bowel ulceration and occasionally perforation.

Diagnosis and assessment of severity

The diagnosis is essentially clinical, supported by the result of investigations in some cases.

Clinical features

Diarrhoea, nausea and vomiting, abdominal pain, tenesmus, and fever occur in various combinations. Pain may be cramp like and transiently relieved by the passage of diarrhoea, but (with *Salmonella* or *Campylobacter* infection) may mimic a surgical acute intra-abdominal emergency.

To make the diagnosis of gastroenteritis there should be a history of diarrhoea **and** vomiting, but this will not always be the case. A history of family or other contacts affected supports a diagnosis of gastroenteritis; foreign travel, ingestion of suspect food and/or immune compromised state may be risk factor(s) for infection. Antibiotic therapy may suggest *C. difficile* colitis. The elderly and patients who are immune compromised are at increased risk from complications of infection with *Salmonella*. Patients with enteric fever may be constipated rather than have diarrhoea at the time of presentation. The diagnosis will depend on evaluation of systemic symptoms and signs in a patient who has potentially been exposed to infection (recent travel to the tropics).

On the secondary assessment look for signs of dehydration which – particularly in the elderly – may be accompanied by circulatory failure, fever, systemic signs of bacteraemia, and abdominal signs. Record the patient's weight and stool output.

> **Key point**
> Do not diagnose gastroenteritis in patients with abdominal pain and vomiting, without diarrhoea. Consider other conditions e.g. acute pancreatitis, appendicitis

Investigations

Stool specimens should be sent for microbiology (to reach the laboratory within 24 hours) for microscopy (leucocytes, red blood cells, ova, cysts and parasites) and culture (particularly for *Salmonella*, *Shigella*, *Campylobacter* and *E. coli* 0157). If amoebiasis is suspected, a "hot stool" specimen should be sent directly to the laboratory (and the laboratory forewarned) to enable detection of trophozoites. Suspicion of *Clostridium difficile* should prompt specific examination for the organism or toxin.

Check the electrolytes, urea and creatinine in any patient with signs of dehydration or requiring intravenous therapy. Request the following investigations in any patient who is febrile or systemically unwell:

- full blood count
- C-reactive protein
- blood cultures
- chest X-ray
- thick and thin blood films for malaria (if history indicates infection possible).

Treatment

The initial treatment of acute gastroenteritis is independent of knowledge of the causative organism, and most patients require only supportive therapy for self-limiting disease.

If there are signs of circulatory failure, treat initially with 1–2 litres of 0.9% saline and reassess. Volume and rate of replacement may be determined clinically (by signs of peripheral perfusion, jugulovenous pulse, auscultation over lung bases and urine output) or in the critically ill patient by central venous pressure measurement. Add potassium once the serum result is known and there is evidence of urine output.

After restoring the circulating volume, correct dehydration gradually, replacing deficit and maintenance requirements for water and electrolytes. The majority of patients with gastroenteritis can be managed with oral rehydration alone, taking advantage of the active, glucose dependent mechanism for absorption of sodium. Proprietary rehydration powders for reconstitution are available.

Antimicrobial therapy should be given for specific indications only:

- cholera
- typhoid
- occasionally those with non-typhoid *Salmonella* or *Campylobacter* (associated bacteraemia and systemic symptoms, immune compromise, significant coexistent medical problem, e.g. malignancy, sickle cell disease, prosthetic device)
- *C. difficile* colitis, particularly if antecedent antibiotic therapy cannot be stopped
- for specific parasitic infections (amoebiasis, giardiasis).

Antidiarrhoeal medication does not either prolong or increase the illness complications. An antiemetic (e.g. prochlorperazine by IM injection) may be helpful.

Surgical intervention is rare, except for complications such as perforation. Inform the local Public Health Department of notifiable diseases. Those whose occupation involves handling food require appropriate advice regarding time away from work.

Acute pancreatitis

The majority of patients with acute pancreatitis have a self-limiting illness and recover with supportive treatment on a general ward. About 20–25% will develop severe acute pancreatitis, require vigorous resuscitation and multidisciplinary care on the intensive treatment unit. These patients are likely to be severely hypovolaemic due to retroperitoneal fluid loss, generalised extravasation of fluid through leaky capillaries, and loss of extracellular fluid from profuse vomiting. They have a mortality of 25–30%.

Aetiology

The common causes are gall stones and alcohol accounting for about 80% of cases. Other causes include metabolic conditions (hyperlipidaemia, hypercalcaemia), drugs, trauma, infection, ischaemia, and hypothermia. In about 10% of patients no cause is found.

Clinical features

Characerically patients with acute pancreatitis report an acute onset of pain in the upper half of the abdomen. The initial pain may be felt in the epigastrium, right or left upper quadrant or rather vaguely in the centre of the abdomen; and it may radiate to the back or encircle the upper abdomen. A small proportion of patients describe pain that is either overwhelming, generalised pain, or localised to the chest. The pain is often severe, aggravated by movement or inspiration, and may be colicky. Nausea is common. During the first 12 hours most patients vomit; this may be profuse and repeated.

Most patients with acute pancreatitis are clinically shocked; tachycardia and tachypnoea may reflect hypoxia, hypovolaemia and pain. Cyanosis may occur early but is less common than in patients who have suffered an intraabdominal vascular problem or myocardial infarction. Jaundice occurs in about one quarter of patients, particularly those who have either gall stone pancreatitis or alcohol related illness.

The abdomen looks normal and mobile on respiration, but distended (particularly in the upper half of the abdomen). A mass may be felt in the upper abdomen. The majority of patients have tenderness over the upper half of the abdomen and occasionally this is restricted to the right upper quadrant. About half of patients have guarding, but rebound tenderness and rigidity are less common. Bowel sounds are reduced or absent in about one third of patients (and duration of ileus is an indicator of severity).

Gall stone pancreatitis is suggested by jaundice, pain and tenderness localised to or maximal in the right upper quadrant, and a positive Murphy's sign. Seriously ill patients with acute pancreatitis may be pyrexial, tachypnoeic and hypotensive (but sometimes peripherally vasodilated), with pleural effusions and ascites, possibly Cullen's and/or Grey Turner's sign, and a prolonged ileus.

Investigations

A serum amylase level greater than 3–4 times the upper limit of normal confirms the clinical diagnosis. However the serum amylase is not always raised in acute pancreatitis. Patients with alcoholic pancreatitis often have a normal amylase as may those presenting late. The amylase level returns to normal soon after the onset of an episode of acute pancreatitis therefore check the urine amylase. Conversely a raised amylase is not specific. A significantly raised (greater than two times normal) serum lipase is considered more specific, but is less commonly available.

A plain abdominal X-ray may show an elevated diaphragm, localised gastroduodenal ileus or a sentinel loop of small bowel, and/or pancreatic calcification indicative of previous disease. In patients where the diagnosis is not clear, ultrasound scan or contrast enhanced CT may be helpful. Both may show a swollen pancreas or fluid in the lesser sac; CT may show non-perfused necrotic areas of pancreas and give information about severity.

Key point
A normal amylase does not exclude acute pancreatitis

Early complications

The most significant early complication is multiple organ failure.

- Cardiovascular collapse: hypovolaemia and myocardial depression
- Respiratory failure: pleural effusions, atelectasis, pulmonary infiltrates, intrapulmonary shunting, adult respiratory distress syndrome
- Acute renal failure
- Coagulopathy
- Metabolic: hypocalcaemia, hyperglycaemia.

Severity and prognosis

Complications, including multiple organ failure, may develop rapidly and unpredictably. Identify patients at increased risk of developing severe acute pancreatitis. This will ensure that they receive high dependency or intensive care, and to avoid potentially unnecessary hazardous interventions in others. Evidence of three or more factors in the modified Glasgow Scoring System (next box) is associated with increased morbidity and mortality; the greater the number of factors present, the worse the prognosis.

228

Adverse prognostic factors in acute pancreatitis

Within 48 hours
- Age > 55 years
- White blood cell count > 15×10^9/l
- Blood glucose > 10 mmol/l (no diabetic history)
- Serum urea > 16 mmol/l (no response to IV fluids)
- PaO_2 < 8 kPa
- Serum calcium < 2.0 mmol/l
- Serum albumin < 32 g/l
- Lactate dehydrogenase > 600 U/l

Management

Baseline investigations should include electrolytes, calcium, glucose, renal function, liver enzymes, coagulation screen, haematology, arterial blood gases, chest X-ray, and ECG.

The priorities are: correct/prevent hypoxaemic and restore.

Treatment Adequate oxygenation and restoration of intravascular volume. This will limit ischaemic damage to the pancreas and reduce the risk of multiple organ failure. Those with severe disease may have a clinical picture similar to that of acute respiratory distress syndrome; if adequate oxygenation cannot be achieved with supplemental oxygen (FiO_2 = 0·85), the patient should be intubated and ventilated.

Rapid infusion of high volumes of crystalloid and synthetic colloid (up to 4–5 litres or more during the first 24 hours) may be required. Monitoring in patients with severe disease should include a urinary catheter and central venous pressure measurement, to guide fluid resuscitation. Blood transfusion may be required for a falling haemoglobin (due to haemorrhagic pancreatitis). Despite adequate fluid replacement patients with persistent circulatory failure may require inotropic support; and those with renal impairment may need haemofiltration or dialysis.

Pain should be treated with intravenous opioids titrated against effect, possibly followed by patient controlled analgesia. A nasogastric tube will reduce nausea and vomiting in those with severe vomiting or an ileus. Address the cause where possible, e.g. discontinuation of drug or alcohol. Arrange ultrasound of the gall bladder and if gall stones are demonstrated in the bile duct, request early endoscopic retrograde cholangiography and sphincterotomy.

Antibiotics are given:

- for the treatment of suspected cholangitis (cholestatic jaundice and fever)
- in severe acute pancreatitis as prophylaxis against infection of necrotic pancreatic tissue from bacterial translocation
- to cover endoscopic retrograde cholangiography.

Early surgery may be performed:

- to debride infected necrotic pancreas
- to exclude other treatable intraabdominal pathology
- or after acute pancreatitis has subsided, to remove gall stones.

TIME OUT 15.2

List eight adverse prognostic factors in patients with acute pancreatitis.

Acute upper gastrointestinal bleeding

Aetiology and clinical presentation

Melaena, haematemesis and symptoms of hypovolaemia and/or anaemia are the common presenting features of acute upper gastrointestinal (GI) bleeding. However, there may be a history of recent abdominal pain due to duodenal ulcer, gastric ulcer, gastric erosions or gastritis. These conditions which together account for about 70% of upper gastrointestinal bleeds. Ingestion of non-steroidal antiinflammatory drugs (NSAIDs) is an important contributory factor in patients with peptic ulcer disease. Other causes of upper gastrointestinal bleeding include varices, Mallory–Weiss tear and tumour.

Haematemesis and/or melaena suggest bleeding from the oesophagus, stomach or duodenum, although black stools may occasionally be due to bleeding into the distal small bowel or ascending colon. Vomiting of fresh as compared with altered blood suggests more serious bleeding. Rapid upper gastrointestinal bleeding can present with dark red blood per rectum, although (particularly in the absence of hypotension) this is more likely to originate in the lower gastrointestinal tract.

Primary assessment and resuscitation

The airway should be managed as described in Chapters 3 and 4. Patients with a reduced level of consciousness (for example those with hepatic encephalopathy) are at risk of aspiration, thus they require endotracheal intubation. Restore intravascular volume, initially with warmed crystalloid (0.9% sodium chloride) and subsequently blood (see Chapter 9 for further details). Packed cells may be preferable in patients with anaemia and vitamin K. Fresh frozen plasma (FFP) may be required for patients with liver disease or on warfarin, and FFP and platelets in those requiring massive blood transfusion. A central venous pressure line should be inserted in patients with evidence of shock, particularly if there is a history of cardiovascular disease or sign(s) of rebleeding or the patient is on a β blocker. Emergency surgery preceded by endoscopy may be required for those with bleeding and hypovolaemia unresponsive to fluid resuscitation and treatment of any coagulopathy. This early surgical consultation is necessary.

Secondary assessment

The history should include details about the duration and severity of bleeding, recent dyspepsia, vomiting, alcohol or drugs (NSAIDs, anticoagulants, β blockers), jaundice, previous gastrointestinal haemorrhage, and other medical problems. Look for signs of family history, chronic liver disease and splenomegaly or malignancy. Melaena may only be apparent on rectal examination. Important early investigations include a full blood count, crossmatch, coagulation screen, biochemistry including liver enzyme profile, hepatitis serology, chest X-ray and a 12 lead ECG if appropriate.

Evidence of rebleeding includes:

- signs of hypovolaemia (fall in central venous pressure, rise in heart rate, fall in systolic blood pressure)
- fresh haematemesis melaema
- fall in haemoglobin (3 g/dl over 48 hours).

Definitive care

After resuscitation, **early** endoscopy (within 12–24 hours) will identify the source of bleeding, provide prognostic information on the risk of rebleeding and offer an opportunity for haemostatic therapy. **Urgent** endoscopy should be sought for patients with severe, continued or recurrent bleeding; persistent or recurrent signs of hypovolaemia; haemoglobin less than 8 g/dl; or suspected varices.

Patients with an increased mortality risk (see next box) should be admitted to a high dependency area.

Adverse prognostic features in patients with gastrointestinal haemorrhage

- Age ≥ 60 years
- Signs of hypovolaemia (systolic blood pressure < 100 mm Hg)
- Haemoglobin concentration < 10 g/dl
- Severe coexistent disease
- Continued bleeding or rebleeding
- Varices

The need for surgery for a bleeding peptic ulcer is determined by the severity, persistence or recurrence of bleeding, and patient risk factors. A surgical team should be informed of all patients especially those at increased risk (see last box). In general, surgery should be considered for patients:

- with severe, continuing gastrointestinal bleeding
- sixty or more years old or with other risk factor(s), who have either persistent bleeding requiring four units of blood **or** one rebleed
- less than 60 years old with no risk factor, who have either persistent bleeding requiring six to eight units of blood **or** two rebleeds.

Key point
Patients with an increased risk of death from a gastrointestinal bleed (e.g. the elderly with persistent or recurrent bleeding) may benefit most from prompt surgery

Vascular causes of acute abdominal pain

Vascular causes of abdominal pain are important because they include conditions which are life threatening but treatable if recognised early. These conditions are relatively uncommon and in the early stages, symptoms – though severe – may be non-specific and "surgical" signs of an acute abdomen relatively lacking. The patients affected are often elderly and have coexistent medical problems. Delay in diagnosis and referral for surgery when appropriate may result in increased mortality and morbidity. The possibility of a vascular cause for abdominal pain should always be considered in patients over the age of 50 and particularly above the age of 70. The three most common vascular causes of abdominal pain are abdominal aortic aneurysm, acute mesenteric ischaemia, and myocardial infarction presenting with abdominal pain.

Abdominal aortic aneurysm
A leaking abdominal aortic aneurysm is the commonest intraabdominal vascular emergency presenting as:

- vague abdominal pain
- a preceding history of back pain for hours or days or a previously diagnosed aneurysm
- shock with a distended tender abdomen (if the patient has not exsanguinated before reaching hospital), atypical abdominal pain
- severe pain of sudden onset in the abdomen radiating to the flank and back, with a pulsatile mass, an abdominal bruit and reduced pulses in one or both lower limbs, accompanied by signs of hypovolaemia.

However, a majority of these patients will not be known to have an aneurysm, pain may not be severe, a mass may be difficult to detect, and signs of hypovolaemia may be minimal. Pain in the abdomen, flank or back in these patients may be misdiagnosed as ureteric colic or acute pancreatitis. Others present with collapse, with neurological symptoms (spinal cord affected) or pain in the lower limbs (distal emboli). Risk factors include age over 65 years, male, hypertension, smoking, known vascular disease, as well as conditions such as Marfan's syndrome. If the diagnosis is not to be missed, the possibility of an aortic aneurysm must be actively considered in any middle aged or elderly patient with a history of abdominal pain, back pain or collapse, even though they are haemodynamically stable.

> **Key point**
> In the patient previously known to have an abdominal aortic aneurysm, beware of attributing pain to another cause, however well the patient may appear

If abdominal aortic aneurysm is suspected, the principles of management are:

- initiate resuscitation, aiming for a systolic blood pressure of about 90 mm Hg (if the patient is conscious)
- carefully titrated IV opioid analgesia
- immediate surgical referral
- crossmatch blood and warn blood transfusion
- portable ultrasound (the aneurysm may be outlined by calcification on an abdominal X-ray)
- rapid transfer to the operating theatre once the diagnosis has been made (because of the possibility of sudden decompensation).

Acute mesenteric infarction

Acute intestinal ischaemia commonly affects the superior mesenteric artery. If diagnosis and treatment are delayed, complications include necrosis of the small bowel, ascending colon and proximal transverse colon. Diagnosis depends on a high index of suspicion particularly in patients at increased risk (see box), and appropriate history and examination.

> **Risk factors for acute mesenteric ischaemia**
>
> - Elderly (older than 50 years, greater risk with increasing age)
> - Known atheromatous vascular disease
> - Source of embolus (atrial fibrillation and other arrhythmias, myocardial infarction, ventricular aneurysm, valvular heart disease, infective endocarditis)
> - Prolonged hypoperfusion
> - Procoagulant disorders

Characteristically the pain is acute, severe and poorly localised out of all proportion to physical signs. There may be a short preceding history of abdominal pain after eating. An alternative presentation is of pain with an insidious onset over 24–48 hours, initially poorly localised and becoming generalised throughout the abdomen. The pain is colicky initially, becoming steady and unrelenting. Vomiting is common, sometimes with haematemesis.

The patient is pale, distressed and usually has diarrhoea with blood. As bowel infarction develops, the abdomen becomes distended with worsening tenderness, guarding and rebound, and absent bowel sounds. Fever and shock due to bacteraemia often occur.

The key to management is clinical suspicion at an early stage when abdominal signs are minimal. An abdominal X-ray can show dilatation of the intestine with multiple fluid levels; the appearance of gas in the portal vein indicates intestinal necrosis.

Treatment includes vigorous fluid resuscitation, opioid analgesia, antibiotics, and urgent surgical referral with a view to laparotomy once the patient has been resuscitated.

Myocardial infarction

Patients with acute myocardial infarction can report upper abdominal pain. If nausea and vomiting are also conspicuous a primary intraabdominal problem may be poorly localised. In acute cardiac failure, distension of the liver capsule causes right upper quadrant pain mimicking a biliary or upper gastrointestinal tract problem. Complete heart block complicating inferior myocardial infarction and causing collapse can be mistaken by the unwary for intraabdominal bleeding. All patients over 40 (and younger if there is any reason to suspect the diagnosis) should have an ECG.

Ulcerative colitis

Ulcerative colitis is an inflammatory disease of uncertain cause affecting the rectum and colon. Many patients experience a gradually progressive illness in which symptoms related to bowel habit are prominent. However, some present with an acute illness characterised by fever, abdominal pain, diarrhoea with blood and mucus, and tenesmus. A proportion of these patients develop fulminant colitis (associated with pancolitis).

Toxic megacolon is a medical emergency and the possibility of this complication should be considered in all patients with severe colitis. In addition to the features of severe colitis (see next box), abdominal X-ray shows dilatation of the colon with a diameter greater than 6 cm and loss of haustrations. Bowel perforation occurs in patients with fulminant colitis, with or without toxic megacolon. Symptoms and signs of perforation may be obvious, but if the patient is on steroids these may be masked and the only clues to this complication may be a deterioration in general condition. Free air may be seen on X-ray.

Features of severe colitis

- Severe diarrhoea (more than six stools a day) with blood
- Systemic features: drowsiness, fever, tachycardia, signs of hypovolaemia, weight loss
- Progressive abdominal pain, distension and tenderness over the colon
- Raised ESR, CRP and white cell count, low haemoglobin and albumin, electrolyte disturbance
- Extraintestinal features related to disease activity (e.g. aphthous ulcers)

Key point
Abdominal signs and leucocytosis may be masked if the patient is on steroids

---

Medical treatment of the patient with severe colitis/toxic megacolon includes resuscitation with fluid and electrolyte replacement, intravenous steroids and antibiotics. Parenteral nutrition is frequently required, as is blood transfusion. A surgical team should be involved early in the patient's management. If surgery is delayed until after the colon has perforated, mortality is significantly increased. In the acutely ill patient colectomy is needed for perforation, features of severe colitis (with or without toxic megacolon) which deteriorate or do not improve after 24–48 hours on medical treatment, and massive continuing haemorrhage.

Crohn's disease

Crohn's disease is a chronic granulomatous inflammatory disease of undetermined cause. Any part of the gastrointestinal tract may be involved, sometimes with "skip lesions", but the ileum is affected in most patients.

The clinical presentation of Crohn's disease is variable, but abdominal pain, diarrhoea, anorexia, weight loss, and fever are common features. Although a chronic illness with recurrent symptoms over years is common, patients with terminal ileitis can present acutely and be misdiagnosed as acute appendicitis. Think of Crohn's disease (as opposed to appendicitis) if the pain is poorly localised to the right lower quadrant and more than 48 hours' duration, a history of previous surgery, pallor and there is no guarding or rebound tenderness (the possibility of an inflamed retrocaecal appendix). Other findings include a palpable mass, perianal signs (more frequently than in ulcerative colitis), scepticaemia and extraintestinal features. Crohn's colitis can also present with a clinical picture similar to that of ulcerative colitis.

Initial investigations include stool samples for microbiology to exclude infectious diarrhoea and abdominal X-ray, haematology and biochemistry, followed by specialist investigation. Treatment includes fluid and electrolyte replacement when required and nutritional supplements, medical treatment, and surgery for complications.

SUMMARY

Abdominal pain is due to a wide variety of conditions, both intra- and extra-abdominal.

Primary assessment and resuscitation

A minority of patients will have a life threatening condition. A rapid diagnosis and immediate treatment are required. Consider:

- is the patient's airway at risk (recurrent vomiting with a depressed level of consciousness)?
- is oxygenation and ventilation adequate (often impaired with chest pathology, severe acute pancreatitis and sepsis)?
- are there signs of circulatory failure (when the abdominal pain is due to a life threatening condition)?

Urgent surgical referral is required, as part of resuscitation, for haemorrhagic shock. Septic shock due to an intraabdominal cause is a multidisciplinary emergency; treatment includes vigorous fluid resuscitation, IV broad spectrum antibiotics, and early specialist consultation.

Secondary assessment and emergency treatment

- A detailed history and careful examination are the most important elements in making a diagnosis.
- Selective imaging and investigation may confirm the diagnosis and/or provide useful supplementary information.
- Careful attention to fluid and electrolyte replacement, analgesia and antibiotics and nasogastric drainage are important, particularly when the patient needs surgery.

Reference

1   Blamey SL, Imrie CW, O'Neill J, Gilmour WH, Carter DC. Prognostic factors in acute pancreatitis. *Gut* 1984; **25**: 1340–6.

Further reading

American College of Emergency Physicians. Clinical policy for the initial approach to patients presenting with a chief complaint of nontraumatic acute abdominal pain. *Annals of Emergency Medicine* 1994; **23**: 906–22.

Bugliosi TF, Meloy TD, Vukov LF. Acute abdominal pain in the elderly. *Annals of Emergency Medicine* 1990; 19: 1383–6.

De Dombal FT. *Diagnosis of Acute Abdominal Pain*, second edition. Edinburgh: Churchill Livingstone, 1991.

De Dombal FT. Acute abdominal pain in the elderly. *Journal of Clinical Gastroenterology* 1994; **19(4)**: 331–5.

Hogan DE. The Emergency Department approach to diarrhea. *Emergency Medicine Clinics of North America* 1996; **14(4)**: 673–94.

Johnson CD. Severe acute pancreatitis: a continuing challenge for the intensive care team. *British Journal of Intensive Care* 1998; **July/August**: 130–7.

Plewa MC. Emergency abdominal radiography. *Emergency Medicine Clinics of North America* 1991; **9(4)**: 827–52.

Report of a joint working group of the British Society of Gastroenterology, the Research Unit of the Royal College of Physicians and the Audit Unit of the Royal College of Surgeons of England. *Upper Gastrointestinal Haemorrhage. Guidelines for Good Practice and Audit of Management.* London: Royal College of Physicians of London, 1992.

Rosen P, Barker R, Danzl DF *et al.*, eds. *Emergency Medicine: Concepts and Clinical Practice*, fourth edition. St Louis: Mosby Year Books Inc, 1998.

Skinner D, Swain A, Peyton R, Robertson C, eds. *Cambridge Textbook of Accident and Emergency Medicine.* Cambridge: Cambridge University Press, 1997.

Steinberg W, Tenner S. Acute pancreatitis. *New England Journal of Medicine* 1994; **330**: 1198–208.

Tintinalli JE, Ruiz E, Krone RL, eds. *Emergency Medicine: a Comprehensive Study Guide*, fourth edition. New York: McGraw-Hill, 1996.

Walker JS, Dire DJ. Vascular abdominal emergencies. *Emergency Medicine Clinics of North America* 1996; **14(3)**: 571–92.

Weatherall DJ, Ledingham JGG, Warrell DA, eds. *Oxford Textbook of Medicine*, third edition. Oxford: Oxford University Press, 1996.

16

The patient with hot red legs or cold white legs

OBJECTIVES

After reading this chapter you will be able to describe:

- the assessment and initial management of common medical problems which arise in the lower limb
- the complications that may arise from limb pathology.

INTRODUCTION

Trauma is the most common condition to affect the lower limb. In addition:

- systemic diseases and dermatological problems often lead to symptoms in the legs
- degenerative diseases may cause pain in the hip and the knee
- oedema usually gravitates to the legs
- chronic venous disease is common in older people.

However, a variety of acute medical problems may also arise in the lower limb. This short chapter describes the assessment and initial management of the most common of these conditions.

Common acute medical problems in the lower limb	
Venous thrombosis	Daily
Phlebitis	Daily
Venous problems in IV drug users	Daily
Cellulitis	Daily
Arterial embolism	Weekly
Intraarterial injection	Monthly
Compartment syndrome	Monthly
Rupture of a Baker's cyst	Monthly

GENERAL PRINCIPLES OF ASSESSMENT OF THE LOWER LIMB

> **Key point**
> Always look at the whole patient before you look at their legs

For a full initial assessment see Chapter 3.

The **history** of a condition that affects the legs takes the same format as any other history. Pain, swelling and loss of function (i.e. inability to weight bear) are usually the most important features. Always consider:

- recent injury
- smoking
- recent infections
- diabetes
- venous or other vascular disease
- pregnancy or use of oral contraception
- known malignancy (may cause coagulopathy)
- drug use
- long distance travel (venous stasis).

The **examination** of the lower limb should follow the sequence of four four-letter words:

> LOOK
> FEEL
> MOVE
> X-RAY

- Look for: site, spread, symmetry, systemic effects
  swelling, bruising and redness.
- Feel for: temperature, tenderness
  oedema and pulses.
- Move for: passive and active range of movements, function (including weight bearing).
- X-ray for: suspected traumatic conditions.

Investigations should usually include blood glucose, full blood count, and plasma chemistry. Special imaging may be appropriate (see later).

VASCULAR CONDITIONS OF THE LOWER LIMB

Venous thrombosis

Facts and figures about deep vein thrombosis

- Around 2–5% of the population have a venous thrombosis at some time during their lives (see later box on incidence)
- Deep venous thrombosis occurs in up to 40% of postoperative patients and increases in incidence with age. Three per cent of such patients progress to pulmonary embolism

- Deep venous thrombosis is estimated to occur in nearly one in every thousand pregnancies and 15–20% of these women will have a pulmonary embolism if left untreated. Pulmonary embolism is the commonest cause of maternal death in the UK and similar developed countries (see later box)

Incidence of venous thromboembolic disease in women

Healthy non-pregnant women (not taking oral contraceptive)	5 cases per 100 000 women per year
Women using a second generation pill (i.e. containing levonorgestrel)	15 cases per 100 000 women per year
Women using a third generation pill (i.e. containing desogestrel or gestodene)	25 cases per 100 000 women per year
Pregnant women	60 cases per 100 000 pregnancies

All of the above numbers increase with age and other known risk factors such as obesity

---

Factors predisposing to thrombosis in pregnancy

- Increased concentrations of clotting factors and fibrinogen
- Production of inhibitors of fibrinolysis by the placenta
- Venous stasis
- Changes in blood vessels and patterns of blood flow
- Relative immobility

TIME OUT 16.1

Make a list of some types of patients who are at a high risk of deep venous thrombosis (DVT).

Thrombosis of the deep veins of the lower limb or pelvis may be caused by changes in:

- blood coagulation (smoking, oral contraceptive, procoagulant conditions)
- blood vessels (pregnancy)
- blood flow (immobility, plaster casts).

There is:

- swelling and oedema distal to the occlusion
- warmth, redness and deep tenderness of the thigh or calf.
- dilated superficial veins

Key points on clinical findings in suspected deep venous thrombosis

- The classic signs depend on venous occlusion. In contrast there may be no signs in the presence of an extensive, non-occlusive but potentially lethal thrombus. Moreover, there is some evidence that non-occlusive thrombi float in the middle of the vein and break free very easily
- Homans' sign cannot be relied upon – it is non-specific and may cause a pulmonary embolus
- Calf muscle tear, ruptured Baker's cyst and superficial phlebitis may all be mistaken for deep venous thrombosis; oedema may occur with ischaemia
- Deep venous thrombosis may be the first sign of occult malignancy – hence the need for abdominal and pelvic examination and investigation

Management

The first line investigation depends on local availability. Plethysmearaphy, and its various modifications, can be used – often for screening. Doppler ultrasound studies are replacing the traditional venogram in many centres. If neither investigation is immediately available the patient must be treated on clinical suspicion alone.

Several bedside D-dimer assays are now available. These tests measure the breakdown products of cross-linked fibrin and are thus more specific for thrombosis than measurement of fibrin degradation products which arise from the breakdown of fibrinogen and fibrin monomer. The clinical sensitivity of these tests approaches 100% but many have low specificity.

Once the diagnosis is confirmed, treatment depends on local protocol. Anticoagulation is required with either an intravenous infusion of standard unfractionated heparin or with one of the newer low molecular weight heparins given subcutaneously (e.g. enoxaparin 1·5 mg per kg every 24 hours). The availability of subcutaneous treatment has led to some patients being treated at home by community nurses. Heparin is discontinued when adequate oral anticoagulation is established. This is continued for a minimum of three months.

Thrombosis of veins distal to the popliteal vein (below-knee deep venous thrombosis) is common because of the venous sinuses present in the soleus muscle of the calf. Clinicians treat below knee DVT with anticoagulant, but the condition is increasingly managed conservatively with:

- elastic stockings
- non-steroidal antiinflammatory drugs
- rest and elevation
- clinic review.

> **Key point**
> At least 5% of below-knee deep venous thromboses spread to the proximal veins and a half of all above-knee venous thromboses embolise to the lungs

For diagnosis and management of suspected pulmonary embolism see Chapter 8.

Phlebitis

Inflammation of the long or short saphenous vein usually occurs in patients with varicose veins. Phlebitis (usually in the arm) can also follow intravenous therapy. The vein is red, hot and tender.

Management

Phlebitis usually settles with topical therapy and oral non-steroidal antiinflammatory drugs. If there is systemic pyrexia, an antibiotic (e.g. co-amoxiclav) can be added. Superficial thrombophlebitis affecting varicose veins is treated with non-steroidal antiinflammatory drugs.

Venous disease in intravenous drug abusers

Repeated injection into the femoral vein causes chronic venous obstruction. There is swelling and oedema of the whole lower limb and dilatation of the superficial vessels; sinuses are often found in the groin. Acute thrombosis may occur, in which case the limb becomes hot, red, and painful.

Management

This deep venous thrombosis is potentially life threatening and should be treated with heparin as described earlier.

Arterial embolism

Thrombi which embolise to peripheral arteries may arise from several sites.

- The left atrial appendage (usually in the presence of atrial fibrillation)
- The left ventricle (invariably on an area damaged by a recent myocardial infarction or dilated ventricle)
- An atheromatous plaque
- An aortic aneurysm
- A thrombosis in a deep vein in a patient with a patent foramen ovale (paradoxical embolism)

All of these possibilities should be considered although the first two are by far the most common.

Emboli tend to lodge at the sites of bifurcation of arteries. Their effects depend on the extent of the occlusion of the circulation and on the degree of collateral circulation that exists. Common sites that involve the lower limb include:

- the aortic bifurcation (bilateral ischaemia to the level of the knees)
- the origin of the deep femoral artery (ischaemia to the mid-calf)
- the bifurcation of the popliteal artery (ischaemia of the foot).

Sudden occlusion of the femoral artery causes the six "P"s:

Findings in arterial occlusion of the lower limb

- Pain
- Pallor
- Pulselessness
- Paraesthesiae
- Paralysis
- Perishing cold

Management

Embolism must be treated within six hours of the onset of symptoms or else propagation of thrombus distal to the embolus will greatly worsen prognosis. Treatment includes:

- oral aspirin (300 mg)
- intravenous analgesia
- intravenous fluids
- referral to a vascular surgeon for embolectomy and/or fibrinolytic therapy.

Intraarterial injection

Irritant substances may cause critical ischaemia if injected into an artery. Intravenous drug users are the commonest sufferers from this problem; temazepam is the drug most usually involved. The ischaemia results from a mixture of vasospasm and multiple small emboli. Severe pain is the prominent symptom but the other signs described above (six "P"s) may be absent.

Management

This is similar to that described earlier for arterial embolism. Drugs that cause arterial dilatation may be considered.

Acute compartment syndrome

Closed compartment syndrome is caused by swollen, contused muscle or bleeding inside a rigid fascial envelope. The onset may be delayed after injury and insidious. Early symptoms are pain – particularly on muscle stretching – and paraesthesiae. The affected part may also (but not inevitably) be pale and cool with a slow capillary refill. Ischaemia results from compression of small blood vessels and so the presence of distal pulses is of no help in excluding the diagnosis.

Compartment syndrome can easily develop unseen under a plaster cast or below an eschar from a burn. The most common site to be affected is the lower leg which has four anatomical compartments but the syndrome is also seen in the forearm (three fascial compartments), buttock, thigh, foot, and the hand.

> **Key point**
> In compartment syndrome, the limb may not be broken, distal pulses may be present and pulse oximetry may be normal

Management

Suspicion of compartment syndrome is an indication for immediate orthopaedic referral. Manometry is useful, particularly in patients with a depressed level of consciousness. There are four compartments in the lower leg and all may require extensive fasciotomy.

> **Key point**
> Arteriography will reveal arterial lesions but will not demonstrate compartment syndrome

OTHER MEDICAL CONDITIONS OF THE LOWER LIMB

Rupture of a Baker's cyst

Bursae in the popliteal fossa occurs either spontaneously or may be connected to the knee joint. An enlarged and isolated popliteal bursa (a Baker's cyst) associated with rheumatoid arthritis, in particular disease. If this cyst bursts, it causes pain in the upper calf as the synovial fluid is squeezed between the calf muscles. The condition is often misdiagnosed as either a muscle injury or a deep vein thrombosis.

> **Key point**
> A popliteal aneurysm may also present as an extraarticular swelling behind the knee

Management

Ultrasound is the initial investigation. Arthrography is diagnostic. The patient should be referred to an orthopaedic surgeon or a rheumatologist.

Cellulitis of the lower limb

Infection of the skin may arise around a wound or without any obvious port of entry. The skin is red, swollen and tender although the degree of pain is very variable. A cause for the infection should be sought but is not usually found. Without treatment cellulitis can progress rapidly, leading to lymphangitis, lymphodenepathy and septicaemia.

Management

Analgesics and antibiotics should be prescribed. The infection may be streptococcal or staphylococcal and so a combination of flucloxacillin and penicillin V is usually appropriate.

Admission for observation and intravenous therapy is indicated for extensive or rapidly progressing lesions. Lesser cases can be treated with oral antibiotics at home but should be reviewed within 36 hours. The limits of the infection should be marked on the skin with a pen so that changes are obvious at review.

Athlete's foot is a fungal infection which gives rise to an itchy whitish area between the toes (usually in the web space between the 3rd and the 4th toes). It may be the cause of an ascending cellulitis and so the toes should always be examined in patients with cellulitis of the leg. If found, athlete's foot is treated with a topical cream such as clotrimazole.

TIME OUT 16.2

Make a list of signs that differentiate arterial embolism from compartment syndrome.

SUMMARY

- A number of serious medical and surgical problems are commonly seen in the lower limb.
- The assessment and management of these conditions follows a logical sequence.
- Trauma is the commonest problem to affect the leg but medical (especially vascular) conditions must always be considered.
- If untreated, some of these conditions can present a threat to life or limb.

FURTHER READING

- Acute extremity ischaemia and thrombophlebitis
  Feldman AJ. In: Tintinalli JE, Ruiz E, Krome RL, eds (on behalf of the American College of Emergency Physicians). *Emergency Medicine*. 4th edn, New York: McGraw-Hill, 1996.
- Vascular emergencies
  Mitchell DC, Wood RFM. In: Skinner D, Swain A, Peyton R, Robertson C, eds. *Cambridge Textbook of Accident and Emergency Medicine*. Cambridge: Cambridge University Press, 1997.

CHAPTER

17

The patient with hot and/or swollen joints

OBJECTIVES

After reading this chapter you should be able to:

- discuss the general principles of recognising, assessing and managing patients presenting with hot and/or swollen joints.

INTRODUCTION

The clinician needs to develop a systematic approach to managing these patients so that appropriate treatment can be provided. This entails:

- recognition that the condition is present
- assessment of the patient
- determining the cause
- appropriate investigation for the suspected diagnosis
- providing appropriate treatment.

> **Key point**
> The aim is to immediately identify and treat septic arthritis.

GENERAL PRINCIPLES OF MANAGING PATIENTS WITH HOT AND/OR SWOLLEN JOINTS

Recognition

This is usually the easy part. The patient presents with any, or all, of the following symptoms and signs related to their joints:

- red joints
- swollen joints
- hot joints

245

- tender joints
- painful joints
- decreased function.

Together these signs and symptoms represent manifestations of inflammation. Swelling indicates organic disease and may be due to intraarticular fluid, synovitis, bone hypertrophy or a swollen periarticular structure.

The nature of the pain can provide you with clues to the cause of the condition. Pain at the end of the day implies a mechanical cause and is therefore often found in patients with osteoarthritis. In contrast, inflammatory disease pain tends to be worse in the morning and after rest, and may improve with exercise.

Loss of function is usually due to the joint being painful and stiff. The latter is most marked in the morning in inflammatory disease. In addition, with chronic joint problems, tendon and articular damage can exacerbate both neurological impairment and muscle weakness.

Assessment

There are many causes for a "hot and/or swollen joint". As treatment varies with the cause, the clinician needs to try to identify the likely causes as soon as possible. Differentiation can be helped greatly in this task by assessing the five "S"s.

The five "S"s of hot joint assessment

- Single or several joints involved
- Site(s)/symmetry
- Sequence of symptoms
- Systemic effects
- Supplementary features

Systemic effects include pyrexia and gastrointestinal upset. Supplementary features include the signs of other organ involvement.

The social impact of the condition needs to be taken into account when developing a management plan. This includes assessment of the patient's current occupational, social and domestic situation and how this is/has been affected following the onset of arthritis.

Causes

One of the most important clues as to the cause of the condition is determining if more than one joint is involved. Before applying this, however, you need to be aware that there are four causes which can potentially manifest as either mono- or polyarthropathies.

Potential causes of both mono- and polyarthropathy

O – Osteoarthritis	Daily
R – Rheumatoid arthritis	Weekly
S – Spondyloarthritis	Annually
C – Connective tissue disease	Annually

Once these have been excluded, you can divide the remaining causes into those which affect a **single** or **several** joints.

Causes of monoarthropathy (Common)

S	– Sepsis	Weekly
I	– Injury	Weekly
N	– Neoplasm	Annually
G	– Gout/pseudo gout	Daily
L	– Loose body	Weekly
E	– Erythrocytes	Monthly

Causes of polyarthropathy (Rare)

S	– Sexually transmitted disease	Anually
E	– Endocrine/metabolic*	Annually
V	– Viral	Monthly
E	– Endocarditis	Only in examinations
R	– Rheumatic fever	Only in examinations
A	– Allergies/drug associated	Only in examinations
L	– Lyme disease	

*e.g. Wilson's Disease, Alkaptonuria

Investigations

Appropriate investigations should now be ordered to confirm or refute your suspected diagnosis. These consist of:

- blood tests
- radiography
- aspiration.

Blood

Though many blood tests can be ordered, it is best initially to concentrate on the base-line measurements given in Table 17.1.

Table 17.1 Blood tests

Test	Condition
Uric acid	Gout
Rheumatoid factor	Present in 50–75% of rheumatoid arthritis and 30% of collagen/vascular disease
Antinuclear factor	Common in connective tissue disorders
Full blood count	Anaemia common in chronic conditions
Erythrocyte sedimentation rate	Reflects severity of inflammation rather than underlying cause
C-reactive protein	Reflects severity of inflammation rather than underlying cause
Urea and electrolytes	Helpful in quantifying the presence of systemic disease

Radiography
During the development of the arthritis, certain radiological features may be evident, varying from nothing to complete disruption (see next box). In addition to these, particular conditions have specific radiological features.

Radiological features of a hot joint

- Normal
- Soft tissue swelling
- Joint space widening
- Underlying bone lucency
- Joint space narrowing
- Bone destruction
- Crystal deposition
- Subluxation/dislocation

Joint aspiration
See practical procedure in Chapter 29. The aspirate should be tested for the following.

- Gram stain
- Culture – bacterial and viral
- Crystals – with polarising microscope
- Red blood cells
- White blood cells
- LDH (Lactate dehydrogenase)
- Glucose
- Protein

Treatment

In the acute phase, all inflamed joints benefit from analgesia and splintage. However, appropriate treatment for the specific cause must also be started.

SPECIFIC TYPES OF HOT JOINTS

Septic arthritis

Causes
Staphylococcus aureus is the causative organism in 80% of cases. It usually spreads via the blood stream but rarely it can result from local osteomyelitis. It is more common in patients with one or more of the following risk factors:

- rheumatoid arthritis
- intravenous drug use
- immunocompromised
- prosthetic joint.

The five "S"s

- Single/multiple joint involved – Single
- Site(s) – Any, **but commonly around the knee in teenagers**

- Sequence of symptoms – **Develops gradually over a matter of hours to days**. In addition to normal signs of a hot joint, there is usually no movement and it is very tender
- Systemic effects – Pyrexial and other signs of bacteraemia
- Supplementary features – Related to the risk factors

Specific investigation

Blood culture may show the causative organism. The joint aspirate shows pus but a Gram stain is necessary to help decide on an immediate antibiotic. This may be modified once the cultures are processed during the following days.

Septic arthritis and pseudogout both give rise to pus in the aspirate and positive birefringent crystals in plane polarised light.

Specific treatment

> **Key point**
> Sepsis can destroy a joint in under 24 hours!

Intravenous antibiotics must be started immediately the diagnosis is suspected. The choice will depend on the local hospital policy but, using the Gram stain, a good initial "blind" combination is given in the box below.

Gram positive cocci	1 g Flucloxacillin – 6 hourly – IV
Gram negative cocci	1·2 g Benzylpenicillin – 6 hourly – IV
Gram negative rods	Gentamicin – dose according to body weight and renal function

Orthopaedic referral is essential as surgical drainage may be required.

Gout

Cause

Normally nucleic acids in cells are metabolised into purines. These, in turn, are converted into uric acid, two thirds of which is eliminated by the kidneys and the remainder by the gut. In gout, sodium monourate accumulates and crystals precipitate into joints, inducing an inflammatory reaction. It follows from this metabolic pathway that uric acid can accumulate following diuretic therapy, starvation, trauma and infection, and renal failure. It can also be secondary to the breakdown of cells as seen in leukaemia, polycythaemia, and some cancers, where it is often precipitated by treatment. A variety of rare congenital conditions are associated with gout.

The five "S"s

- Single/multiple joint involved – Single
- Site(s) – Metatarsophalangeal joint of the hallux (other joints can be involved)
- Sequence of symptoms – Comes on abruptly, typically at night
- Systemic effects – None usually
  - Urate nephropathy
  - Uric acid stones
- Supplementary features – chronic tophaceous gout: tophi (urate deposits) develop in avascular areas after repeated attacks. Sites include pinna, tendons, and the elbows.

Specific investigations
Aspirate – Negative birefringent needle shaped crystals

> **Key point**
> Even in acute gout, the serum urate may be normal

Specific treatment
Remove the precipitating cause and provide analgesia. Usually this takes the form of a non-steroidal antiinflammatory drug, but be aware of gastrointestinal complications, particularly in the elderly. It is therefore advisable to co-prescribe a proton pump inhibitor for gastromucosal protection. After three weeks consider using allopurinol to reduce the plasma urate level. In patients unable to use non-steroidal antiinflammatory drugs, colchicine can be helpful.

> **Key point**
> Aspirin in high doses (300 mg tds) can be used to treat gout. In contrast low doses (<150 mg) can cause gout

Pseudogout

Cause
Sporadic, hereditary, metabolic disease associated. Pseudogout results from the precipitation of calcium pyrophosphate crystals in joints. This is more likely when any of the following risk factors are present: old age; dehydration; illness; hypothyroidism; diabetes mellitus; any arthritis; high serum calcium and low serum magnesium or phosphate.

> **Tip**
> Pseudogout is the commonest cause of an acute monoarthropathy in the elderly

The five "S"s
- Single/multiple joint involved – Single
- Site(s)/symmetry – Mainly the knee
- Sequence of symptoms – Less severe and longer lasting than gout. In chronic form it leads to destructive changes like osteoarthritis
- Systemic effects – Usually none, unless associated with a metabolic condition, for example, haemochromatosis
- Supplementary features – Usually none

Specific investigations
Aspirate the joint and check the fluid for weakly positive birefringent rod shaped crystals in plane polarised light. Calcium pyrophosphate deposits in cartilage, ligaments, and joint capsules may also be seen on X-ray. This can occur in any cartilaginous joint but the knee is classically involved. There may also be joint destruction.

Specific treatment

Correct any cause and provide analgesia. As this is usually a non-steroidal antiinflammatory drug, the same cautions need to be applied as described for gout.

Rheumatoid arthritis (disease)

Cause

The cause is unknown but is linked to HLA DR4. Rheumatoid disease is more common in females (3:1) and peaks in the fourth decade. It affects approximately 1% of the adult population.

The five "S"s
- Single/multiple joint involved – Multiple usually, rarely single
- Site(s) – Hands and feet initially. Symmetrical
- Sequence of symptoms – Tends to affect the hands and feet initially, with pain and stiffness most marked in the mornings. Fusiform swellings of the interphalangeal and metacarpophalangeal joints are noticeable early on, with larger joints becoming involved later. Eventually ulnar deviation and volar subluxation of the metacarpophalangeal joints occur along with swan neck, and boutonnière deformities of the fingers, and Z-deformities of the thumbs. Some changes in the feet, especially subluxation of the metatarsophalangeal joints. In addition there can be extensor tendon rupture and intrinsic muscle wasting of the hands and feet. It is important to remember that the atlantoaxial joint can also be involved. Rheumatoid changes here can lead to subluxation and potential spinal cord compression during airway maneouvres.
- Systemic effects – Anaemia, weight loss
- Supplementary features – These include:
  - lungs – pulmonary fibrosis, pleuritis, bronchiolitis obliterans
  - cardiovascular system – vasculitis, pericarditis
  - liver – hepatitis
  - central nervous system – carpal tunnel, multifocal neuropathies
  - eyes – episcleritis, scleritis, dry eyes, scleromalacia
  - kidney – amyloid
  - reticuloendothelial – lymphadenopathy, splenomegaly
  - skin – rash, nodules

Key point
Rheumatoid disease affects multiple systems

Specific investigation
- Rheumatoid factor (50–75%)
- Antinuclear factor (30%)
- A chest X-ray may show pulmonary fibrosis, nodules and rarely pleural effusions

Non-specific treatment
- Regular exercise
- Household aids

Specific treatment
- Disease modifying anti-rheumatic drugs (DMARDS)

The dose of non-steroidal antiflammatory drug can be reduced by combining it with paracetamol. Disease modifying drugs are used if there is no response to the non-steroidal antiflammatory or synovitis has persisted for more than six months. Examples include methotrexate, gold, penicillamine, and sulphasalazine. Remember that these drugs have many side effects including marrow suppression (all), oral ulcers (all), proteinuria (all), myasthenia (penicillamine), hepatitis (sulphasalazine/penicillamine). Nevertheless early use of these drugs in appropriate cases can reduce long-term disability.

- Refer to rheumatologist
- Intra-articular injection
- Surgery

Gonococcal arthritis (*Neisseria gonorrhoeae*)

Cause
This occurs most frequently in young people. A purulent effusion is rare (<30%).

The five "S"s
- Single/several joints involved – Multiple
- Site(s)/symmetry – Involves midsized joints such as knee, wrist, and elbow
- Sequence of symptoms – Usually migratory arthralgia
- Systemic effects – Skin rash and other symptoms associated with gonococcal infection
- Supplementary features – Associated with red rash/vesicles over the distal part of the limbs. May also get tenosynovitis of the wrist and hands

Specific investigations
- Aspirate – send for GCFT (gonococcal fixation test and serum)
- Serum for GCFT
- Urethral or high vaginal swab

Specific treatment
- Antibiotics
- Refer to genitourinary medicine for treatment, contact tracing and screening for other sexually transmitted diseases

Spondyloarthritis

This represents a collection of conditions which are seronegative (for rheumatoid factor) and have several common symptoms. The types you are most likely to see can be remembered by the acronym "PEAR".

P – Psoriatic arthritis
E – Enteropathic arthritis
A – Ankylosing spondylitis
R – Reiter's syndrome

The five "S"s common presentation
- Single/several joint involved – Multiple or monoarthritis of large joints (small joints involved in psoriatic arthritis); characterised by enthesopathy i.e. develop inflammation at the site of ligamentous insertion into bone
- Site(s)/symmetry – Spine and sacroiliac joints; asymmetrical when involves several joints
- Sequence of symptoms – Depends upon the specific type of spondyloarthritis (see later)

- Systemic effects – Can include uveitis
- Supplementary features – Depends upon the specific type of spondyloarthritis but can include: calcification of tendon insertions; uveitis; aortic regurgitation; upper zone pulmonary fibrosis; and amyloidosis

Psoriatic arthritis

Commonly, this involves the terminal interphalangeal joints asymmetrically but there are many different presentations. The patient usually also has the skin and nail manifestations of psoriasis.

Enteropathic arthritis

Typically this person has associated inflammatory bowel disease.

Ankylosing spondylitis

Typically seen in young males presenting with back stiffness especially in the morning. Although rare, they may eventually get the "question mark" spinal posture (kyphotic spine with hyperextended neck) due to progressive spinal fusion; a fixed spinocranial ankylosis and restricted respiration. In 50% of cases, the hip is involved and in 25%, the knee and ankle are affected.

Reiter's syndrome

This is made up of a triad of urethritis, conjunctivitis, and seronegative arthritis. In the UK this typically presents in young male patients. A recent history of non-specific urethritis or diarrhoea can occasionally be elicited.

Specific investigations

HLA B-27 is present in 88–96% of patients with ankylosing spondylitis. The spinal X-ray may also show "bamboo spine" as well as squaring of the vertebra and erosions of the apophyseal joints. Obliteration of the sacroiliac joint is also commonly visible in established cases. Bilateral sacroiliitis is the characteristic radiological feature.

Specific treatment

Early rheumatological referral is necessary. Exercise must be started early to maintain as much mobility and posture as possible. In the other types of spondyloarthritis, exercise should be started once the acute symptoms have settled. Treat the underlying condition.

TIME OUT 17.1

Construct an algorithm to include the important steps in the diagnosis and management of a hot swollen joint.

SUMMARY

A hot joint is a condition easy to recognise but it has many causes. A systematic approach is therefore needed. This includes a well "phrased" history followed by a five "S" assessment and appropriate investigations.

Key point
Do **not** leave a septic joint until the next day – infection can destroy a joint in under 24 hours

253

CHAPTER

18

The patient with a rash

OBJECTIVES

After reading this chapter you will be able to:

- understand the common terms used in dermatology
- discuss cutaneous manifestations of life threatening illness
- apply a structured approach to the assessment and management of the patient with a rash.

INTRODUCTION

The skin is a large organ which may be affected by a primary disorder or manifest signs of systemic illness. It may also provide the signs required to diagnose immediately life threatening illnesses. Careful assessment using a structured approach is necessary to distinguish the serious from a coincidental rash. Early recognition of these signs will allow prompt, potentially lifesaving, disease specific therapy to be initiated.

This chapter will provide you with a structured approach to common dermatological problems – some of which are life threatening.

USEFUL TERMINOLOGY

- **Angiooedema**
  Similar to urticaria but involves the subcutaneous tissues, especially the face, lips and tongue. Presents with swelling rather than wheals. It is rarely life threatening but be wary of laryngeal compromise. Hypotension/anaphylaxis can occur (uncommonly), as can bronchospasm and gastrointestinal disturbance. ABC treatment should include intravenous hydrocortisone, intramuscular adrenaline, antihistamines, reassessment.
- **Bulla**
  A fluid-filled blister greater than 1 cm in diameter, e.g. as in pemphigoid
- **Ecchymoses**
  Bruises (i.e. confluent petechiae)
- **Erosion**
  Partial epidermal loss (no scar usually)

255

- **Erythema**
  Redness that blanches on pressure, indicating dilated capillaries. It should be distinguished from purpura which can be red, orange, purple or brown but does not fade on firm pressure
- **Erythroderma**
  Widespread erythema (i.e. greater than 90% body surface area affected)
- **Macule**
  Flat lesions, any colour, e.g. a freckle, and less than 5 mm in diameter
- **Nikolsky's sign**
  Gentle rubbing of the skin causes the epidermis to separate from the underlying dermis with subsequent erosions
- **Nodule**
  A raised rounded lesion greater than 1 cm diameter
- **Papule**
  A raised rounded lesion less than 1 cm in diameter, e.g. a mole
- **Patch**
  Larger version of a macule (greater than 5 mm in diameter)
- **Petechiae**
  Pin-point haemorrhage
- **Plaque**
  A raised patch, e.g. a plaque of psoriasis on an elbow. Therefore a maculopapular rash consists of raised and flat lesions. These are often less than 1 cm diameter, e.g. as seen in a penicillin rash
- **Purpura**
  A condition that can be red, orange, purple, or brown but does not fade on firm pressure (unlike erythema)
- **Pustule**
  A pus filled blister, usually less than 1 cm in diameter, e.g. as in a furuncle (i.e. boil)
- **Ulcer**
  Full loss of epidermis and some dermis (scar possible)
- **Urticaria**
  Formation of pruritic, transient (< 24 hours) wheals (like nettle rash). These are collections of dermal oedema surrounded by erythema. Systemic symptoms are extremely rare
- **Vesicle**
  A fluid-filled blister less than 1 cm diameter, e.g. as in herpes labialis

IMMEDIATELY LIFE THREATENING EMERGENCIES

Life threatening illnesses involving the skin may present with signs relating to airway, breathing or circulation.

Immediately life threatening illnesses with signs in the skin		
Airway	Obstruction	Anaphylaxis
		Angiooedema
Breathing	Bronchospasm	Anaphylaxis
Circulation	Shock	Meningococcal septicaemia
		Gonococcal septicaemia
		Cellulitis
	Shock	Anaphylaxis
		Erythroderma

These conditions can be usefully grouped into four different areas by the type of rash associated with the underlying condition. These are:

- urticaria
- erythema
- purpura and vasculitis
- blistering disorders.

URTICARIA

Anaphylaxis may present with predominantly dermatological features including pruritus and urticaria. These features are usually florid but may be subtle. They may be associated with airway obstruction, bronchospasm, shock, and gastrointestinal disturbance. The specific management of this condition is considered in detail in Chapter 9.

Angiooedema is a related condition that may present with some similar features. It is characterised by swelling of the subcutaneous tissues, predominantly affecting the face. Notably these lesions are rarely itchy in contrast to the intense pruritus often associated with urticaria. Involvement of mucous membranes or the tongue, larynx or pharynx may result in airway obstruction. Angiooedema may herald the onset of anaphylaxis. Frequently no cause is apparent and attacks may be recurrent. Angiooedema should be treated in the same manner as anaphylaxis. Rarely patients may have angiooedema resulting from C1 esterase inhibitor deficiency. This should be treated similarly to other causes of angiooedema but may require specific treatment with either fresh frozen plasma or C1 esterase inhibitor concentrate where available.

A flow diagram for the diagnosis of urticaria is given in Figure 18.1.

ERYTHRODERMAA AND EXFOLIATION

This may result from a number of causes (see box) although the common link is resulting marked vasodilatation. Shock may occur from a number of mechanisms including vasodilatation, fluid loss, and endotoxin related. A striking clinical feature is the heat radiated by these patients which may result in problems with thermoregulation.

Causes of erythroderma and exfoliation

- Psoriasis
- Toxic epidermal necrolysis
- Drug eruptions
- Staphylococcal scalded skin syndrome
- Toxic shock syndrome
- Lymphoma
- Seborrhoeic dermatitis
- Contact dermatitis
- Idiopathic

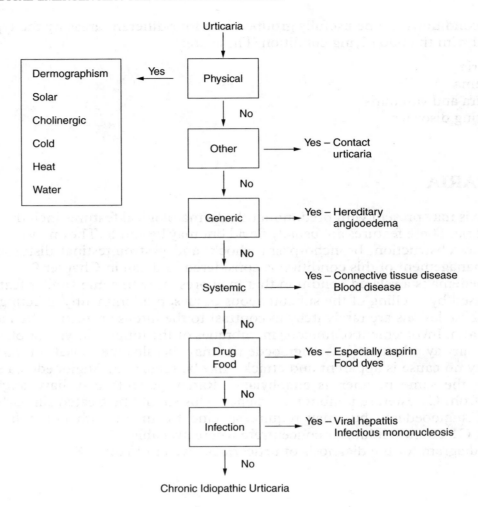

Figure 18.1 The diagnosis of urticaria

The patient with red skin (erythema)

Erythema is defined as **redness that blanches on pressure** and indicates dilated capillaries. It should be distinguished from purpura which can be red, orange, purple or brown but does not fade on firm pressure. Erythroderma means widespread erythema (i.e. greater than 90% of the body surface area affected).

During the primary assessment it is important to ensure a high inspired oxygen concentration as oxygen consumption is greatly increased. Hypovolaemia should be corrected with crystalloid as described in Chapter 9. Patients with erythroderma, especially where the skin has peeled leaving a large moist area, will continue to lose large amounts of fluid. This fluid should be replaced. The amount of fluid required can be calculated with standard formulae used for burn injuries. Inotropic support or vasoconstrictor drugs may occasionally be required to treat the shock after adequate fluid resuscitation. This step should be undertaken in conjunction with specialist advice.

The secondary assessment will often reveal the underlying cause for erythroderma. A well "phrased" history may help to identify:

● Previous skin disease. The patient will often be aware of preexisting atopic dermatitis, seborrhoeic dermatitis or psoriasis. Enquiry should be made about the recent use of systemic or topical steroids as abrupt withdrawal may precipitate an acute flare-up.

- Drug use. A full drug history must be obtained, including all topical medications. This enquiry must not be limited to prescribed medications but should include over the counter medications, herbal remedies, and cosmetic use. The reaction to topical applications may be local or systemic.
- General review. Enquiries of current or recent infections, tampon use and recent burns should be made as each of these predisposes to toxic shock syndrome. Systemic features of lymphoma may include night sweats, weight loss, and pruritus.

Pain and skin tenderness are unusual symptoms in erythroderma but their presence should highlight staphylococcal scalded skin syndrome or toxic shock syndrome as more likely causes. Pruritus is a common feature and rarely helps to discriminate the underlying cause although severe pruritus may suggest cutaneous lymphoma.

Specific treatment can be started after resuscitation has been initiated and a working diagnosis made. This may include:

- Covering weeping or open lesions with saline soaked dressings. This may reduce subsequent contamination and secondary infection. If large areas are to be dressed dry sterile dressings should be used to reduce heat loss in the early stages. It may be useful to photograph the rash before covering it.
- Intravenous flucloxacillin should be given (unless contraindicated) if staphylococcal infection is suspected. Topical and prophylactic antibiotics are of no benefit and may cause later complications.
- Intravenous opioid analgesia may be required.

Disease specific treatment should be initiated on the basis of specialist advice.

Summary

The assessment and management of an erythematous patient is shown in Figure 18.2.

> **Key point**
> Nikolsky's sign – sheering stress on epidermis causes new blisters

PURPURA AND VASCULITIS

The patient with purpura

Purpura is caused by red cells leaking out of blood vessels into the dermis. Although the main cause is inflammation and leakiness of these blood vessels, i.e. vasculitis (see later), there are other causes to be considered.

> **TIP**
> Remember, unlike erythema, purpura does not blanch on firm pressure
> Petechiae are pinpoint haemorrhages
> Ecchymoses are bruises (i.e. confluent petechiae)

Purpura may be part of a rapidly progressive septic illness or, in contrast, may be a component of a longstanding stable vasculitis. The hallmark of a purpuric rash is the failure to blanch with pressure. This is best seen by pressing on the rash with a microscope slide or a clear drinking glass.

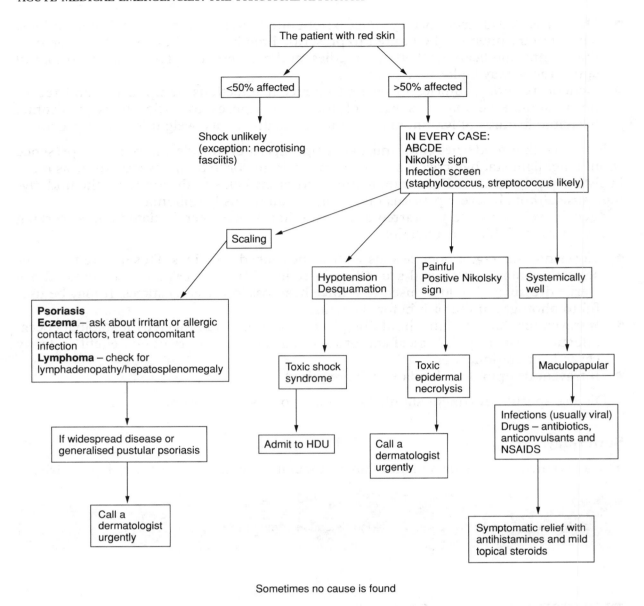

Figure 18.2 Assessment and management of the erythematous patient

Purpura may be caused by an abnormality of the blood or the vessels. These points are summarised in Figure 18.3.

Key point
The presence of a purpuric rash in an ill patient is due to overwhelming septicaemia until proven otherwise

Primary assessment
There are a number of infections which produce a characteristic clinical picture of a purpuric rash associated with shock.

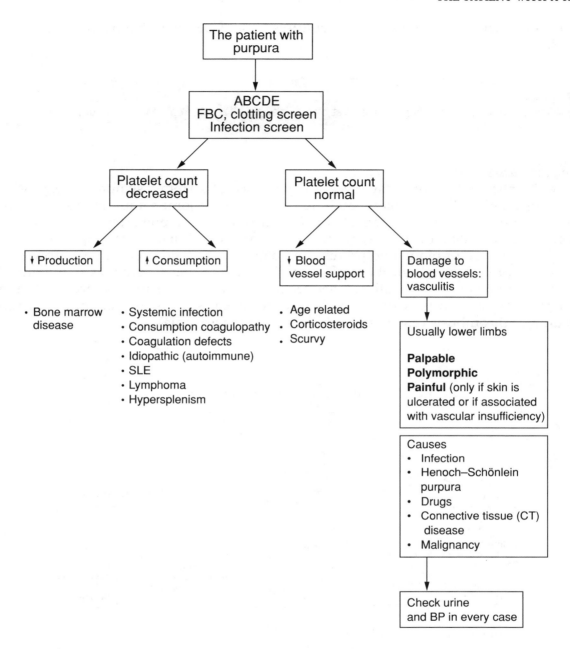

Figure 18.3 The patient with purpura: an algorithm to aid differential diagnosis

Infections associated with shock and purpura

- Meningococcus
- Gonococcus
- *Staphylococcus aureus*
- *Rickettsia*
- Arbovirus

The most common cause is meningococcal septicaemia. It is important to remember that this can occur without any symptoms or signs of meningitis. Its management is discussed fully in Chapters 9, 11, and 14 but remember that benzylpenicillin should be given immediately. If possible blood cultures should be taken before the first dose of antibiotics.

Key point
If in doubt, treat with benzylpenicillin first and investigate for alternative causes later

---

Secondary assessment

The well "phrased' history may reveal the presence of systemic symptoms, e.g. urinary symptoms, and abdominal pain combined with fever or joint symptoms may suggest a systemic vasculitis such as Henoch–Schönlein purpura or polyarteritis or a systemic infection. A detailed drug history must be obtained. Further investigations should include urinalysis for blood and protein, full blood count, and urea and electrolytes.

The comprehensive physical examination should seek specific clues as to the underlying cause of purpura or vasculitis. Changes to the mental state may be present but may be subtle. This can occur with meningitis, connective tissue diseases or with intracranial bleeding or thrombosis (e.g. in thrombotic thrombocytopenia).

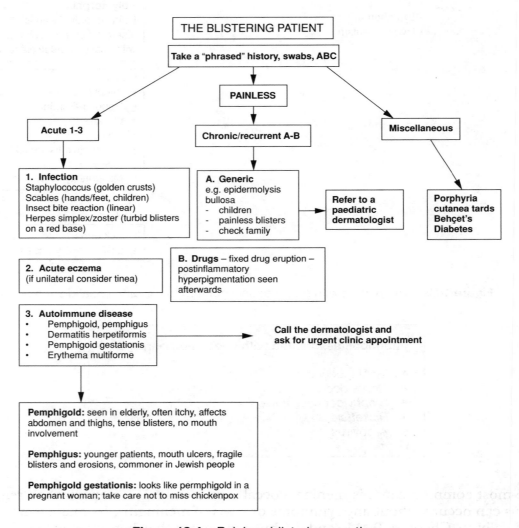

Figure 18.4   Painless blistering eruptions

Definitive care of the underlying problem will frequently involve the input of a number of specialities including haematology, immunology, rheumatology, general medicine, and intensive care. Do not delay resuscitative treatment for a specialist opinion.

BLISTERING ERUPTIONS

Blisters are accumulations of fluid that occur in two common sites.

- Within the epidermis (intraepidermal) – often having a thin roof.
- Under the epidermis (subepidermal) – often thick walled.

Any may contain blood. Although there are more comprehensive classifications, the differential diagnosis of blistering eruptions is based on whether they are painless (Figure 18.4) or painful (Figure 18.5).

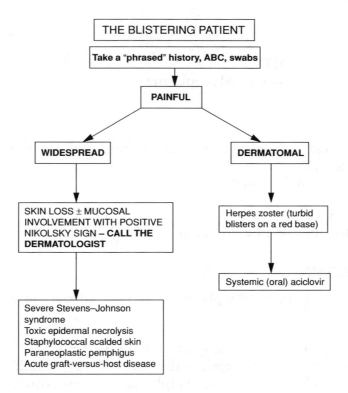

Treatment

Treat impetigo with flucloxacillin not ampicillin
Treat all affected family members if you suspect impetigo or scabies
Insect bite reactions resolve spontaneously but pruritus is helped by antihistamines
Acute eczema responds to topical steroids
For widespread herpetic infection or shingles, treat with systemic aciclovir
If herpetic infection near the eyes, discuss management with an ophthalmologist

Figure 18.5 Painfull blistering eruptions

IS THIS STEVENS–JOHNSON SYNDROME (SJS) OR TOXIC EPIDERMAL NECROLYSIS (TEN)?

Terminology in these conditions can be confusing. SJS is considered to be erythema multiforme in association with mucous membrane (ocular, oral, genital) involvement. However, erythema multiforme is rarely classically targetoid and often appears maculopapular. To help differentiate it from the usual maculopapular eruptions, there is the aforementioned mucosal involvement, pain is a feature and if it progresses to TEN, this is heralded by the development of the Nikolsky sign.

TEN, where there is full thickness loss of the epidermis, presents with tenderness and redness of the skin followed by exfoliation (like a scald). It may follow Steven–Johnson or appear *de novo*. It often starts in the flexures. It is a dermatological emergency and requires swift recognition and treatment as it carries a mortality of 30% which increases in the elderly (who are usually on the most medication). Management needs to be on a high-dependency unit.

Causes of SJS

- Sulphonamides and NSAIDS
- Herpes simplex, streptococcus, Mycoplasma

Causes of TEN

- Any drug but most commonly anticonvulsants, antibiotics (especially sulphonamides), and NSAIDS
- Infection (bacterial, viral, fungal)
- Idiopathic
- As a sequel to SJS
- Rarely as a paraneoplastic phenomenon

If you suspect SJS/TEN

1. ABC (IVI should be peripherally placed in uninvolved skin; oral intake of fluids may be impossible)
2. Pain relief++
3. Take a detailed drug history and stop any offending drugs
4. Perform an infection screen as sepsis is the main cause of death
5. Don't use flamazine (crossreacts with sulphonamides and causes neutropenia)
6. Don't give steroids
7. Call the dermatologist on call urgently to confirm the diagnosis and supervise treatment

Differential diagnosis of TEN

1. Staphylococcal scalded skin – seen in children, may see evidence of impetigo, especially around the mouth and nose
2. Paraneoplastic pemphigus – usually associated with haematological malignancy; may look very similar to SJS with subsequent TEN, but responds to steroids; characteristic histology
3. Acute graft-versus-host disease

INFECTION AND THE SKIN

The skin may be directly involved in an infective process. Cellulitis is a common problem that can occasionally become life or limb threatening if necrotising fasciitis develops or septicaemia ensues. The infecting organism causing cellulitis is usually a group A streptococcus. First line treatment should be with a penicillin.

Primary herpes zoster (chicken pox) is an unpleasant illness. However, it may become life threatening in immunocompromised patients (e.g. post transplant, high dose steroids, acquired immunodeficiency syndrome). The rash is characterised by the simultaneous presence of vesicles, pustules, and crusted lesions. It is important in the immunocompromised patient to recognise the illness as early as possible, when only a handful of vesicles may be present. The illness may be complicated by pneumonitis. Immunocompromised patients with primary herpes zoster should be treated with an intravenous antiviral agent, such as aciclovir.

TIME OUT 18.1

a. List the four categories of dermatological conditions that can be immediately life threatening.
b. Draw the algorithm for each condition.

SUMMARY

- Life threatening skin conditions are rare but may be rapidly fatal.
- Resuscitation may involve specific treatments including adrenaline for anaphylaxis and benzylpenicillin for meningococcal septicaemia.
- A careful history and examination may be required to elicit subtle features in the early stages of life threatening illness.
- Seek specialist advice early.
- Most dermatological conditions presenting as an emergency are not life threatening.

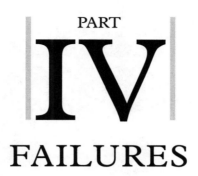

PART

IV

FAILURES

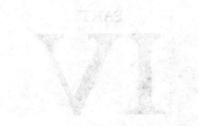

CHAPTER

19

Organ failure

OBJECTIVES

After reading this chapter you will be able to:

- understand the concept of organ failure and its impact on other body systems
- describe the structured approach to management.

INTRODUCTION

Organ failure is a common medical problem. It is, however, only a manifestation of a variety of underlying disease processes. Thus, organ failure is not a diagnosis but the final stage of a progressive pathology. This chapter will focus on:

- respiratory failure
- cardiac failure
- brain failure
- renal failure
- liver failure
- "endocrine" failure.

    For each group, the common precipitants will be discussed and integrated with relevant clinical signs. It is important to realise how organ failure has an effect on other systems.

RESPIRATORY FAILURE

Acute respiratory failure

This is uncommon in general medicine but is most often seen in patients with either a severe asthma attack, tension pneumothorax, pulmonary embolus or severe pneumonia (see Chapter 8). The management, irrespective of the cause (see box), is to clear and secure the airway followed by ventilation with high flow oxygen. Acute respiratory failure necessitates immediate collaboration with colleagues in the intensive care unit.

> **Causes of acute respiratory failure**
>
> | | |
> |---|---|
> | Pulmonary | Asthma, pulmonary embolus |
> | Cardiac | Dysrhythmia, failure, arrest |
> | Neurological | Status epilepticus, unconsciousness |
> | Neuromuscular | Myasthenia gravis |
> | Trauma | Head, neck, chest |

Chronic respiratory failure

Many patients present with an acute exacerbation of their chronic pulmonary disease. The common underlying causes, often seen on acute medical wards, are listed in the box below.

> **Causes of chronic respiratory failure**
>
> | | | |
> |---|---|---|
> | Parenchymal disease | Chronic bronchitis | Daily |
> | | Emphysema | Daily |
> | | Pulmonary fibrosis | Weekly |
> | | Bronchiectasis | Weekly |
> | | Pulmonary vascular disease | Weekly |
> | Obstructive sleep apnoea | | Monthly |
> | Chest wall problems | Kyphoscoliosis | Weekly |
> | | Extreme obesity | Weekly |
> | Neuromuscular disorders | Motor neurone disease | Annually |
> | | Cervical cord lesion | Annually |

Chronic bronchitis and emphysema (chronic obstructive pulmonary disease – COPD), pulmonary fibrosis, and pulmonary vascular disease are frequently encountered in both emergency and general medicine. All three can cause hypoxaemia whilst chronic obstructive pulmonary disease is the commonest cause of hypercapnic ventilatory failure.

Pathophysiology

Chronic obstructive pulmonary disease (COPD)

This is a collective term referring to patients who have chronic bronchitis and/or emphysema. Chronic bronchitis is a common disorder manifested by chronic inflammation both in the bronchi and also bronchioles. The major cause is cigarette smoking, although inhalation of other gases may give rise to a similar problem. These noxious compounds stimulate increased mucous production and airway narrowing secondary to mucous gland hypertrophy, oedema, bronchoconstriction and subepithelial airway fibrosis. Furthermore, the chronic chemical irritant increases mucous production and also impairs the ciliary escalator, preventing clearance. Hence coughing is a major symptom.

In chronic bronchitis the inflammatory changes affecting the large airways have minimal effect. However, those affecting the smaller airways produce a fixed obstruction affecting both inspiration and expiration. Consequently hypoxaemia predominates and this may lead to pulmonary vasoconstriction. These patients often hypoventilate, hence predisposing to an elevated $PaCO_2$. In addition, chronic hypoxaemia will lead to an increase in erythropoietin production by the kidneys culminating in secondary polycythaemia. The combination of pulmonary vasoconstriction and increased blood viscosity adversely influences right heart function. It is not surprising, therefore, that pulmonary hypertension and right heart failure are common sequelae.

In contrast, emphysema affects alveolar walls and is attributed to enzyme degradation of both collagen and elastin. This in turn destroys the alveolar walls and hence the alveolar spaces coalesce. Again cigarette smoking is a common cause of this condition. Whilst the changes have patchy distribution throughout the lung they mainly affect the apex. This is related to greater mechanical stress at the apex due to the weight of the remaining lung tissue. In comparison, α-1-antitrypsin deficiency (a rare condition) causes similar changes in the dependent areas. This is likely to reflect higher blood flow and unchecked enzyme degradation because of the lack of the protective antiprotease compound – α-1-antitrypsin.

The forces influencing lung volume are normally a balance between the chest wall attempting to spring out whilst the lung tends to collapse or recoil. In emphysema the enlarged parenchymal air spaces, formed by alveolar coalescence, cause two major structural problems. The first is loss of elastic recoil and hence increase in size, functional residual capacity, and compliance. The second is destruction of the framework that attaches the alveoli to the airway.

As the forces that exert traction to maintain a patent airway have been disrupted, small airways and particularly those without cartilaginous support will collapse during expiration and cause air trapping. As a result the residual volume increases and expiration is prolonged.

> **Key point**
> In emphysema there is a marked collapse of small airways

In chronic obstructive pulmonary disease there is impaired ventilation and reduced perfusion of areas with inadequate ventilation. The latter are referred to as shunts. The end result is a rise in $PaCO_2$ and a fall in PaO_2. However, some patients with emphysema can maintain reasonably normal gases due to an increase in both rate and effort of breathing.

Pulmonary fibrosis

Diseases associated with diffuse pulmonary fibrosis are shown in the box.

> **Diseases associated with diffuse pulmonary fibrosis**
>
> - Cryptogenic fibrosing alveolitis
> - Occupation, e.g. asbestosis/pneumoconiosis
> - Extrinsic allergic alveolitis (usually upper lobe and late in the disease)
> - Drug, e.g. busulphan, bleomycin, paraquat
> - Rheumatoid disease
> - Systemic sclerosis
> - Systemic lupus erythematosus
> - Sarcoid

Hypoxaemia is often severe and present at rest whilst the $PaCO_2$ is generally normal or low. The latter is attributed to hyperventilation increasing the elimination of carbon dioxide.

271

Bronchiectasis

This condition is characterised by chronic dilatation of at least some of the bronchi. The bronchial wall is irreversibly damaged as a consequence of early inflammation or infection of either the bronchus or adjacent lung parenchyma. The normal transport of mucus is impaired and chronic local suppuration ensues.

A variety of conditions are associated with bronchiectasis and they are shown in the box.

Conditions associated with bronchiectasis	
Infection:	Measles pneumonia
	Whooping cough
	Tuberculosis
Immune related:	Immunoglobulin deficiency
	Complement deficiency
Inhalation:	Gastric aspiration
	Ammonia inhalation
	Foreign body inhalation
Others:	Immotile cilia
	Kartagener's syndrome
	α1 antitrypsin deficiency

The pathophysiology of bronchiectasis is poorly understood. Despite the wide variety of conditions associated with bronchiectasis there are certain common features.

Firstly a severe infection causes extensive tissue damage mediated by persistent inflammation. The repair processes, however, are inadequate, for example, with immunoglobulin deficiency or lack of major inhibitors of proteolytic enzymes, i.e. α-1-antitrypsin deficiency. If the inflammation is left unchecked extensive tissue destruction, inadequate repair scarring and tissue distortion occur. As focal areas of the lungs framework are destroyed the associated bronchoalveolar units become dilated.

Assessment

Usually the patient with respiratory failure will be unable to complete sentences. Accessory muscle use is prominent and the patients are often either hyperventilating or cyanosed with plethoric facies and laboured respiration. A tachycardia is invariably present.

Immediate management

In all of these patients it is important to:

1. treat hypoxaemia
2. identify and treat the reason for the acute exacerbation
3. assess the severity of the respiratory failure
4. monitor the response to treatment.

Hypoxaemia kills. Therefore patients should receive high flow oxygen especially when the underlying cause of their breathlessness is unknown. The major cause of hypercapmia in patient with COPD is impaired ventilation/perfusion matching. Patients will compensate by increasing the rate of ventilation but this increases the work of breaking (the pink puffer; type one respiratory failure).

In contrast, patients with severe chronic obstructive pulmonary disease and hypercapnoea usually have lower tidal volumes due to a short inspiratory time and an increased respiratory rate ("blue bloater", type two respiratory failure). There is little evidence to support the theory that supplemental oxygen in COPD patients "removes the hypoxic drive", causing alveolar hypoventilation and hypercapnia. The major effect is to increase dead space ventilation, probably secondary to worsening V/Q monitoring due to a loss of hypoxic pulmonary vasoconstriction. Therefore, oxygen therapy should be given to ensure a saturation of 90–92% to reduce hypoxaemia and prevent further hypercapnia. However, in the acute situation, especially when the diagnosis remains in doubt, high flow oxygen should be given and adjusted according to arterial blood gas results. In patients who respond appropriately, it is only necessary to increase the flow to ensure a PaO_2 of greater than 8 kPa. If , however, life threatening hypoxaemia persists without increasing hypercapnia the patient will require some form of assisted ventilation.

The reason for clinical deterioration is usually bronchospasm further impairing ventilation. Nebulised β_2 agonists will reduce this burden as will therapy with steroids and antibiotics. These will also help to reduce the luminal inflammatory response and infected secretions. Aminophylline is often beneficial in patients who have an acute exacerbation of chronic obstructive pulmonary disease. This bronchodilator has other benefits including inotropic stimulation, increased cardiac output, and improved renal perfusion. This is of particular benefit in patients who have coexistent ventricular failure.

As a consequence of the acute and chronic respiratory compromise, the central nervous system drive to respiration increases. However, in a patient with dangerous hypercapnia and acidosis, the respiratory drive can be enhanced by temporary stimulants such as doxapram. (Doxapram is not a specific stimulant for the respiratory centre and often produces profound agitation.) If the patient does not respond appropriately to treatment, reassessment is required to identify any of the possible causes listed in the box below.

Causes of treatment failure in respiratory failure

Untreated bacterial infection
Sputum retention
Coexistent pneumothorax
Inadequate bronchodilator therapy
Coexistent pulmonary oedema
Underlying dysrhythmia
Inappropriate sedation
Wrong diagnosis

It is essential that the patient is assessed regularly after treatment to detect either a failure to respond or a deterioration. Thus there is a need to include frequent blood gas monitoring in the acute phase. Should the patient fail to progress, early liaison with an intensivist and respiratory physician is necessary.

Summary

Acute on chronic respiratory failure is a common medical emergency. All patients should initially receive high flow oxygen and this should be titrated according to the results of blood gas analysis. Early intervention is required by either a respiratory physician or intensivist, if the patient fails to respond to treatment with bronchodilators, steroids, antibiotics, and respiratory drive stimulants.

CARDIAC FAILURE

Introduction

Cardiac failure in most circumstances is failure of the pump. This may be due to problems with the muscle, electrical conduction, valves or inappropriate filling. Both left and biventricular failure are commonly seen in acute medical emergencies. The major manifestation that causes concern, from a clinical point of view, is pulmonary oedema.

Pulmonary oedema

The lung has a framework of interstitial connective tissue that extends from the large airways and blood vessels distally to form a delicate interface between the alveolar cell and the associated capillary endothelium. This space is so thin that it does not interfere with gas transfer. The normal plasma oncotic pressure ensures that fluid does not enter this space. It follows, therefore, that any increase in capillary pressure may result in fluid accumulating in this space, i.e. interstitial oedema. This is normally limited by lymphatic drainage. Further increases in capillary pressure, however, may lead to substantial oedema of the interstitial space. Consequently, the alveoli and associated capillaries become surrounded by oedema. Continued increases in capillary pressure overwhelm the lymphatic drainage, resulting in alveolar oedema that can occasionally accumulate in the airways (see next box).

Summary of the pathophysiology of pulmonary oedema

Increased hydrostatic pressure
Increased capillary permeability
Reduced interstitial pressure
Impaired lymphatic drainage
Reduced oncotic pressure

As a consequence of this process, the following changes may occur.

- Small airways become either narrowed by interstitial oedema or filled with oedema.
- The lung becomes firm and less compliant; consequently less air enters during inspiration and when the airways eventually open they do so with a click which is represented clinically as a fine crackle.
- During expiration early airway closure occurs, producing wheezing.
- Reduced ventilation in less compliant areas leads to local hypoxaemia and reflex arteriolar constriction. This reduces perfusion and diverts blood to less affected areas.
- Reflex hyperventilation is due to stimulation of vagal sensory "J receptors" because of distortion of the lung tissue by oedema.

Symptoms

Breathlessness is the major symptom due to a combination of hyperventilation, hypoxaemia, bronchospasm, and intraalveolar oedema. This is often accompanied by tachypnoea, cough, orthopnoea and paroxysmal nocturnal dyspnoea. Severe cases can be associated with cyanosis, a cough productive of frothy, often blood-stained sputum or frank haemoptysis. Cheyne–Stokes (periodic) respiration is seen occasionally.

The primary function of the heart is to provide body tissues with a continuous flow of oxygenated blood sufficient for their metabolic needs. Heart failure occurs when this demand can no longer be met and control of intracardiac pressures is lost. The volume of blood expelled during systole is determined by the force and the velocity of myocardial cell contraction (see Chapter 9 for further details). These two important factors are in turn governed by:

- the extent to which the myocardium is stretched before contraction – **the preload**
- the load imposed on the ventricle during contraction – **the afterload**
- the **contractile state of the myocardium**.

Considering these three mechanisms the causes of left ventricular failure can therefore be classified as:

- **Increased preload** or **volume overload** where the ventricle has to expel more blood per minute than normal, e.g. aortic incompetence, mitral incompetence, and patent ductus arteriosus.
- **Increased afterload** or **pressure overload** where resistance to outflow from the left ventricle is increased, e.g. aortic stenosis and systemic hypertension.
- **Myocardial dysfunction** due to either loss of contractile tissue following a myocardial infarction or diminished contractility with a cardiomyopathy.

As a consequence of myocardial failure the fall in cardiac output is responsible for both a reduction in effective arterial blood volume as well as an increase in venous pressure. These responses are known to lead to the release of antidiuretic hormone (ADH).

With an acute reduction in left ventricular performance there is a rapid increase in left ventricular filling pressure and hence pulmonary venous pressures. This will lead to fluid accumulation within the lung. The lung compliance as well as vital capacity is reduced, resulting in an increase in the work of breathing. This may be increased further by bronchoconstriction secondary to oedema of the bronchi. Furthermore, with increasing pulmonary venous hypertension the alveolar membrane becomes thickened and oedematous, impairing gas transfer and leading to arterial hypoxaemia.

The combination of engorged vascular systems, interstitial oedema, and alveolar fluid is responsible for the mixed obstructive and restrictive function defects. The restrictive component, which predominates, is secondary to reduced compliance from vascular congestion.

Orthopnoea occurs either when pulmonary oedema first appears or is exacerbated on lying flat. This change in posture causes a shift of blood to the pulmonary circulation from the systemic. The resultant increase in intracapillary hydrostatic pressure produces oedema. It is believed that both further elevations in pulmonary capillary pressure due to pulmonary venoconstriction and pulmonary venous hypertension due to severe systemic vasoconstriction are responsible for paroxysmal nocturnal dyspnoea.

From a cardiac point of view, there is one basic measurement that will influence the treatment of pulmonary oedema and that is the blood pressure. The patient with left ventricular failure and a systolic blood pressure of 90 mm Hg or above can be treated with any vasodilator such as nitrates, loop diuretics or opioids. The main concern, however, is that whilst these may reduce the preload, they may also initially precipitate hypotension.

In contrast, in the hypotensive patient (systolic less than 90 mm Hg) inotropic therapy is required and dopamine is the favoured initial agent. This drug will not only increase heart rate but also augment renal perfusion.

Pathophysiological response to heart failure

Cardiac

The initial response of the heart to increased workload, either volume and/or pressure, is an increase in the rate and force of contraction – as one would see in the physiological response to exercise. As the condition progresses, however, compensatory mechanisms are invoked and these can initially be regarded as physiological but eventually become pathological. They include:

- Dilatation of the heart, increasing the volume of the left ventricle usually due to a combination of volume overload and myocardial disease.
- Hypertrophy of the heart (left ventricle) due to chronic increasing afterload with aortic stenosis and/or systemic arterial hypertension. This leads to hypoxia of the myocardial cell, in particular at its centre.
- Impaired myocardial contractility.
- Redistribution of cardiac output. Sympathetic mediated vasoconstriction ensures that the cardiac output is diverted away from the skin, splanchnic circulation and kidneys. Renal arterial and vasoconstriction may reduce the renal blood flow by as much as 75%.
- The neural response to the dilating/failing heart is mediated by the sympathetic nervous system which also induces and stimulates vasoconstriction, as described earlier. The result is:
  - increased rate and force of contraction
  - vasoconstriction
  - renin secretion.

Renal

Renal retention of sodium and hence water is responsible for an increase in extracellular and plasma volume. This response is primarily mediated by the kidneys, but also by the neuroendocrine system (see next section).

- Reduced renal blood flow – as described earlier.
- Reduced glomerular filtration. Although glomerular filtration is reduced in cardiac failure, it is disproportionate when compared with renal blood flow.
- Increased absorption of sodium, mainly mediated by the action of aldosterone.

Neuroendocrine

- Sympathetic nervous system – as described earlier.
- Renin–aldosterone–angiotensin system – in response to a falling cardiac output, both the increase in sympathetic activity and renal arterial vasoconstriction are effective stimuli for renin secretion. The renin is responsible for an increase in angiotensin mediated vasoconstriction and stimulating aldosterone secretion which in turn stimulates tubular reabsorption of sodium (as described earlier) and hence blood volume expansion. Whilst this will have the beneficial effect of increasing preload it will also increase the total circulating volume.

TREATMENT SUMMARY

A – clear; $FiO_2 = 0.85$
B – consider nebulised salbutamol
C – systole BP ≥ 90 mm Hg – venodilate
                  < 90 mm Hg – inotropes
Consider the use of Frusemide to clear "lung water."
Establish underlying cause.
Early discussion with cardiologist/intensivist for the minority of patients who need more intensive therapy and monitoring.

Causes of pulmonary oedema.
Left ventricular failure – see Chapters 8 and 9 for further details.

Valvular disease

Mitral stenosis

Pathophysiology
Chronic rheumatic heart disease is by far the most common cause. The mitral valve cusps are thickened and often fused with associated thrombus on the atrial surface. Calcification may also occur. The left atrium is characteristically enlarged and mural thrombus may be present proximal to the posterior mitral valve cusp.

Mitral stenosis reduces left ventricular filling. Consequently, cardiac output falls and pulmonary vascular resistance increases. Left ventricular cavity size usually remains normal. In contrast, the left atrium enlarges and chronic left atrial hypertension induces a rise in pulmonary capillary pressure and hence pulmonary oedema formation. Furthermore, reactive pulmonary hypertension, repeated pulmonary emboli, frequent chest infections or even haemosiderosis may occur.

Treatment
Pulmonary oedema associated with mitral stenosis responds well to diuretic therapy. If the patient is in atrial fibrillation with a rapid ventricular response then appropriate treatment is with digoxin. In addition, intravenous heparin should be started as either a prelude to cardioversion or formal anticoagulation because of the high incidence of embolism.

Rarely left atrial myxomas (present in two per 100,000 of the population) may present as progressive breathlessness, orthopnoea, paroxysmal nocturnal dyspnoea or fluid retention. The acute management is described under mitral stenosis. As there is a significant risk of emboli, surgery is the definitive treatment.

Mitral regurgitation

Pathophysiology
Of the many causes of mitral regurgitation (Table 19.1) the most is the floppy mitral valve. Irrespective of the cause, however, the main physiological disturbance is an increase in left ventricular output. The pressure within the aorta is significantly greater than that in the left atrium so the majority of the left ventricular ejection fraction enters the left atrium. The left ventricular output is maintained, however, by a sinus tachycardia. If severe, mitral regurgitation can lead to pulmonary oedema and/or a low output state.

Table 19.1 The causes of mitral regurgitation

Structure affected	Pathogenesis
Valve cusps	Floppy mitral valve, infective endocarditis, rheumatic heart disease
Chordae	Floppy mitral valve, connective tissue diseases, infective endocarditis
Papillary muscle	Acute myocardial infarction, cardiomyopathy
Valve ring	Left ventricular dilatation

During diastole there is a large flow of blood from the left atrium to the left ventricle, comprising blood received from the pulmonary circulation combined with that regurgitated during the preceding systole. This increased volume will lead to left ventricular failure, raised pulmonary capillary pressures and hence pulmonary venous hypertension.

Treatment
Medical treatment does not differ from that described for mitral stenosis. Vasodilatation to reduce afterload is also helpful, especially in acute mitral regurgitation.

Aortic stenosis

Pathophysiology
The causes of aortic stenosis are listed in the box.

Causes of aortic stenosis

Congenital bicuspid (fused commissure)
Rheumatic heart disease
Calcified "senile" valve
Infective endocarditis

Aortic stenosis gives rise to left ventricular hypertrophy. This produces diastolic stiffness of the myocardium, higher end diastolic pressures and, eventually, pulmonary oedema. As the disease progresses, the left ventricular cavity becomes dilated, especially in severe cases.

Treatment
Aortic stenosis is a mechanical problem that will, in most cases, require surgical intervention. Acute pulmonary oedema, in this context, can be managed by diuretic therapy and bed rest before surgery. This, however, is only a temporising measure.

Aortic regurgitation

Pathophysiology
The causes of aortic regurgitation are listed in the box.

Causes of aortic regurgitation

Infective endocarditis
Rheumatic heart disease
Trauma
Rheumatoid disease
Marfan's syndrome
Dissecting aneurysm
Syphilis
Ankylosing spondylitis

Aortic regurgitation is associated with an increase in left ventricular stroke volume. The regurgitant flow is greatest in early diastole when the difference in pressure between the aorta and left ventricle is maximal. The volume of regurgitated blood is determined not only by the severity of the aortic valve disease, but also by the compliance of left ventricle and systemic vascular resistance. The left ventricular output may be more than double.

The end diastolic pressure in the aorta is low and the resistance to ejection of blood by the left ventricle is reduced. This reduction in resistance, allied to a large stroke volume, is responsible for the rapid upstroke and wide pulse pressure.

Treatment

Acute aortic regurgitation is a surgical emergency. It is nearly always secondary to infective endocarditis in the presence of acute pulmonary oedema. Vasodilatation, as with acute mitral regurgitation, is the treatment of choice whilst plans are being made for emergency aortic valve replacement.

> **Key point**
> All patients must receive appropriate advice and treatment, where relevant, for infective endocarditis – irrespective of the valvular problem

ACUTE HYPERTENSION

Pathophysiology

Increased left ventricular load, possibly augmented by increased sympathetic nerve activity, is responsible for left ventricular hypertrophy. The consequent increase in muscle mass may be responsible for the development of ischaemia and also ventricular dysfunction, both predisposing to left ventricular failure.

Treatment

Sodium nitroprusside is the agent of choice as its action can be immediately reversed by discontinuation (50 mg of sodium nitroprusside added to 500 ml of 5% dextrose gives a solution of 100 micrograms per millilitre). Intraarterial pressure monitoring is necessary. An infusion of sodium nitroprusside at 10 micrograms per minute (6 ml per hour) should be started with increments of 10 micrograms per minute every 5 minutes until a maximum dose of 75 micrograms per kilogram.

RIGHT VENTRICULAR FAILURE

Pathophysiology

The commonest cause of right ventricular failure is an inferior myocardial infarction. Failure of the ventricle to contract appropriately reduces forward flow into the pulmonary circulation and manifests as low output left ventricular failure. This may be the first clue to the underlying diagnosis. Further signs include tachycardia, hypotension, and a third heart sound. However, there is no pulmonary oedema. Features of systemic venous hypertension predominate. This clinical picture may initially be confused with a pericardial effusion or constrictive pericarditis but Kussmaul's sign is negative and there is no pulsus paradoxus.

Treatment

This comprises a fluid challenge to increase the right ventricular filling pressure. Often inotropes have to be added. Under ideal circumstances these patients should be monitored on the coronary care unit and their treatment facilitated by readings from a pulmonary arterial flotation catheter.

> **Key point**
> Cardiac tamponade and constrictive pericarditis are rare

Summary

Left and biventricular failure are common medical emergencies. The underlying cause is usually ischaemic heart disease. A critical feature in the management of these patients is blood pressure. This will dictate whether venodilatation or inotropic support is the management of choice.

BRAIN FAILURE

Introduction

Brain failure is defined as intellectual dysfunction, loss of intelligence or loss of intellectual capacity. This condition must be differentiated from learning difficulties where there is a subnormal intellectual capacity from the outset that is often caused by brain disease acquired during prenatal or early life.

Differential diagnosis of brain failure

In this context brain failure is not a medical emergency, but it is considered because the differential diagnosis often causes concern (see box).

> **Differential diagnosis of brain failure**
>
> Dementia
> Pseudodementia   Acute confusional state
>   Inattention
>   Depression

All of these conditions will affect the mental state but in the context of acute medicine the important diagnosis to establish is that of an acute confusional state. This is the commonest condition that affects the mental state and the commonest form of pseudodementia.

In a patient who is acutely confused, the abnormality in mental state is due to reduced cerebral function commonly secondary to a toxin, i.e. the patient has an encephalopathy. Furthermore, brain failure can occur acutely, but this is associated with global cerebral dysfunction – as described in Chapter 11.

The confused patient is unable to maintain a coherent stream of thought or action. Thus the serial sevens are used to establish this diagnosis. However, this is even difficult for the doctor. An alternative method is to do the so-called one-tap two-tap test, i.e. the doctor instructs the patient that if he taps once the patient should respond by tapping twice; however, if he taps twice the patient should not tap. A similar test is to ask the patient to recite rapidly all the letters of the alphabet that rhyme with tree. This ensures that they have to keep the task in mind whilst reciting the appropriate letters. This is a good assessment of mental attention.

Mental state examination comprises four critical components as shown in the box.

Critical components of mental state examination

- Level of consciousness
- Language
- Memory
- Visuospatial skills

- Level of consciousness – there is always an abnormality in the conscious state and the patient may be inattentive, confused, delirious or even drowsy.
- Language abnormalities are common and fluent aphasia is a characteristic problem with Alzheimer's disease.
- Memory – formal assessment can be done, for example, with a Folstein 30 point assessment. In the context of meaningful clinical review, the best method is to casually involve the patient in a conversation about a recent event ensuring that it is compatible with their social, cultural, and economic background. This will easily identify problems with both language and memory.

Key point

Do not focus on "overlearned" knowledge such as details of the family as even the most demented patient may still be able to recollect some relevant details

---

- To document visuospatial skills, ask the patient to write their name, address, and a sentence about the weather. Do not dictate the sentence otherwise you will miss language problems. In addition, draw a circle and tell the patient that this is the face of a clock. Ask them to put the numbers on the clock and set the clock at, e.g. 4.30 pm. It is important that you draw the circle to identify any problems in the patient's visual field (if they draw the circle, it will be confined to their limited vision).

If you suspect a diagnosis of dementia then help should be sought from either a neurologist or a geriatrician. This is a chronic disabling disease and, therefore, before a firm diagnosis is made it is important not to miss a treatable condition. These are rare but should be sought. A computed tomography scan is therefore essential to exclude a meningioma, chronic bilateral subdural haematoma without trauma and hydrocephalus. Other potential treatable causes are vitamin B12 deficiency, syphilis, and hypothyroidism. These should easily be detected with a spectrum of clinical signs. Thus there is no need, unless clinical features dictate, to request either a serum T4 or syphilis serology. Although a large number of neurological diseases can cause dementia the majority are very rare, and Alzheimer's disease is by far the commonest.

Summary

Brain failure commonly presents as an acute confusional state. The differential diagnosis includes dementia, acute confusion, inattention, and depression, and is facilitated by a comprehensive medical history and search for an underlying treatable cause. In the context of acute confusional state, this is usually a toxin. In contrast treatable causes for dementia include meningioma, chronic bilateral subdural haematomata, hydrocephalus and vitamin B12 deficiency.

ACUTE RENAL FAILURE

Objectives

Introduction

This usually occurs as part of a circulatory disturbance. However, approximately 5% of emergency admissions have transient disturbance in renal function.

Definition

- Rapidly rising plasma urea or creatinine (over hours).
- Urine output of less than 400 ml per day or less than 30 ml an hour for three consecutive hours or excessive urine output in the face of deteriorating renal function (non-oliguric renal failure).

Causes

Although the causes of renal failure are divided into three groups (see box) those grouped as prerenal are the commonest. Often, you will suspect that renal failure is likely from either the clinical features or the history. Occasionally, however, it will come to light when laboratory results are examined.

Causes of acute renal failure	
Prerenal	Hypotension, e.g. following shock
	Hypovolaemia, e.g. gastrointestinal haemorrhage, persistent vomiting or diarrhoea, diuretic or hyperglycaemic states
	Selected renal ischaemia, e.g. hepatorenal syndrome
Intrinsic renal disease	Glomerular, e.g. primary part of a systemic disease
	Vascular, e.g. vasculitis, coagulopathy
	Tubular, e.g. acute tubular necrosis
	Interstitial, e.g. drug related acute interstitial nephritis
Postrenal	Urethral obstruction, e.g. prostatic pathology
	Ureteric obstruction, e.g. carcinoma of the bladder

Either way you need to consider the treatable causes (see box) and institute appropriate therapy. In addition check that the necessary urgent investigations have been requested.

Potentially reversible causes of renal failure	
Hypovolaemia	Hypercalcaemia
Heart failure	Nephrotoxic drugs
Sepsis	Urinary tract obstruction
Hypotension	Urinary tract infection
Hypertension	

> **Urgent investigations in suspected acute renal failure**
>
> 1. Plasma sodium, potassium, urea, creatinine, and glucose
> 2. Urine stick test, microscopy, biochemistry, and culture
> 3. Arterial blood gases
> 4. ECG
> 5. Renal ultrasound scan

Urine analysis is useful in the differential diagnosis of acute renal failure. Table 19.2 provides a summary of the relevant biochemical features.

Table 19.2   Urine biochemistry in renal failure

	Prerenal	Acute tubular necrosis
Urine sodium (mmol/l)	<20	>40
Urine osmolality (mosmol/kg)	>500	<350
Urine: plasma osmolality	>1·5	<1·2
Urine: plasma urea	>8	<2
Urine: plasma creatinine	>40	<20

The values in Table 19.2 assume previously normal renal function. It is important to remember that these values can be affected by pre-existing renal disease, and diuretic therapy (increases urinary sodium excretion). Tubular function may be altered in the elderly and those with liver disease. In contrast, sodium excretion is reduced in patients with intrinsic renal disease, e.g. glomerulonephritis.

Both stick testing and microscopy of urine also provide useful information in the differential diagnosis of acute renal failure. The presence of red cells, red cell casts, and proteinuria is suggestive of acute glomerulonephritis. In contrast, a positive urine stick test for blood, but negative microscopy for red cells is indicative of rhabdomyolysis. The presence of tubular cell casts, tubular cells, and granular casts is highly suggestive of acute tubular necrosis.

Management

In addition to the primary and secondary assessments, specific therapy should correct the cause of acute renal failure, quickly to deal with any life threatening problems (see box) or oliguria.

> **Life threatening complications**
>
> - Hyperkalaemia
> - Pulmonary oedema

Hyperkalaemia of greater than 6·5 mmol/l should be treated with a combination of intravenous dextrose and soluble insulin (10 units). If ECG changes are present add in addition to 10 ml of 10% calcium chloride. In contrast, if the plasma potassium is between 5·5 and 6·5 mmol/l, calcium resonium should be given either orally or per rectum.

Frusemide is of little value in treating the pulmonary oedema associated with acute renal failure. Opiates provide symptom relief. Fluid removal by haemodialysis is the management of choice.

In suspected prerenal failure always ensure that the patient is fully hydrated and has a urinary catheter *in situ*. Exclude potentially reversible causes for renal failure. If the patient has failed to respond to a fluid challenge give intravenous frusemide (250 mg over one hour). If urine output remains less than 40 ml/hour over the next hour give a further 500 mg over two hours. Failure to respond to this regime indicates that the patient needs dopamine at 2·5 microgram/kg/min via a central vein combined with continuous infusion of frusemide (50 mg/hour).

It is important to monitor:

- hourly   urine output
  clinical examination
- 4 hourly pulse, blood pressure
- daily   serum, urea, electrolytes and creatinine
  arterial blood gases

If after this treatment the patient has still failed to respond then urgent liaison with a nephrologist is required as the patient may need urgent dialysis.

Indications for early dialysis in acute renal failure

- Hyperkalaemia refractory to treatment
- Pulmonary oedema
- Severe metabolic acidosis refractory to treatment

Summary

In the management of renal failure:

- always consider potentially reversible causes.
- ensure the patient is fully hydrated and receives a fluid challenge.
- ensure a postrenal cause is excluded by catheterisation and abdominal ultrasound.
- always do a rectal/vaginal examination to exclude a pelvic tumour.
- intrinsic renal disease as a cause of acute renal failure is rare, but clues to this diagnosis will be obtained from the patient's history and urine microscopy.

LIVER FAILURE

Introduction

The incidence of both acute and acute on chronic liver failure is increasing. However, they are still rare presentations as acute medical emergencies. The immediate management of these two conditions is virtually identical.

Definition

Liver failure is a syndrome that follows severe impairment of the hepatocyte function – hence it is also referred to as hepatocellular failure.

Clues to the diagnosis

The history from a patient with liver disease can be clouded by associated encephalopathy. Nevertheless it is always of paramount importance to be aware of your own safety, and enquiries regarding viral hepatitis and at-risk groups are necessary. Other symptoms that predominate are often non-specific and include tiredness and occasionally dark urine and pale stools.

A history of drug use, both proprietory and street related (especially paracetamol and ecstasy), should be actively sought along with details of foreign travel and alcohol consumption.

Cardinal signs of hepatocellular dysfunction

> **Cardinal signs of hepatocellular dysfunction**
>
> Jaundice
> Hepatic encephalopathy
> Ascites
> Coagulopathy

Jaundice indicates impaired release of conjugated bilirubin and its intensity is proportional to the extent of hepatocellular necrosis.

Hepatic encephalopathy is manifest by a broad spectrum of neuropsychiatric features that are epitomised by an impaired mental state and neuromuscular dysfunction.

> **Key point**
> Hepatic encephalopathy is reversible

This form of neurological dysfunction occurs when blood is shunted from the portal venous system into the systemic circulation without hepatic extraction of substances such as ammonia, phenols and GABA (γ aminobutyric acid)-like glycoprotein. These compounds are believed to act as inhibitory neurotransmitters depressing both motor function and the conscious level. This may easily be assessed using the Glasgow Coma Score, but hepatologists in particular prefer to use Childs grading.

> **Childs grading of hepatic encephalopathy**
>
> Grade
> 1   Prodromal phase – euphoria or irritability
> 2   Impending coma – drowsiness, lethargy and confusion interspersed
>   with agitated or aggressive behaviour
> 3   Stupor – somnolent but rousable
> 4   Coma

Patients with encephalopathy can present with a variety of neurological signs ranging from flexor, equivocal or extensor plantars (positive Babinski response) to extrapyramidal features. However, the classic sign is asterixis, a non-specific "flapping" tremor associated with liver failure, carbon dioxide retention and uraemia. This is due, in part, to neuromuscular incoordination of the wrist flexors and extensors.

Key point
Hepatic encephalopathy is the great neurological mimic

The differential diagnosis of hepatic encephalopathy is summarised in the next box and a useful acronym is "three Hs and four Is".

Differential diagnosis of hepatic encephalopathy

Hypoxia
Hypovolaemia
Hypoglycaemia
Alcohol
Neurodegenerative conditions
Drugs
Infection
Impaction of faeces
Intracranial haemorrhage
Imbalance of electrolytes

Ascites occurs primarily due to a raised portal venous pressure secondary to distortion and destruction of the sinusoids with supraadded impaired venous drainage.

Coagulopathy, the bleeding tendency associated with liver failure, is multifactorial. It is primarily due to impaired synthesis of all coagulation factors (factor VIII is predominantly produced by the endothelium). This is often exacerbated by thrombocytopenia secondary to hypersplenism or platelet dysfunction. Therefore, it is advisable to check both the prothrombin and activated partial thromboplastin times. Occasionally disseminated intravascular coagulation can supervene so D-dimers or fibrin degradation products should be quantitated.

In addition, two other features worth mentioning are foetor hepaticus and immunocompromise. Foetor hepaticus is a characteristic smell of the patient's breath which is due to sulphur compounds. All patients with liver failure are relatively immunocompromised and severe infection may be present without coexistent pyrexia or leucocytosis.

Critical clinical features

- Hypoxaemia – this is multifactorial in origin and is primarily related to the widespread peripheral pulmonary vasodilatation. This results in approximately two thirds of patients becoming hypoxaemic, but the precise cause remains unknown. It is exacerbated by abnormalities in ventilation, perfusion and transfer factor. However, it is important to realise that a resultant shunt hypoxaemia is readily reversible with high flow oxygen.

    If this sequence of events is left untreated it will progress to pulmonary oedema and a poor prognosis.
- Hypotension – this is a manifestation of systemic vasodilatation combined with a hyperdynamic circulation. Patients therefore exhibit a bounding pulse, prominent left ventricular impulse and a flow murmur. Of interest is the fact that whilst the systemic blood flow is increased renal perfusion is reduced along with urine output.

Key point
Fifty per cent of patients with acute liver disease will have coexistent gastrointestinal haemorrhage

Hypotension associated with liver disease is therefore a combination of systemic vasodilatation and hypovolaemia. The situation can be compounded by the fact that patients can have a coexistent dysrhythmia.

- Hypoglycaemia – this is extremely important and easy to miss. Hepatic glucose synthesis and release is impaired and this process is exacerbated by raised levels of circulating insulin.

> **Key point**
> Hypoglycaemia is common in patients with liver dysfunction and may mimic hepatic encephalopathy

It is important to be aware of the potential for acute hypoglycaemia. Failure to recognise this condition can lead to irreversible brain damage – unlike the situation with hepatic encephalopathy.

> **Key point**
> Hypoxaemia, hypovolaemia and hypoglycaemia are the common cardinal features of liver failure

Other key features include:

- Cerebral oedema – this is attributed to arterial vasodilatation and failure of cellular osmoregulation with reduction in cerebral oxygen consumption. The crucial factor is how to distinguish cerebral oedema from hepatic encephalopathy. Often this is impossible. However, in patients with grade 4 coma both cerebral oedema and hepatic encephalopathy coexist. Thus early discussion with a hepatologist and intensivist is required.
- Renal failure – this is very common in patients with liver failure, but only a minority are associated with true hypovolaemia. Most patients have a "functional" renal failure.

> **Key point**
> In patients with liver failure remember that urea and creatinine are not reliable indicators of renal function as hepatic synthesis of urea is reduced and tubular excretion of creatinine is increased

Impaired water clearance, sodium pump failure, intravenous fluids, and diuretics can give rise to hyponatraemia. These may also contribute to hypokalaemia and the coexistent metabolic alkalosis. Other acid–base disturbances include centrally driven respiratory alkalosis associated with hypovolaemia and metabolic acidosis due to anaerobic metabolism from lactate accumulation and tissue destruction.

> **Key points**
> Abnormalities in electrolytes and arterial blood gases have a profound effect on already compromised physiology, in particular precipitating or exacerbating hepatic, neurological, and cardiac dysfunction
> Both the major systemic manifestations of liver failure and the pathophysiology are related to hypoxaemia, hypovolaemia, and hypoglycaemia

MANAGEMENT OF LIVER FAILURE

Management of liver failure

1. Universal precautions
2. High inspired FiO_2
3. Secure IV access and treat hypovolaemia
4. Recognise and proactively treat the potential for hypoglycaemia

---

Urgent investigations in liver failure

Full blood count	Liver enzyme profile
Prothromibin time	Viral serology
Urea and electrolytes	Serum/urine for toxicology
Glucose	Urine – microscopy/culture
Arterial blood gases	Ascites – microscopy/culture
Blood cultures	protein/amylase
Paracetamol level	cytology

Ideally, fluid replacement should be a combination of dextrose and blood as any solution containing sodium chloride will result in the formation of ascites. However, if the patient has, or is suspected of having, haemorrhagic shock then resuscitation should follow the structured approach of two litres of balanced salt solution followed by blood. The ascites can be treated later. The use of fresh frozen plasma or vitamin K should be governed by the clotting screen results.

Thus the initial management of the shocked patient with acute liver failure follows conventional guidelines. Providing that airway breathing, and circulation are adequately dealt with then no new disability problems will arise. If, however, there is a deterioration in the neurological status and hypoglycaemia has been excluded, the patient should be treated for hepatic encephalopathy with oral lactulose in sufficient quantities to produce several loose stools per day. The patient should be managed in a high dependency or intensive treatment unit in combination with an intensivist.

In the patient with acute liver disease there is no difference in either monitoring or requested investigations when compared with the structured approach. However, it is prudent to request acute virology and paracetamol levels. Liaise with gastroenterologists or hepatologists regarding other tests to identify the cause of the liver dysfunction. Furthermore, if acute liver dysfunction is associated with pregnancy then an obstetrician needs to be part of the management team.

Key point
Initial management of a patient with liver failure includes treating hypoxaemia, hypovolaemia, and hypoglycaemia. Specialist personnel should also be requested depending upon the potential underlying problem.

DEFINITIVE CARE

Early liaison with a specialist hepatology unit will be guided by the local gastroenterologist. The important issues in this final stage of management are listed in the box.

> **Important issues in the definitive care of liver failure**
>
> 1. Treatment of vasodilatation and increasing oxygen uptake
> 2. Prevention or treatment of cerebral oedema
> 3. Treatment of coexistent renal failure with haemofiltration
> 4. Temporary hepatic support versus emergency transplant

Outcome measures

Many features will dictate the outcome.

- The shorter the interval between onset of jaundice and hepatic encephalopathy, the better the outcome.
- Severe hepatic encephalopathy is associated with a poor prognosis.

Summary

Irrespective of the cause of either acute or acute on chronic liver failure, the initial management is the same. Treat hypoxia, hypovolaemia, and hypoglycaemia (the three Hs). Early liaison with a gastroenterologist/hepatologist is necessary.

ENDOCRINE FAILURE

Introduction

Of all conditions that are associated with endocrine failure the two that cause most concern are related to hyperglycaemia and adrenocortical insufficiency. The latter may be related to either a primary adrenal problem or secondary to pituitary pathology.

HYPERGLYCAEMIC STATES: DIABETIC KETOACIDOSIS

> **Causes of diabetic ketoacidosis**
>
> - New presentation of insulin dependent diabetes
> - Known insulin dependent diabetes – inappropriate reduction in insulin
>   coexistent infection
>   surgery
>   myocardial infarction
>   emotional stress

> **Key point**
> Consider ketoacidosis in any ill diabetic especially if there is vomiting or tachypnoea
>
> - Never diagnose primary hyperventilation until diabetic ketoacidosis has been excluded
> - Always exclude ketoacidosis in patients who are confused, comatosed or have a metabolic acidosis

Initial management

This follows the structured approach. The patient will be receiving oxygen and appropriate fluid therapy, especially if they are hypotensive. An initial glucometer reading will be confirmed with a formal blood glucose. Urine testing for ketones is necessary.

> **Key point**
> Suspect hyperosmolar non-ketotic coma (HONK) in patients who are hyperglycaemic with low urinary ketones

As soon as an elevated blood glucose is identified the patient should receive 10 units of intravenous soluble insulin whilst an infusion is being prepared. Subsequent management is facilitated by central venous access.

Additional treatment in the primary assessment

- Insulin infusion: make up a solution of 50 units of soluble insulin in 50 ml of normal saline, i.e. one unit per millilitre. This should be administered intravenously at a rate of 6 ml per hour. The blood glucose usually falls by approximately 5 mmol/hour.

> **Key point**
> In the presence of persistent ketonuria ensure that 10% dextrose is the fluid replacement of choice combined with insulin at six units per hour to ensure total metabolic correction

Once the blood sugar is less than 15 mmol/l then the patient can be changed to soluble insulin three times per day or the normal regime restarted, ensuring an adequate intake of calories.

- Fluid replacement: patients with diabetic ketoacidosis are profoundly dehydrated and an initial fluid challenge of 1 litre of normal saline should be given over 30 minutes. This should be followed by a second litre over one hour and then followed by litre bags over two, four and eight hours. When the patient's serum glucose is less than 15 mmol/l the infusion should be changed to 10% dextrose unless the patient has coexistent hypovolaemia when saline should also be administered.
- Potassium replacement: potassium should not be given in the first 2 litres of fluid. However, subsequently 20 mmol should be added to each bag but only if the serum potassium is less than 5 mmol/l. In contrast if the serum potassium is less than 3 mmol/l then 40 mmol of potassium should be added.

> **Key point**
> Hypokalaemia is a potential cause of death in patients being treated for diabetic ketoacidosis

- Bicarbonate: this should only be given if the arterial pH is less than 6·9. A 50 ml aliquot should be administered over 30 minutes followed by arterial blood gas samples.
- Antibiotic therapy: always examine carefully for the presence of an underlying infection. Never forget to check the feet and perineum.

If sepsis is suspected, but no primary site found then give a broad spectrum antibiotic such as ceftriaxone 1 g. The subsequent choice of antibiotic will be influenced by the results of urine and blood cultures.

Key point

A raised white count in a patient with diabetic ketoacidosis does not indicate an underlying infection

Patients who have diabetic ketoacidosis are at an increased risk of thromboembolic complications. They should therefore be anticoagulated with heparin according to local policy.

Monitoring

In addition to that described in the primary assessment, the minimum specific monitoring of a patient with diabetic ketoacidosis is summarised in the box.

Monitoring progress in diabetic ketoacidosis

- 15 minute checks: Glasgow Coma Scale, pulse and blood pressure
- 1 hourly checks: glucometer, urine output and central venous pressure
- 2 hourly checks: blood glucose until less than 20 mmol/l
- 4 hourly checks: plasma potassium, arterial pH or venous bicarbonate

---

Change over from insulin infusion to subcutaneous injection

The insulin infusion should be continued until urinary ketones are negative. Most patients will be tolerating a normal diet by this stage and it is therefore safe to convert to subcutaneous insulin. However, the infusion should be continued for approximately 60 minutes after the first subcutaneous dose. In the newly diagnosed diabetic, start with short acting soluble insulin three times per day before meals. After 24 hours it should be possible to estimate the total daily insulin dose. This should then be subsequently administered as two thirds of the daily dose before breakfast and the remainder before supper. Each dose should comprise half of soluble insulin and half of intermediate acting insulin. Glucometer readings should be taken before breakfast, lunch, and dinner, and the insulin should be adjusted accordingly.

In contrast, known diabetic patients can be restarted on their normal insulin regime; however, they should be monitored in case this has to be amended.

HYPEROSMOLAR NON-KETOTIC HYPERGLYCAEMIA

Key point

This diagnosis is considered in any patient with severe hyperglycaemia, dehydration, and drowsiness

Key point
Hyperosmolar non-ketotic coma is differentiated from diabetic ketoacidosis by:

- blood glucose greater than 30 mmol/l but only 1+ or absence of ketonuria
- plasma osmolality greater than 350 mosmol/kg

The patient with hyperosmolar non-ketotic hyperglycaemia is usually elderly but the management should follow the guidelines for diabetic ketoacidosis with the following exceptions.

- Half normal saline is used for fluid replacement if the plasma sodium is greater than 145 mmol/l. Insulin sensitivity is greater in the absence of severe acidosis, therefore, the infusion should be started at 3 ml per hour.
- The risk of thromboembolism is high; therefore the patient should be formally anti-coagulated with heparin according to local policy unless there are contraindications.
- Total potassium is low and plasma level is more variable.

ACUTE ADRENAL INSUFFICIENCY

Key point
This diagnosis should be considered in any patient with:

- unexplained hypotension
- mild hyponatraemia
- corticosteroid therapy
- pigmentation
- preceding anorexia, vomiting, diarrhoea, and weight loss

The causes of adrenal insufficiency are listed in the box.

Causes of acute adrenal insufficiency

- Rapid withdrawal of chronic corticosteroid therapy
- Sepsis or surgical stress in patients with chronic adrenal dysfunction from:
    chronic corticosteroid therapy
    autoimmune adrenalitis
- Rare causes such as tuberculosis, age related infection with cytomegalovirus and adrenal metastases
- Bilateral adrenal haemorrhage (rare) secondary to fulminant meningococcal septicaemia or anticoagulant therapy
- Sepsis or surgical stress in patients with hypopituitarism

Key management issues

The patient will be treated appropriately by the structured approach, according to their presenting symptoms especially if they are comatosed, hypotensive or confused. Remember that the patient may be hypoglycaemic. As soon as the diagnosis of acute adrenal insufficiency is suspected give 100 mg of intravenous hydrocortisone immediately followed by 100 mg three times per day.

The urgent investigations will not differ from those normally requested in the primary assessment. A random cortisol and adrenocorticotrophic hormone (ACTH) measurement may provide supportive evidence of the clinical diagnosis, but the latter should be confirmed by a short Synacthen® test providing the patient is receiving dexamethasone and not hydrocortisone.

The typical biochemical findings in acute adrenal insufficiency are low sodium (120–130 mmol/l), raised potassium (5–7 mmol/l), raised urea (>6.5 mmol/l), and low glucose.

Key point
Patients with acute adrenal insufficiency do not always exhibit classic biochemical features

---

Intravenous fluid replacement, dextrose and hydrocortisone should continue until the patient is asymptomatic. A maintenance therapy can then be instituted with hydrocortisone 20 mg in the morning and 10 mg at night. Fludrocortisone is not always necessary and will be co-prescribed according to local policy or if the patient is hypotensive.

SUMMARY

Diabetic emergencies are common in medical practice. Consider hyperglycaemia in all patients who are hyperventilating, confused, comatosed or acidotic. Fluid replacement and intravenous insulin are the essential therapy.

Acute adrenal insufficiency should be suspected in any patient who has unexplained hypotension, mild hyponatraemia, corticosteroid therapy, pigmentation or preceding anorexia, nausea, vomiting, and weight loss. The mainstay of therapy is to provide adequate inspired oxygenation and fluid replacement while increasing the serum glucose (if required) and providing intravenous hydrocortisone replacement.

TIME OUT 19.1

List the causes of:
(i)   respiratory failure
(ii)   cardiac failure
(iii) brain failure
(iv)   renal failure
(v)   liver failure
(vi)   endocrine failure
For each cause list the underlying problems, e.g. hypoxaemia, hypovolaemia.
Note how common problems occur, irrespective of the cause, and how and when these problems will be treated in the initial assessment.

SUMMARY

Organ failure is a common medical emergency. Initial treatment is directed at the manifestations of failure, rather than at the underlying cause.

SPECIAL CIRCUMSTANCES

CHAPTER

20

The elderly patient

OBJECTIVES

After reading this chapter you will be able to understand:

- why age does not influence the structured approach to patient assessment
- how age influences the disease pathophysiology
- how age influences homeostasis
- the special considerations that have to be taken when assessing and managing an acutely ill elderly patient.

INTRODUCTION

Defining "elderly" is not easy. Some patients in their 60s are physiologically older than those in their 80s. In general, "elderly" characteristics become more prevalent after the age of 75 years.

When the elderly become acutely unwell, assessment and treatment will follow the structured approach previously described. However, the elderly differ in a number of ways which may affect assessment and treatment.

MULTIPLE CONDITIONS

The prevalence of most disease increases with increasing age. The elderly, therefore, tend to have multiple conditions. In addition to any acute presenting problem, there are usually other coexisting chronic disorders. These make assessment more difficult and may influence prognosis and management.

Key point
Multiple pathology is the rule in the elderly

NON-SPECIFIC/ATYPICAL PRESENTATION

Illness in the elderly often presents with confusion, falls, immobility or incontinence, rather than the typical pattern seen in a younger population, e.g.

- pneumonia is equally as likely to present with either confusion or pleuritic pain and breathlessness
- cardiac failure may present with confusion or falls rather than breathlessness.

The reasons for this are multiple. The physiological and pathological changes associated with ageing produce a reduction in physical and mental reserves. Under normal circumstances, the elderly person is able to function satisfactorily with these limited reserves, remaining mobile, continent, and mentally clear. However, with the additional stress of an acute illness these abilities may be overcome. Consequently, confusion, falls, immobility, and incontinence are common presenting features.

Acute myocardial infarction, pleurisy or acute abdominal emergencies may not present with pain in the elderly. Possible reasons for this include:

- reduced perception of visceral pain
- multiple pathology – diminished awareness of a symptom amongst a complex of symptoms
- associated mental impairment or communication difficulties.

> **Key point**
> Any acute medical problem in the elderly can present with confusion, falls, immobility or incontinence. An acute abdomen or acute myocardial infarction may be painless

POLYPHARMACY AND ALTERED DRUG HANDLING

Adverse drug reactions are an important cause of morbidity, even mortality, in older people.

> **Key point**
> Approximately one in ten older patients will experience an adverse drug reaction. This may either precipitate their admission to or follow treatment in hospital

Factors underlying adverse drug reactions are complex (see Figure 20.1). Old people usually have multiple conditions which gives more opportunity for prescribing and may lead to polypharmacy.

The elderly may have impaired hearing, eyesight, memory, and manual dexterity which can affect their ability to follow a prescribed drug regime (reduced compliance).

Polypharmacy, especially if the drug regime is complex, is also associated with reduced compliance.

A number of changes in pharmacokinetics and pharmacodynamics occur with increasing age.

- Reduced renal clearance – increases the risk of toxicity for water soluble drugs excreted by the kidney (especially digoxin, gentamicin).

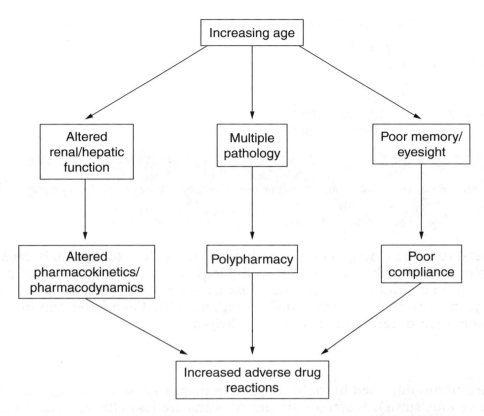

Figure 20.1 Factors underlying adverse drug reactions in the elderly

- Reduced hepatic clearance – reduces first-pass metabolism for certain drugs, increasing the likelihood of adverse effects (important for propranolol and morphine). Reduced activity of hepatic mixed-function oxidase causes a decline in clearance of diazepam and chlordiazepoxide.
- Altered body composition – there is a relative increase in body fat and a reduction in body water (associated with the reduction in lean body mass) with increasing age. This results in a reduced volume of distribution for water soluble drugs and an increased volume of distribution for lipid soluble drugs. Therefore, following a given dose of digoxin (based on body weight), a higher serum level is achieved in the elderly compared with the young. The increased volume of distribution for lipid soluble drugs (diazepam, chlordiazepoxide, thiopental) increases the amount of drug bound in body fat and increases the half-life of these drugs.
- Reduced protein levels – may be important with some drugs which bind to albumin.
- Increased sensitivity – has been demonstrated with opiates and benzodiazepines. The elderly require lower doses of warfarin to achieve anticoagulation, without any demonstrable changes in warfarin pharmacokinetics.

Some drugs which are commonly associated with adverse effects in the elderly include the following.

Digoxin

There is an age related decline in renal function. Therefore the body is less able to excrete digoxin and hence levels may rise. The levels required to produce both a therapeutic effect and toxicity are very close. Thus, there is a significant risk of toxicity with increasing age and any intercurrent illness.

The adverse effects of digoxin are multiple and may be life threatening, for example:

- cardiac   arrhythmias
- gastrointestinal   anorexia
  nausea/vomiting
  diarrhoea
- neurological   confusion/agitation
  visual disturbance.

> **Key point**
> Be suspicious of digoxin toxicity in any patient on digoxin who develops anorexia, vomiting or confusion

As a general rule, the elderly require a reduced loading dose of digoxin because of the reduced volume of distribution (0·5 mg compared with 1·0 mg in younger patients). They also require a reduced maintenance dose because of the reduced renal clearance (125 micrograms or 62·5 micrograms daily compared with 250 micrograms in a younger patient). Estimation of serum digoxin levels is helpful.

Diuretics

Diuretics are commonly used in the elderly, often inappropriately (for leg oedema associated with venous stasis). Homeostatic mechanisms are less efficient (see later). Thus patients taking diuretics are more prone to dehydration, metabolic disturbances, and postural hypotension, especially when there is intercurrent illness.

Antihypertensives

The use of antihypertensives is increasing in the elderly. These drugs are more likely to cause adverse effects, particularly postural hypotension, because of impaired homeostasis.

Non-steroidal antiinflammatory drugs

Non-steroidal antiinflammatory drugs (NSAIDs) are responsible for a quarter to a third of hospital admissions for gastrointestinal bleeding in older people. They can cause renal failure, fluid retention, and worsening of heart failure.

Sedatives and hypnotics

Drowsiness and falls are caused by sedatives and hypnotics. Their half-life tends to be prolonged (due to increased volume of distribution and reduced hepatic clearance of diazepam and chlordiazepoxide). The elderly are more sensitive to the effects of sedatives and hypnotics. Withdrawal reactions are common if these drugs are stopped abruptly. An acute confusional state a couple of days after admission may be the first indication that the patient had been taking sleeping tablets.

Antidepressants

Common side effects from tricyclic antidepressants include postural hypotension, confusion, dry mouth, and also urinary retention in males. The newer selective seretonin reuptake inhibitors (SSRI) antidepressants are less likely to cause side effects.

Major tranquillisers

Phenothiazines and haloperidol commonly cause side effects including drowsiness, unsteadiness, postural hypotension, constipation, and drug-induced Parkinsonism.

Treatment for Parkinson's disease

Levodopa preparations are associated with a high prevalence of side effects, mainly postural hypotension, confusion, and dyskinesia. Anticholinergic drugs are even more likely to cause confusion.

Key points
- An accurate drug history is essential
- Always be suspicious that any new problem may be a side effect of an existing medication, rather than an indication for additional drug therapy
- The drug regime should be as simple as possible (in terms of the number and the frequency of dosing) to improve compliance and reduce the risk of adverse reactions
- When introducing new drugs, start with a low dose and increase slowly. Review regularly. Always question whether a particular drug is needed. If it is, what would be the correct dose?

IMPAIRED HOMEOSTASIS

This is important in a number of ways. Postural hypotension due to impaired blood pressure control is mentioned in Chapter 12. Two other important areas are fluid and electrolyte imbalance and temperature homeostasis.

Fluid and electrolyte imbalance

A number of changes occur with increasing age which affect sodium and water homeostasis increasing the risk of fluid and electrolyte disturbance. These changes include:

- a reduction in renal blood flow
- loss of nephrons
- impaired ability to
    excrete an extreme sodium load
    conserve sodium, etc.
    concentrate urine
    excrete a water load
- total body water decreases with age (associated with the reduction in lean body mass)
- thirst declines with age
- levels of plasma renin and aldosterone are reduced (although no changes in angiotensin II concentrations have been found). This probably contributes to the reduced ability to preserve sodium when necessary

Fluid and electrolyte imbalance can be exacerbated by increased fluid loss (diarrhoea and/or vomiting) and reduced fluid intake (which is more likely to cause serious metabolic disturbance). Water replacement is less effective because of the reduced sensation of thirst. The elderly have impaired water conservation. In addition the reduced total body water means the patient starts from a lower baseline and that dehydration occurs more readily.

Temperature homeostasis

Core body temperature is held within a narrow range around 37°C. Heat is generated in most tissues of the body and lost by radiation, convection, conduction, and evaporation. The balance between heat production and heat loss is regulated by the hypothalamus.

If the core temperature rises, the hypothalamus is perfused by "heated" blood and responds by causing cutaneous vasodilatation and sweating. This allows increased heat loss.

In contrast if the core temperature falls, the hypothalamus increases core heat production (increased muscle tone with shivering) and reduces heat loss from the skin (cutaneous vasoconstriction). In the elderly these processes are impaired because of:

- a delayed vasoconstrictor response to cold
- a smaller increase in metabolic heat production (probably due to the reduced muscle bulk)
- a decline in the perception of cold, which affects behavioural responses, for example wearing extra clothes, seeking shelter.

Key point

Homeostatic mechanisms are less efficient in the elderly. The stress of an acute illness, or the effects of drugs, are more likely to be associated with postural hypotension, fluid and electrolyte disturbance, and temperature control

The main clinical manifestation of impaired temperature homeostasis seen in the United Kingdom is hypothermia.

HYPOTHERMIA

Introduction

Hypothermia is defined as a core body temperature of 35°C or less. The true prevalence is unclear. Mortality is high, especially in the elderly, with estimates varying from 30 to 75%.

Multiple factors usually contribute to hypothermia. The elderly are at particular risk because of impaired temperature homeostasis. Other important factors include:

- physical – poor mobility, risk of falling
- social – living alone, inadequate heating
- medical conditions – affecting heat production, heat loss or temperature control
- drugs/alcohol – phenothiazines cause vasodilatation and act directly on the temperature control centre in the hypothalamus. Benzodiazepines, antidepressants, and opioids act centrally and may increase the risk of falling. Alcohol will predispose to hypothermia by inhibiting shivering, impairing hepatic gluconeogenesis, and inducing peripheral vasodilatation.

The causes of hypothermia are listed in the box.

Causes of hypothermia

- **Excessive heat loss**
  - environmental exposure
  - increased cutaneous blood flow
- **Inadequate heat production**
  - malnutrition
  - hypoglycaemia
  - hypothyroidism
  - diabetic ketoacidosis
  - adrenal insufficiency
  - hepatic failure
  - uraemia
- **Altered thermoregulation**
  - hypothalamic dysfunction
  - spinal cord injury T1 or above
- **Drugs**
  (i) Central effects
  - alcohol
  - phenothiazines
  - barbiturates
  - opioids
  - benzodiazepines
  (ii) Peripheral vasodilatation
  - alcohol
  - phenothiazines

Pathophysiology

Mild hypothermia (35–32°C)

The initial response to a fall in temperature is to increase the metabolic rate by shivering and to reduce heat loss by peripheral vasoconstriction. Even at this early stage, psychomotor function can be impaired, especially in the elderly, manifested by confusion, dysarthria, and incoordination.

Moderate hypothermia (32–28°C)

As the core temperature falls below 32°C, cardiac conduction becomes impaired, heart rate falls and cardiac output decreases. Atrial fibrillation with a slow ventricular response is common. In addition shivering stops and is replaced by hypertonia. Coma may develop.

Severe hypothermia (below 28°C)

There is a high risk of ventricular fibrillation. As the temperature continues to fall, hypotension results and eventually asystole occurs. In severe hypothermia, coma may be associated with a flat electroencephalogram but this is not indicative of brain death and may be reversible.

In addition to these cardiovascular and neurological effects, hypothermia has other important effects.

Respiratory

Respiratory effects include tachypnoea in the early stages, followed by hypoventilation as hypothermia becomes more severe. Loss of cough and gag reflex predisposes to aspiration pneumonia.

Renal

A "cold diuresis" occurs, due to increased central blood volume (peripheral vasoconstriction shunting blood from peripheral to central circulation) and associated release of antidiuretic hormone. There may be additional sodium and water losses due to impaired function of epithelial transport mechanisms in the kidney. The result is severe volume depletion and hypotension.

Gastrointestinal

Hypomotility is common and gastric dilatation may occur with increased risk of aspiration. Hypothermia may cause acute pancreatitis and acute peptic ulceration with haematemesis.

Haematological

The haemoconcentration associated with the reduced plasma volume may predispose to thrombotic complications. In addition there may be bleeding problems. Clotting factors work less efficiently at lower temperatures and thrombocytopenia may occur due to sequestration of platelets.

Impaired oxygen delivery

As the temperature falls, the haemoglobin oxygen dissociation curve shifts to the left. Thus oxygen delivery to hypothermic tissues is impaired. However, hypothermia also reduces the tissues' oxygen requirements.

Hyperglycaemia

Moderate to severe hypothermia inhibits the action of insulin. This leads to reduced glucose utilisation and hyperglycaemia.

Assessment

Primary assessment and resuscitation
Airway

- Airway may be obstructed due to depressed conscious level.

Breathing

- Respiratory rate reduced with moderate/severe hypothermia.
- May be evidence of aspiration pneumonia (although slow shallow breathing may make clinical signs difficult to detect).

Circulation

- Check blood pressure. Treat hypotension due to hypovolaemia ("cold diuresis"). Caution with rate of fluid replacement as the cold myocardium does not tolerate excessive fluid loads.
- Check core temperature with a low reading thermometer or rectal thermocouple probe. Initiate rewarming measures.
- Check pulse for 60 seconds.
- ECG monitoring (risk of atrial fibrillation (AF), ventricular fibrillation (VF), asystole).

Disability

- Neurological dysfunction may be either the cause or the effect of hypothermia.
- Check glucose.

Rewarming

Rewarming techniques can be active or passive, and active rewarming can be external or internal. Which method is most appropriate will depend on a number of considerations including the degree of hypothermia, the rate of development of hypothermia, the age of the patient and the patient's cardiovascular status. A young person who is hypothermic due to cold exposure will usually tolerate rapid, active, surface rewarming. In contrast, this will lead to circulatory collapse in an elderly patient. An ideal rate of rewarming is 0.5°C per hour. In the presence of cardiac arrest, core temperature must be raised as rapidly as possible. However, if the patient does not have a life threatening arrhythmia, interventions aimed at rapid rewarming should be used with caution to minimise the risk of precipitating arrhythmias.

Key point
The hypothermic myocardium is very sensitive. Any physical manipulation of the patient (central lines, nasogastric tubes, endotracheal tubes, rapid rewarming techniques) increases the risk of developing ventricular fibrillation. This is resistant to defibrillation until the core temperature has risen to 32°C.

Passive rewarming

This uses the patient's own heat production to raise core temperature. Any wet clothing is removed and the patient is dried and then insulated with blankets. It is important to keep the head covered as up to 30% of body heat can be lost from this site. Warm humidified oxygen minimises respiratory heat loss.

Active external rewarming

Immersion in warm water (40°C) can be appropriate in conscious uninjured patients with a core temperature of greater than 30°C, where hypothermia has been of short duration and rapid onset. However, it is inappropriate and impractical for the majority of hypothermic patients. Circulating water blankets, electric blankets, warm air blankets, and heating cradles are less efficient than warm water immersion but more practical. There are a number of potential dangers with active external rewarming. When hypothermia has developed slowly and has been prolonged, there is hypovolaemia due to "cold diuresis" and profound acidosis in the underperfused peripheral tissues. The vasodilatation caused by external heating may therefore cause hypotension and a metabolic acidosis. Active external rewarming also causes a significant "afterdrop" in core temperature that can potentially trigger arrhythmias.

Active internal rewarming

Intravenous fluids should be heated to 40°C but their small volume means that they have a minimal effect on core temperature. Inspired humidified air heated to 42°C minimises respiratory heat loss but contributes little to active rewarming. Irrigation of hollow organs (stomach, bladder) and body cavities (pleura, peritoneum) with warm fluid (40°C) can be used in extreme conditions, such as cardiac arrest, but may need to be continued for several hours. Irrigation fluids should be isotonic and potassium free. Haemodialysis and cardiopulmonary bypass can bring about rapid rewarming but they require specialised skills and availability is limited.

Management of arrhythmias

Atrial arrhythmias are common and usually reversible with rewarming alone; specific antiarrhythmic therapy is rarely needed. Ventricular arrhythmias in the hypothermic patient are usually refractory to drugs and defibrillation. Antiarrhythmic drugs should not be used until the body temperature is normal. Below 32°C, defibrillation is unlikely to succeed. Therefore, the initial three shocks of the ventricular fibrillation algorithm should be given but, if unsuccessful, further attempts should be withheld until the temperature is greater than 32°C. Repeated defibrillation in the hypothermic patient will simply cause myocardial damage.

It is difficult to distinguish reversible from irreversible hypothermia. Apnoea, asystole and absence of brain activity are usually signs of death but can also be present in severe reversible hypothermia. Patients should continue with cardiopulmonary resuscitation until a deep body temperature of at least 32°C has been achieved or the temperature has failed to rise despite effort. Only then can a definite diagnosis of death be made.

> **Key point**
> The patient is not dead until both warm and dead

Secondary assessment

In all hypothermic patients chest X-ray and 12 lead ECG are essential. ECG may show "J" waves although they have no prognostic significance. Check urea and electrolytes, amylase, glucose, and thyroid function, together with drug screen and alcohol estimation. Arterial blood gases will need to be corrected for the low core temperature. Take blood cultures and start empirical broad spectrum antibiotic therapy, as the usual signs of infection may be masked.

Once rewarming has been initiated and the patient stabilised, reassess for any underlying condition that may have precipitated the hypothermia.

Summary

- Hypothermia is a life threatening condition.
- It is often associated with other life threatening conditions.
- Assessment and treatment follows the structured approach previously described.
- The rate of rewarming needs to be adjusted according to the clinical situation.
- Ventricular fibrillation or circulatory collapse can be precipitated by rapid rewarming techniques.
- The patient is not dead until both warm and dead.

TIME OUT 20.1

The percentage of elderly hospital admissions associated with drug side effects is:

(a) 1%
(b) 4%
(c) 10%

SUMMARY

In the elderly patient:

- assessment follows the structured approach.
- multiple conditions are common.
- disturbances in mobility, mental function, and continence are common presentations of many conditions.

CHAPTER

21

Transportation of the seriously ill patient

OBJECTIVES

After reading this chapter you will be able to:

- discuss the principles necessary for the safe transfer and retrieval of critically ill patients
- describe the systematic "ACCEPT" approach for managing such patients.

INTRODUCTION

Key point
Transport is a potential period of instability

There is an increasing need to transfer patients who are medically ill. Historically, patients are often transferred from home to hospital by ambulance and this will continue. However, with changes in the provision of health care more patients are being transferred because of the following:

- reduction in number of and increased pressure on hospital beds
- transfer for tertiary care, e.g. neurosurgery, cardiothoracic surgery
- intensive care treatment either for supraspecialist care or beds.

Thus it is common for patients to be transferred between hospitals, because of a bed shortage in one region or throughout the United Kingdom. It is important to remember that the transfer distance is irrelevant. Movement from one ward to another is just as important, and can be associated with just as many problems, as a transfer over 500 miles.

PRINCIPLES OF SAFE TRANSFER

The aim of a safe transfer policy is to ensure that there is continuing medical treatment for the patient without any detrimental effect. To achieve this the **right** patient has to be

309

taken at the **right** time, by the **right** people, to the **right** place by the **right** form of transport. This requires a systematic approach that incorporates a high level of planning and preparation **before** the patient is moved.

The systematic approach to patient transfer

A – assess the situation
C – control the situation
C – communication
E – evaluate the need for transfer
P – package and prepare
T – transportation

By following the ACCEPT approach, appropriate procedures are done in the correct order and are not forgotten. The acronym also emphasises the need for a great deal of preparation before the patient is transported.

ASSESSMENT

The clinician involved with patient management does not always accompany the patient during transfer. It is therefore important that the transportation procedure begins with assessing the situation. This is helped by answering several key questions.

Assessment questions

- What are the patient's basic details?
- What is the problem?
- What has been done?
- What was the effect?
- What is needed now?

The clinician should also determine the lines of responsibility, not only for the patient before transfer, but also during any future transportation. In practice this is usually jointly held by the referring consultant clinician, the receiving consultant clinician and the transfer personnel. However, there should be a named person with overall responsibility to organise the transfer.

Conditions requiring transfer

There is an increasing need to transfer patients who require active resuscitation. Some of the more frequent medical conditions needing transfer between hospitals are listed in the box.

Conditions requiring transfer

Breathing	Asthma
	Respiratory failure
	Pneumothoraces
Circulation	Unstable angina – awaiting angioplasty
	Myocardial infarction
	Dysrhythmia (either brady or tachy)
	Sepsis
	Variceal haemorrhage
	Acute liver failure
	Renal failure necessitating dialysis
Disability	Carbon monoxide poisoning
	Poisoning/overdose
	Intracerebral haemorrhage
	Intracranial abscess
	Intracranial tumour
	Myasthenia gravis
	Guillain–Barré syndrome

Potential problems during transfer

From the above list of conditions requiring transfer, one can predict potential problems that may arise – as in any clinical practice. For reference these will be listed in the following seven boxes.

Potential cardiac problems

	Primary
Airway	Hypoxaemia
Breathing	Hypercarbia
Circulation	Myocardial infarction
	Dysrhythmia
	Cardiac failure (either left or right or biventricular)
	Rupture of papillary or ventricular muscle
	Cardiac tamponade
	Pulmonary embolus
Disability	Deterioration in Glasgow Coma Score
	Secondary
	Pain
	Peripheral embolus

Most cardiac patients requiring transfer will receive appropriate analgesia and anti-coagulation or thrombolysis before transfer. The two most likely problems during transfer are either dysrhythmia, including cardiac arrest, or cardiac failure. Management of any dysrhythmia should follow the guidelines specified by the European and United Kingdom Resuscitation Councils (see Chapter 6). In contrast, the presence of cardiac failure would require either treatment with venodilators or inotropes (left or biventricular failure) or with a fluid challenge (right ventricular failure).

311

Potential respiratory problems	
Airway	Hypoxaemia
Breathing	Hypercarbia
	Severe bronchospasm
	Acute/chronic respiratory failure
	Respiratory arrest
Circulation	Cardiac arrest

It is unusual for patients to develop these problems during transfer, as the potential for deterioration should have been recognised. Thus most patients are sedated, paralysed, and ventilated – but this is not always the case.

Patients with neurological conditions are commonly transferred to a tertiary referral centre, as most hospitals do not have the relevant facilities. The potential problems encountered are listed in the box.

Potential neurological problems	
Airway	Hypoxaemia
Breathing	Hypercarbia
	Respiratory arrest
Circulation	Cardiac arrest
	Hypoglycaemia
	Hyponatraemia
Disability	Deterioration in Glasgow Coma Score
	Fit
	Subarachnoid haemorrhage

Similarly, most hospitals do not have facilities for managing patients with renal or hepatic disease. The relevant potential problems are listed in the next two boxes.

Potential renal problems	
Airway	Hypoxaemia
Breathing	Hypoxaemia
Circulation	Hypovolaemia
	Fluid overload
	Hypertension
	Dysrhythmia
	Metabolic acidosis
	Hyperkalaemia
Disability	Deterioration in Glasgow Coma Score
	Fit

Potential hepatic problems

Airway	Hypoxaemia
Breathing	Hypercarbia
Circulation	Hypovolaemia
	Hyponatraemia
	Hypokalaemia
	Hypoglycaemia
	Lactic acidosis
	Dysrhythmia
	Haemorrhage
Disability	Deterioration in Glasgow Coma Score
	Fit

Two other groups of patients that often require transfer are those who have taken an overdose or who are septic, and the associated problems are listed in the next two boxes.

Potential problems associated with overdose

Airway	Hypoxaemia
Breathing	Hypercarbia
Circulation	Hypovolaemia
	Haemorrhage
	Hypokalaemia
	Hypotension
Disability	Dysrhythmia
	Reduced Glasgow Coma Score
	Fit

Potential problems associated with a septic patient

Airway	Hypoxaemia
Breathing	Pulmonary oedema
Circulation	Hypovolaemia
	Haemorrhage
	Hypoglycaemia
	Disseminated intravascular coagulation
Disability	Reduced Glasgow Coma Score
	Fit

Although there is a broad spectrum of clinical conditions, there are clearly defined common potential problems, notably hypoxaemia, fluid balance, fitting, changes in Glasgow Coma Score and electrolyte disturbances. Thus once the patient's condition has been stabilised there is only a limited number of common complications. These will be prevented or reduced by ongoing treatment and monitoring. There are three major principles.

1. Do no further harm
2. Ensure ABCDE are maintained during transport
3. The most important assessment is the reassessment.

313

CONTROL

The person in charge needs to take control of the situation following the primary assessment (Chapter 3).

All immediately life threatening conditions need to be identified and treated and the patient monitored. The responsible clinician should also decide the most appropriate place for further management, for example, either in the resuscitation room or ward, or whether to move the patient to an area in the hospital with greater resources. A common example of this is moving a patient from the ward to a high dependency unit.

The secondary assessment includes a head to toe survey, perusal of the medical notes, and formulating a management plan by considering the clinical findings, response to treatment, and the results of any investigations. At the end of this phase it should be clear if transportation will be necessary.

COMMUNICATION

Moving ill patients from one place to another obviously requires the cooperation and involvement of several people. Therefore key personnel need to be informed when transportation is being considered, as shown in the next box.

Communication

- The patient's consultant
- Your consultant (if different from above)
- The intensive care unit consultant
- The patient's relatives
- The accepting consultant
- Ambulance control
- Special transportation controls (when appropriate)

It can be quite time consuming if all communication is delegated to one person. Therefore delegate the tasks up to appropriate people, taking into account their expertise and the local policies. In all cases it is important that information is passed on clearly and unambiguously. This is particularly true when talking to people over the telephone. A useful tip is to plan what you wish to say before telephoning and use the systematic summary shown in the box.

Communication plan

- Who you are
- What is needed from the listener
- What are the patient's basic details
- What is the problem
- What has been done
- What was the response
- What is needed

The second statement is repeated at the end to help summarise the situation and inform the listener what is required. The response to all these points should be documented in the patient's notes. The person in overall charge can then assimilate this information so that a proper evaluation of the patient's requirements for transportation can be made. In doing this, the clinician has to balance the risks involved in transfer against the risks of staying and the potential benefits of treatment from the receiving unit.

EVALUATION

Critically ill patients require transfer because of the need for:

- specialist treatment, such as haemodialysis
- specialist investigations unavailable in the referring hospital
- intensive care or high dependency unit facilities
- a bed.

Having identified the need for transfer, the responsible clinician has to triage the patient considering their priority in relation to other patients on the intensive care or high dependency unit, the urgency of transfer and the nature of the medical support required. Following acute life threatening illnesses or injuries, the patient may require urgent transfer after resuscitation, for example, the movement of a patient with a sub-arachnoid haemorrhage to the neurosurgical centre. In contrast, patients with organ failure may require less urgent transfer to a tertiary hospital. Under these circumstances, it may be possible to use the transfer team from the specialist centre. On occasions, when empty beds are scarce, it is possible to transfer a less critically ill patient rather than the one currently being dealt with. This obviously requires formal triage of the patients involved and it needs to be done by the consultants in charge of their care.

Triage

- Intensive care treatment
- Critical/ill – unstable
- Ill – stable
- Unwell
- Well

PACKAGE AND PREPARATION

Patient

Key point
Inadequate resuscitation will result in instability during transfer

---

To avoid complications during any journey, meticulous resuscitation and stabilisation should be done **before** transfer. This may involve procedures requested by the receiving hospital or unit. The transferring team must also ensure that the patient's airway is cleared, and appropriate respiratory support is being provided. In many cases this will mean intubating the patient if it has not been done previously. Blood gases should be taken following this procedure, or after a change in ventilator setting, to make sure that

315

the patient is maintaining an adequate PaO_2 (ideally more than 13 kPa) and $PaCO_2$ of 4·0–4·5 kPa.

> **Key point**
> Remember a patient with pulmonary pathology may take up to 15–20 minutes to stabilise on a new ventilator or ventilator setting

The ventilator obviously needs to be portable. In addition, it must be able to provide the functions the patient requires. This includes variable FiO_2, inspiratory/expiratory (I/E) ratio, respiratory rate, tidal volume and positive end expiratory pressure (PEEP). For safety there should also be a disconnect alarm and an ability to measure airway pressure. Those requiring intubation should be connected to an end tidal carbon dioxide monitor in addition to the basic monitoring equipment required for all patients.

> **Basic monitoring equipment**
>
> - Pulse oximetry
> - Suction
> - ECG, defibrillator
> - Blood pressure – preferably direct intraarterial monitoring
> - Thermometer
> - Urinary catheter
> - Naso/orogastric tube

Chest drains should be secured and unclamped with any underwater attachment being replaced by a Portex drainage bag.

> **Key point**
> Chest drains need to be inserted prophylactically if the patient has a simple pneumothorax or is at risk of developing one as a result of fractured ribs

Venous access is essential and preferably should be by two large bore cannula. The patient must receive adequate fluid resuscitation to ensure an optimal tissue oxygenation because this enables them to tolerate transfer better. Preferably the haematocrit should be over 30%. In some patients inotropic support may also be necessary. Before transfer invasive central monitoring may have been used to optimise volume replacement. During transfer, however, these lines become unreliable.

Appropriate drugs must be available to maintain the patient's airway, breathing, and circulation. This will require, in some circumstances, infusion pumps (with a backup power source).

The transfer team should confirm that all equipment is functioning, including battery charge status and oxygen availability, against what is calculated as necessary. The oxygen supply should be sufficient to last the maximum expected duration of the transfer with a reserve of 1–2 hours. There should also be a non-invasive blood pressure device and a self-reinflating bag (such as an Ambu Bag) so that resuscitation can be maintained in the event of either a power or gas failure. A member of the team should also be given the task of ensuring that all the patient's documents are taken. These include case notes, results of any investigations, and the transfer form. All lines and drains should then be secured to the patient and the patient secured to the trolley. The trolley should then be secured to the ambulance and positioned such that all monitors are visible and lines are accessible.

Transport – time/mode

The choice of transport needs to take into account several factors.

> **Factors involved with transport**
>
> - Nature of illness
> - Urgency of transfer
> - Mobilisation time
> - Geographical factors
> - Weather
> - Traffic conditions
> - Cost

Road ambulances are by far the most common means used in the United Kingdom. They have a low overall cost, rapid mobilisation time and are less affected by weather conditions. They also give rise to less physiological disturbance. Air transfer is used for journeys over 50 miles or two hours in duration or if road access is difficult. Although this mode of transport is fast, this has to be balanced against the organisational delays and the inter-vehicle transfer at the beginning and end of the journey. Helicopters are used for distances of approximately 50–150 miles and are particularly useful when road or fixed winged air ambulances are not possible. They are, however, often cramped, noisy and uncomfortable. Fixed winged aircraft should ideally be pressurised and are used for transfers of distances greater than 150 miles. Depending on the geographical location other forms of transport are used, particularly outside the United Kingdom. These include anything from a boat to horseback.

Personnel

In addition to the ambulance crew, a minimum of two attendants should accompany a critically ill patient. One attendant should be an experienced medical practitioner who is competent in resuscitation and organ support. Ideally this doctor should have received training in intensive care and transportation medicine. The Intensive Care Society (ICS) recommend at least two years' experience in anaesthesia, intensive care medicine or other equivalent specialties. The clinician must be accompanied by another experienced attendant who is usually a nurse. This person should be qualified with, ideally, two years' intensive care experience. All personnel should be competent in the transfer procedure and familiar with the patient's clinical condition. They should have adequate insurance to cover both death and disability occurring during transfer.

Personal equipment

In addition to the medical equipment described previously, the transfer team needs their own personal equipment.

Personal equipment

P – phone
E – enquiry number and name
R – revenue
S – safe clothing
O – organised route
N – nutrition
A – A–Z
L – lift home

This equipment will ensure that the journey is more comfortable and that a number of contingencies are available should problems occur. The telephone will enable direct communication with both the receiving and home unit. However, they should be given contact names and numbers before leaving. All personnel require appropriate clothing to ensure safety and enough money to enable them to get home should the ambulance be re-diverted to other duties. They also require a planned route and food if a long journey is envisaged.

TRANSPORTATION

Physiological problems during transfer can arise from both the patient's condition as well as the effects of movement. The latter include tipping, vibration, acceleration and deceleration forces, as well as barometric pressure and temperature changes seen with air transport. Adequate preparation can minimise many of these effects.

The standard of care and monitoring before transfer needs to continue. This will include SaO_2, ECG and arterial pressure monitoring. The end tidal carbon dioxide recording needs to be maintained in all patients who are intubated. Non-invasive arterial pressure monitor is sensitive to motion artefacts and therefore the intraarterial route is recommended. As mentioned previously, many of the central monitoring devices, such as central venous pressure or pulmonary artery wedge pressure, may be inaccurate due to movement of the ambulance.

The patient should be well covered and kept warm during the transfer. With ground transfer, road speed decisions depend both on clinical urgency and the availability of limited resources such as oxygen. Ambulance staff should therefore be advised whether a particularly smooth ride is required or a short journey time is important.

With adequate preparation, the transportation phase is usually incident free. Occasionally, untoward events occur; thus the patient must be reassessed using the structured approach. Appropriate corrective measures should then be taken. This reassessment has to be thorough and cannot be done when faced with excessive vehicular motion. Therefore, in the case of land vehicles ask the driver to stop at the first available place. Following such events it is important to communicate with the receiving unit. They can then be adequately prepared and may be able to provide ongoing advice. Again this communication should follow the systematic summary described previously. A continuous record of the patient's condition during the transfer should be made. This can be helped by having monitors with memory functions, which can be accessed later.

At the end of the transfer, the team should make direct contact with the receiving team. A verbal, succinct, systematic summary of the patient can then be provided. This must be accompanied by a written record of the patient's history, vital signs, treatment, and significant clinical events during transfer. All the other documents which have been taken with the patient should also be handed over. Whilst this is going on, the rest of the transferring team can help move the patient from the ambulance trolley to the receiving unit's bed. A copy of the transfer sheet should then be handed over with one copy retained by the transfer team who can then retrieve all their equipment and personnel for the return journey.

The data collection sheets should be subjected to regular audit by a designated consultant in each hospital. This will ensure transfers are appropriate and to the correct standards. Problems can also be addressed and corrected.

TIME OUT 21.1

A 27 year old mechanic presented with an occipital headache. A clinical diagnosis of subarachnoid haemorrhage is confirmed by CT scan and lumber puncture. The local neurosurgical centre is 30 miles away by road. The patient's vital signs are:

A – patent (FiO$_2$ 0·85)
B – rate 14 per minute
C – sinus tachycardia 110 per minute
BP 120/70
(IV access secured)
D – GCS 15/15; PERLA, no lateralising signs
glucose 7·0 mmol/l

Write down an outline of how you, as the doctor in charge, would arrange this patient's transfer to the neurosurgical centre.

SUMMARY

The safe transfer and retrieval of a patient requires a systematic approach. By following the ACCEPT method, important activities can be done at the appropriate time.

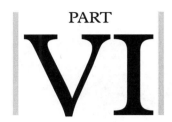

PART

VI

INTERPRETATION OF EMERGENCY INVESTIGATIONS

CHAPTER

22

Acid–base balance and blood gas analysis

OBJECTIVES

After reading this chapter you will be able to:

- describe the meanings of the common terms used in acid–base balance
- describe how the body removes carbon dioxide and acid
- explain the cause of an increased anion gap
- understand the system for interpreting a blood gas result.

TERMINOLOGY

It is important to understand the meaning of the terms commonly used when discussing acid–base balance.

Acids and bases

Originally the word "acid" was used to describe the sour taste of unripe fruit. Subsequently many different meanings have led to considerable confusion and mis-understanding. This was not resolved until 1923 when the following definition was proposed.

> An acid is any substance which is capable of providing hydrogen ions (H⁺)

A strong acid is a substance that will readily provide many hydrogen ions and conversely, a weak acid provides only a few. In the body we are mainly dealing with weak acids such as carbonic acid and lactic acid.

The opposite of an acid is a **base** and this is defined as any substance that "accepts" hydrogen ions. One of the commonest bases found in the body is bicarbonate (HCO_3^-).

The pH scale, acidosis/acidaemia, alkalosis and alkalaemia

The concentration of hydrogen ions in solution is usually **very** small, even with strong acids. This is particularly true when dealing with acids found in the body where the hydrogen ion concentrations are in the order of 40 nanomoles/litre (nmol/l).

> 1 nanomole = 1 billionth of a mole

To place this low concentration in perspective compare it with the concentration of other commonly measured electrolytes. For example, the plasma sodium is around **135 mmol/l**, i.e. 3 million times greater!

Dealing with such very small numbers is obviously difficult and so in 1909 the pH scale was developed. This scale has the advantage of being able to express any hydrogen ion concentration as a number between 1 and 14 inclusively. The pH of a normal arterial blood sample lies between 7·36 and 7·44 and is equivalent to a hydrogen ion concentration of 44–36 nanomoles/litre respectively.

It is important to realise that when using the pH scale, the numerical value **increases** as the concentration of hydrogen ions **decreases** (Figure 22.1). This is a consequence of the mathematical process that was used to develop the scale. Therefore an arterial blood pH below 7·36 indicates that the concentration of hydrogen ions has increased from normal. This is referred to as an **acidaemia**. Conversely, a pH above 7·44 would result from a reduction in the concentration of hydrogen ions. This condition is referred to as an **alkalaemia**.

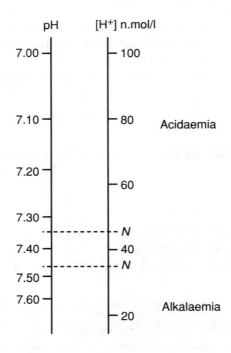

Figure 22.1   The hydrogen ion scale

Another important consequence of the derivation of the pH scale is that **small changes in pH mean relatively large changes in hydrogen ion concentration**; for example, a fall in the pH from 7·40 to 7·10 means the hydrogen ion concentration has risen from 40 to 80 nanomoles/litre, i.e. it has doubled.

Summary

- Hydrogen ions are only present in the body in very low concentrations.
- As the hydrogen ion concentration increases the pH falls.

- As the hydrogen ion concentration falls the pH rises.
- An acidaemia occurs when the pH falls below 7·36 and an alkalaemia occurs when it rises above 7·44.

> **Key point**
> Small changes in the pH scale represent large changes in the concentration of hydrogen ions

Buffers

Many of the complex chemical reactions occurring at a cellular level are controlled by special proteins called enzymes. These substances can only function effectively at very narrow ranges of pH (7·36–7·44). However, during normal activity the body produces massive amounts of hydrogen ions which if left unchecked would lead to significant falls in pH. Clearly a system is required to prevent these hydrogen ions causing large changes in pH before they are eliminated from the body. This is achieved by the "buffers". They "take up" the free hydrogen ions in the cells and in the blood stream, thereby preventing a change in pH.

There are a variety of buffers in the body. The main intracellular ones are proteins, phosphate, and haemoglobin. Extracellularly there are also plasma proteins and bicarbonate. Proteins "soak up" the hydrogen ions like a sponge and transport them to their place of elimination from the body, mainly the kidneys. In contrast, bicarbonate reacts with hydrogen ions to produce water and carbon dioxide.

$$H^+ + HCO_3^- \Leftrightarrow H_2O + CO_2$$

The carbon dioxide is subsequently removed by the lungs.

With these common terms defined, let us now consider why people can become acidaemic and how this can be corrected by the body.

ACID PRODUCTION AND ITS REMOVAL

All of us, whether we are healthy or ill, produce large amounts of water, acid, and carbon dioxide each day. A healthy adult will normally produce 15 000 000 nanomoles of hydrogen ions each day as waste products generated when food is metabolised to release energy. This process occurs at a cellular level where these products initially accumulate. If this was left unchecked irreparable cellular damage would result.

The first acute compensatory mechanism is the intracellular buffering system. As described previously, this provides the cell with a temporary way of minimising the fluctuations in acidity. Subsequently, these waste products (i.e. carbon dioxide and hydrogen ions) are excreted into the blood stream where they are taken up by the extracellular buffers (Figure 22.2).

However, this is only a temporary solution because there is only a limited amount of buffer. If this was the sum total of the body's defence to acids and carbon dioxide then the buffers would soon be exhausted, thereby allowing the products of metabolism to accumulate in the blood stream. A system is, therefore, needed to remove these harmful substances from the body so that they do not reach toxic levels and, at the same time, regenerate the buffers. Fortunately the body can eliminate these waste products removed by the lungs and the kidneys. Let us look at each of these in turn.

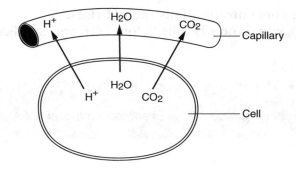

Figure 22.2 Removal of waste products from cells

Carbon dioxide removal (the respiratory component)

Carbon dioxide (CO_2) released from cells is transported in the blood to the lungs and, after diffusing into the alveoli, it is ultimately removed from the body during expiration (Figure 22.3).

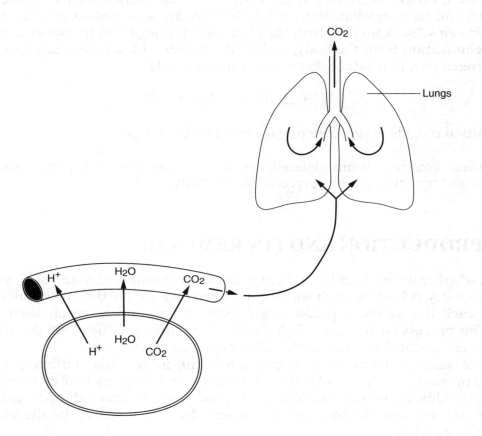

Figure 22.3 Removal of carbon dioxide by the lungs

If carbon dioxide is produced faster than it can be eliminated or there is a blockage to its removal, then it will accumulate in the blood stream. Here it reacts with water in the plasma to produce hydrogen ions (H^+) and bicarbonate (HCO_3^-):

$$CO_2 + H_2O \Leftrightarrow H^+ + HCO_3^-$$

The greater the amount of carbon dioxide, the more hydrogen ions are produced. If this increase in plasma concentration of hydrogen ions causes the pH to fall below 7·36 then an **acidaemia** has been produced. As the cause of the acidaemia in this case is a problem in the respiratory system, it is known as a **respiratory acidosis**.

If a sample of arterial blood was taken immediately this occurred then the result given in Table 22.1 would be obtained.

Table 22.1 Effect of a respiratory acidosis on blood gas analysis

	Normal values	Effect of a respiratory acidosis
pH	7·36–7·44	↓↓
$PaCO_2$	4·8–5·3 kPa	↑↑↑
	36–40 mm Hg	
HCO_3^-	21–27 mmol/l	↑

As a by-product of the reaction between carbon dioxide and water, the bicarbonate concentration also increases by the same amount as the hydrogen ions. However, this increase is usually in the order of several nanomoles. As the normal concentration is 21–27 mmoles (i.e. 21–27 **thousand** nanomoles) the net increase in bicarbonate is very small. Consequently these changes in concentration are enough to change the pH scale but are not large enough to alter significantly the plasma bicarbonate concentration.

In a normal person at rest, the respiratory component will excrete at least 12 000 000 nanomoles of hydrogen ions per day. It is therefore easy to see that there can be a rapid onset of acidosis during episodes of hypoventilation.

Acid removal (the metabolic component)

As has already been described, acids are continuously produced as a result of cellular metabolism. The amount produced from normal metabolism is approximately 3 000 000 nanomoles/day. This acid load is soaked up by buffers in the blood stream so that they can be transported safely for elimination (Figure 22.4).

One of the buffers is bicarbonate. This is generated by the kidneys and released into the blood stream where it reacts with free hydrogen (Figure 22.5).

In certain circumstances, so much acid is produced by the cells that it exceeds the capacity of the protein buffers and bicarbonate. If this results in an accumulation of free hydrogen ions in the plasma so that the pH falls below 7·36 then an acidaemia has been produced. As this is a result of a defect in the metabolic system, it is termed a metabolic acidosis.

If a sample of arterial blood was taken when this occurred then the result given in Table 22.2 would be obtained.

Table 22.2 Effect of a metabolic acidosis

	Normal values	Effect of a metabolic acidosis
pH	7·36–7·44	↓↓
$PaCO_2$	4·8–5·3 kPa	4·8–5·3 kPa
	36–40 mm Hg	36–40 mm Hg
HCO_3^-	21–27 mmol/l	↓

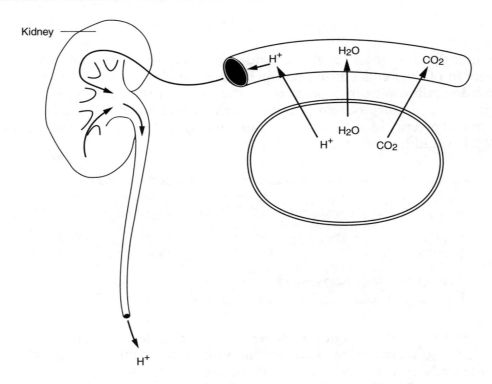

Figure 22.4   Removal of hydrogen ions by the kidney

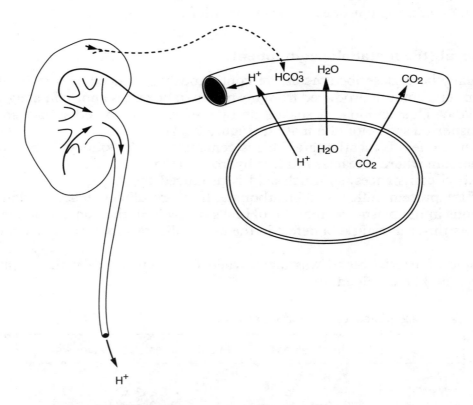

Figure 22.5   Release of bicarbonate into the blood

The bicarbonate level has fallen as a consequence of reacting with the free hydrogen ions to produce carbon dioxide and water.

Summary

- Carbon dioxide and acids are being produced continuously by cellular metabolism.
- The removal of carbon dioxide by the lungs is termed the **respiratory component**.
- The removal of acid by the kidneys is termed the **metabolic component**.

The respiratory–metabolic link

Thus, it can be seen that the body has two distinct methods of preventing the accumulation of hydrogen ions and the subsequent development of an acidaemia. As a further protection these two components are in balance (or equilibrium) so that each can **compensate** for a derangement in the other.

This link between the respiratory and metabolic systems is due to the presence of **carbonic acid** (H_2CO_3) (Figure 22.6). The ability for each system to compensate for the other becomes more marked when the initial disturbance in one system is prolonged.

The production of carbonic acid is dependent upon an enzyme called carbonic anhydrase that is present in abundance in the red cells and the kidneys. It is therefore ideally placed to facilitate the link between the respiratory and the metabolic systems.

Let us consider how this link can help the body respond to an excess of either carbon dioxide or acid.

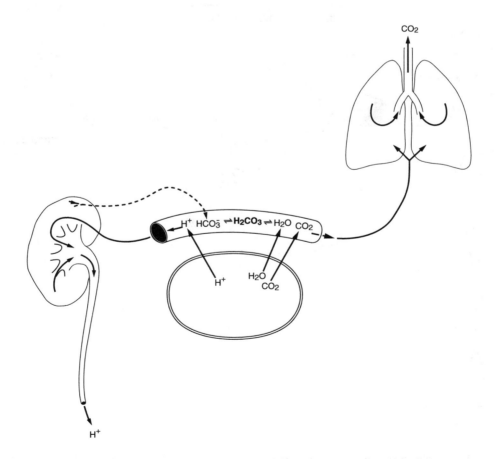

Figure 22.6 Carbonic acid–bicarbonate buffers: acid production and its removal

Example 1

In a patient with inadequate alveolar ventilation, e.g. chronic bronchitis, carbon dioxide accumulates. As we have seen this will tend to cause a respiratory acidosis. Rather than the body existing in a chronic state of acidosis, the metabolic system can help compensate by increasing bicarbonate production by the kidneys. Utilising the carbonic acid link enables the removal of some of the excess carbon dioxide (Figure 22.7). However, this takes several days to become effective as it is dependent upon the increased production of enzymes in the kidney.

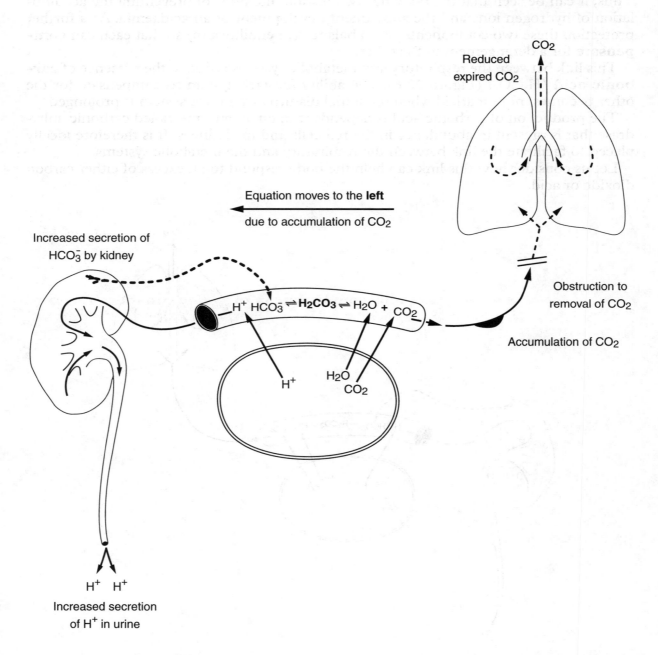

Figure 22.7 Metabolic compensation for a respiratory acidosis (i.e. the metabolic system is compensating for the respiratory system)

It is important to realise that in the acute situation the **body does not fully compensate**. Consequently, if an arterial blood sample is taken at this time, it will demonstrate that there is still a persistent but slight underlying acidaemia (Table 22.3).

Table 22.3   Underlying acidaemia

	Normal values	Effect of a respiratory acidaemia	Effect of metabolic compensation
pH	7·36–7·44	↓↓	↓
$PaCO_2$	4·8–5·3 kPa	↑	↑
	36–40 mm Hg		
HCO_3^-	21–27 mmol/l	↑	↑↑

Example 2

Diabetic patients sometimes develop a state of excess acid production known as **diabetic ketoacidosis**. The excess cellular acid is released into the plasma to be transported to the kidney for excretion. However, the kidneys are only able to excrete the additional acid load slowly and a metabolic acidosis develops. The kidneys are slowly stimulated to increase bicarbonate production. This will counteract the acidaemia but it takes several days. In the meantime, because of the carbonic acid link, some of the excess acid can be converted to carbon dioxide and eliminated by the respiratory system (Figure 22.8).

This compensation occurs quickly because excess hydrogen ions are detected by special receptors in the brain which, in turn, increase the respiratory rate and depth within minutes (compare this with the slow response of the kidneys). This process enables the body to eliminate the extra carbon dioxide, providing that there is no obstruction to ventilation. The lowering of carbon dioxide levels in the blood encourages further free acid to be converted into carbonic acid and eventually carbon dioxide.

However, the body does not fully compensate in the acute situation. Therefore even after several hours, respiratory compensation will only be partial and the patient will still be slightly acidaemic (Table 22.4).

Table 22.4   Slight acidaemia

	Normal values	Effect of a metabolic acidosis	Effect of respiratory compensation
pH	7·36–7·44	↓↓	↓
$PaCO_2$	4·8–5·3 kPa	4·8–5·3 kPa	↓
	36–40 mm Hg	36–40 mm Hg	
HCO_3^-	21–27 mmol/l	↑	↓

It must also be remembered that the degree to which the respiratory system can compensate is dependent upon the work involved in breathing and the systemic effects of a low arterial concentration of carbon dioxide.

Summary

- The metabolic component of the body's acid elimination mechanism can compensate for a respiratory acidosis by increasing the production of bicarbonate by the kidneys.

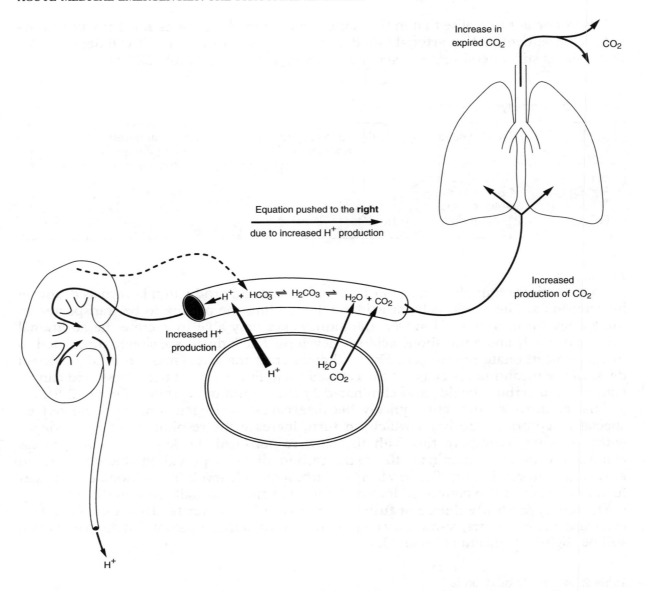

Figure 22.8 Respiratory compensation for a metabolic acidosis (i.e. the respiratory system is compensating for the metabolic system)

- Compensation by the metabolic component usually takes days to achieve.
- The respiratory component of the body's acid elimination mechanism can compensate for a metabolic acidosis by increasing ventilation of the lungs and eliminating carbon dioxide.
- Compensation by the respiratory component usually takes place within minutes.
- In the acute situation the body never overcompensates; therefore the underlying acidaemia will remain.

Combined metabolic and respiratory acidosis

It follows from the earlier description that should both the metabolic and respiratory systems be defective or inadequate to the body's needs, then the accumulation of acid and carbon dioxide will be unchecked. An example of this particularly dire situation is seen in patients following a cardiorespiratory arrest. This results in the cells of the body producing lactic acid because they are being starved of oxygen. In addition carbon dioxide accumulates in the cells and blood because it can no longer be excreted by the lungs due to the failure of ventilation (Figure 22.9).

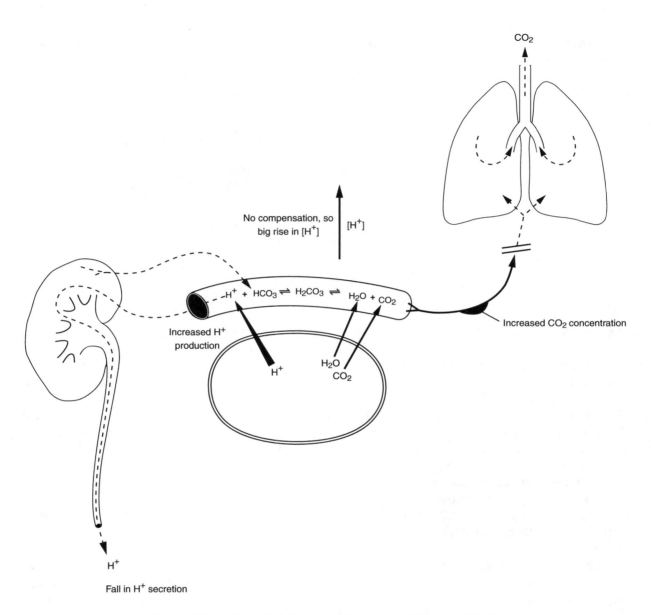

Figure 22.9   Combined metabolic and respiratory acidosis

An arterial blood sample taken at this time would therefore demonstrate a combined respiratory and metabolic acidaemia (Table 22.5).

Table 22.5   Combined respiratory and metabolic acidaemia

	Normal values	Effect of respiratory and metabolic acidosis
pH	7·36–7·44	↓↓↓↓
$PaCO_2$	4·8–5·3 kPa	↑↑
	36–40 mm Hg	
HCO_3^-	21–27 mmol/l	↓↓

CENTRAL VENOUS AND ARTERIAL BLOOD SAMPLES

So far we have concentrated on arterial blood analysis. This is blood that has had the benefit of passing through the lungs, where carbon dioxide can be eliminated and oxygen taken up. In contrast, central venous blood (i.e. blood in the right atrium) represents a mixture of all the blood returning to the heart from the body's tissues. It therefore has a high concentration of the body's waste products and low levels of oxygen (Table 22.6).

Table 22.6 Comparison of the composition of arterial and central venous blood

	Arterial blood	Central venous blood
pH	7·36–7·44	7·31–7·40
PCO_2	4·8–5·3 kPa	5·5–6·8 kPa
	36–40 mm Hg	41–51 mm Hg
HCO_3^-	21–27 mmol/l	25–29 mmol/l
PO_2 on air	Over 10·6 kPa	5·1–5·6 kPa
	Over 80 mm Hg	38–42 mm Hg

Compare these results with those following a cardiorespiratory arrest. In the absence of cardiopulmonary resuscitation no blood will go through unventilated lungs. Therefore the arterial sample and central venous sample will be **approximately the same**.

In contrast following endotracheal intubation, artificial ventilation, and external chest compression, the carbon dioxide delivery to the alveoli is resumed. This is easily cleared by mechanical ventilation and some oxygen is taken up. The removal of carbon dioxide can be so effective that there is a marked reduction in arterial carbon dioxide and the development of a paradoxical respiratory alkalosis (i.e. low arterial carbon dioxide despite high venous carbon dioxide and acidosis). Consequently, the arterial pH can be neutral, mildly acidotic or even alkalotic depending upon how much carbon dioxide is being removed. In contrast, severe arterial acidosis in a patient receiving cardiopulmonary resuscitation indicates that resuscitation is inadequate, i.e. there is either inadequate blood flow to the lungs or inadequate ventilation or a combination of both.

The arterial sample taken during the resuscitation of a patient with a cardiorespiratory arrest is simply demonstrating the clinician's ability to remove carbon dioxide and add oxygen. The patient's true "acid" state (i.e. pH, carbon dioxide and bicarbonate) is more accurately deduced from analysis of blood from a central vein.

A SYSTEMATIC APPROACH FOR ANALYSING A BLOOD GAS SAMPLE

There are many similarities between analysing a blood gas result and interpreting a rhythm strip. In both cases it is important to assess the patient first and to be aware of the clinical history and current medications. A review of the other laboratory investigations is also helpful. In the emergency situation, however, this data may not be immediately available. Consequently you will have to interpret the initial results with caution and follow trends whilst the rest of the information is being obtained.

The system

History
- Any symptoms due to the cause of an acid–base disturbance?
- Any symptoms as a result of an acid–base disturbance?

Results
- Is there an acidaemia or alkalaemia?
- Is there evidence of a disturbance in the respiratory component of the body's acid–base balance?
- Is there evidence of a disturbance in the metabolic component of the body's acid–base balance?
- Is there a single or multiple acid–base disturbance?
- Is there any defect in oxygen uptake?

Integration
- Do the suspicions from the history agree with the analysis of the results?

Is there an acidaemia or alkalaemia?

In most patients you will come across, there will be an acute single acid–base disturbance. In these circumstances the body rarely has the opportunity to completely compensate for the alteration in hydrogen ion concentration. Consequently the pH will remain outside the normal range and thereby indicate the underlying acid–base disturbance.

---

pH less than 7·36 = underlying acidaemia
pH greater than 7·44 = underlying alkalaemia

In acute, single acid–base disturbances the body usually does not have time to fully compensate. The pH will therefore indicate the primary acid–base problem

---

Nevertheless a normal pH does not necessarily mean the patient does not have an acid–base disturbance. In fact there are three reasons for a patient having a pH within the normal range:

- there is no underlying acid–base disturbance
- the body has fully compensated for a single acid–base disturbance
- there is more than one acid–base disturbance with equal but opposite effects on the pH.

Using your knowledge of the patient's history and examination you will have a good idea which of these options is the true answer. However, to confirm or refute your suspicions you will need to see if there is any evidence of alterations in the respiratory and metabolic components of the body's acid–base balance. This entails reviewing the $PaCO_2$ and standard bicarbonate (or base excess) respectively.

Is the abnormality due to a defect in the respiratory component?

Checking the $PaCO_2$ gives a good indication of the ventilatory adequacy because it is inversely proportional to alveolar ventilation. When combined with pH it can be used to determine if there is either a problem with the respiratory system or if the respiratory component is simply compensating for a problem in the metabolic component.

Take, for example, an arterial sample with a pH of 7·2 and a $PaCO_2$ of 8·0 kPa (60 mm Hg). A pH of 7·2 indicates that there is an acidaemia. As the $PaCO_2$ is raised, this indicates that there is a **respiratory acidosis**. Consider now a patient with a similar pH but a $PaCO_2$ of 3·3 kPa (25 mm Hg). There is still an acidosis but as the $PaCO_2$ is lowered, it would imply there is **respiratory compensation to a metabolic acidaemia**. To confirm this the metabolic component would need to be assessed.

Is the abnormality due to a defect in the metabolic component?

To determine the metabolic component, the concentration of bicarbonate is measured. In a similar situation to that described earlier, when the bicarbonate concentration is combined with pH one can determine if there is either a primary metabolic or compensatory metabolic problem.

Using the second example above, the bicarbonate was found to be 9·5 mmol/l. This is below the normal range (22–27 mmol/l). Consequently, a pH of 7·2 and a $PaCO_2$ of 3·3 kPa (25 mm Hg) is in keeping with the idea that this patient has a **respiratory compensation to a metabolic acidaemia**.

It is important to realise that not all laboratories measure bicarbonate. Instead the base excess is calculated. This is defined as the number of moles of **bicarbonate** which must be added to the equivalent of one litre of the patient's blood so that a pH of 7·4 is produced. Respiratory influences are eliminated by keeping the partial pressure of carbon dioxide constant at 5·3 kPa (40 mm Hg). The value should be zero but a normal range is −2 to +2 mmol/l.

For example, an arterial blood sample with a pH of 7·25, a $PaCO_2$ of 3·3 kPa (25 mm Hg) and a base excess of −15 indicates that there is a metabolic acidaemia with a compensatory respiratory alkalosis.

The base excess is used to help to calculate the dose of bicarbonate that should be given to a patient to correct the metabolic acidaemia. However, it is important to realise that a slight metabolic acidosis is beneficial because it facilitates the release of oxygen from the haemoglobin molecule to the tissues.

Is there a single or multiple acid–base disturbance?

To narrow down the diagnosis even further we need to consider how much the $PaCO_2$ and bicarbonate (base excess) concentration has changed. If these changes fall within certain limits then there is usually only a single acid–base disturbance. Alternatively if they are outside this range then it is likely that the patient has more than one acid–base disturbance.

There are two methods of assessing these changes. As both systems work, it is entirely up to you to choose the one you prefer. For those who like looking at pictures we would recommend using a graph. Alternatively, for those who prefer to do mental arithmetic, we would recommend the memorising of certain numbers.

Graphical method
Take a moment to familiarise yourself with the layout of Flenley's graph (Figure 22.10). In particular note the following.

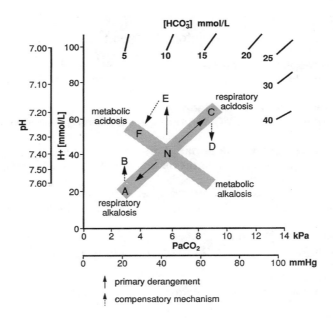

Figure 22.10   Flenley's graph

- The graph is showing how the pH alters with changes in $PaCO_2$.
- Cutting diagonally across the graph are lines which indicate the concentration of bicarbonate. These are known as isopleths.
- As the concentration of standard bicarbonate increases the gradient of the isopleths falls.
- Fanning out from this box are the possible ranges of normal responses you could expect with single acid–base disturbances.
- The bands representing the acute respiratory disturbances run approximately parallel to the isopleths. Respiratory acidaemia and alkalaemia will alter the pH and $PaCO_2$ but have little effect on the bicarbonate concentration. These bands do not include patients who have had long enough to develop metabolic compensation and so altered their bicarbonate concentrations. Such patients are represented in the chronic respiratory acidosis group.
- The band representing the metabolic disturbances runs across the isopleths. Therefore metabolic acidaemia and alkalaemia will alter the bicarbonate concentration as well as the pH and $PaCO_2$. These bands include the patients who are using respiratory compensation to counteract the pH changes. However, it does not include those patients who have had long enough to develop metabolic compensation (i.e. those who have a chronic metabolic disturbance).

Using this graph you can plot the results from the blood gas analysis. If it lies within one of these bands then there is likely to be only one acid–base disturbance. However, if the results lie outside these normal ranges then there is likely to be more than one acid–base disturbance.

Arithmetic method
This system has the disadvantage of using the older units for $PaCO_2$, i.e. mm Hg. Nevertheless by applying the numbers listed below you will be able to determine if the changes in $PaCO_2$ and bicarbonate are appropriate for a single acid–base disturbance. If there is an inconsistency between the actual results and those derived by calculation then it is likely that the patient has more than one acid–base disturbance.

Expected changes *

Acute respiratory acidaemia:
a 1·0 mm Hg rise in $PaCO_2$ produces a 0·1 mmol/l rise in HCO_3

Chronic respiratory acidaemia:
a 1·0 mm Hg rise in $PaCO_2$ produces a 0·5 mmol/l rise in HCO_3

Acute respiratory alkalaemia:
a 1·0 mm Hg fall in PaCO2 produces a 0·2 mmol/l fall in HCO_3

Chronic respiratory alkalaemia:
a 1·0 mm Hg fall in $PaCO_2$ produces a 0·4 mmol/l fall in HCO_3

Metabolic acidaemia:
a 1·0 mmol/l fall in HCO_3 produces a 1·0 mm Hg fall in HCO_2

Metabolic alkalaemia:
a 1·0 mmol/l rise in HCO_3 produces a 0·6 mm Hg rise in HCO_2

* All these values are taken from the middle of the normal ranges.

You have now finished the interpretation of the parameters in the blood gas analysis which provide information on the patient's acid–base balance. There is, however, one more important value which needs to be assessed in an arterial sample and that is the partial pressure of oxygen. This is important because a failure to take up oxygen can lead to many adverse conditions including hypoxia. With regard to the acid–base balance, hypoxia can give rise to metabolic acidosis because it causes the cells to change to anaerobic metabolism and so produce excessive quantities of lactic acid.

Defect in oxygen uptake

By knowing the FiO_2 it is possible to predict what the PaO_2 would be if the patient was ventilating normally.

Since atmospheric pressure is 100 kPa (approximately 760 mm Hg), 1% is 1 kPa or 7·6 mm Hg. This would mean that inspiring 30% oxygen from a facemask would produce an inspired partial pressure of oxygen of 30 kPa (228 mm Hg). This should lead to an arterial concentration of around 20–25 kPa (152–257·6 mm Hg) because there is a normal drop of about 7·5 kPa (57 mm Hg) between the partial pressure of oxygen inspired at the mouth and that in the alveoli. A drop of significantly greater than 10 kPa (76 mm Hg) would imply that there is a mismatch in the lungs between ventilation of the alveoli and their perfusion with blood.

For example, an arterial PaO_2 of 32·9 kPa (250 mm Hg) in a patient breathing 40% oxygen is within normal limits. In contrast, an arterial $PaCO_2$ of 23·7 kPa (180 mm Hg) in a patient breathing 50% oxygen indicates that there is a defect in the take-up of oxygen.

- Using kPa
  An inspired oxygen of 50% will have a partial pressure of approximately 50 kPa. This would mean the expected $PaCO_2$ would be at least 50 − 10 = 40 kPa.

- Using mm Hg
  An inspired oxygen of 50% will have a partial pressure of 380 mm Hg (i.e. half the normal atmospheric pressure). This would mean that the expected $PaCO_2$ would be at least 380 − 76 = 304 mm Hg.

Example

Using this system for interpreting blood gases let us now consider the following case.

History

A 17 year old girl who is normally in good health is found at home by her parents in a restless and confused state. She is pale, sweaty, and hyperventilating.

Results

Whilst she was breathing room air, an arterial sample was taken for blood gas analysis. The results are given in Table 22.7.

Table 22.7 Example arterial blood sample

	Normal values	Patient's values
pH	7·36–7·44	7·10
$PaCO_2$	4·7–6·0 kPa	2·4 kPa
	35–45 mm Hg	18 mm Hg
HCO_3	21–28 mmol/l	5·5 mmol/l
Base excess	± 2 mmol/l	–14 mmol/l
$PaCO_2$	Over 12·0 kPa	14 kPa
	Over 90 mm Hg *	105 mm Hg

* On room air

Analysis

History

The hyperventilation may be a primary problem (e.g. anxiety) or compensation for an underlying metabolic acidaemia. You would therefore suspect from the history that there could be either a respiratory alkalaemia or a metabolic acidaemia with respiratory compensation. With regard to acid–base balance you can also deduce from the history that this is an acute event. It is therefore unlikely that there would be sufficient time for any metabolic compensation in either of the possible acid–base disturbances suspected.

Systematic analysis of the blood gas results

- Is there an acidaemia or alkalaemia?
  As the pH is below 7·36 there is an acidaemia.
- Is there evidence of a disturbance in the respiratory component of the body's acid–base balance?
  Yes, the $PaCO_2$ is low. In the light of the pH this indicates there is either respiratory compensation to a metabolic acidaemia or a combination of a big metabolic acidaemia and smaller primary respiratory alkalaemia.
- Is there evidence of a disturbance in the metabolic component of the body's acid–base balance?
  Yes, the bicarbonate concentration is low and the base excess is very negative. In the light of the pH and $PaCO_2$ this supports the two possibilities suggested in the previous question.
- Is there a single or multiple acid–base disturbance?
  Using Figure 22.10 you can see that the results lie within the metabolic acidaemia band. This would imply that the patient has a metabolic acidaemia with respiratory compensation and has not had time to develop metabolic compensation.

339

Using the arithmetic model:

if the patient had a metabolic acidaemia, a 1 mmol/l fall in actual HCO_3 produces a 1·0–1·3 mm Hg fall in $PaCO_2$.

Therefore:

a 18·5 mmol/l fall in HCO_3 would produce a 18·5–24·1 mm Hg fall in $PaCO_2$.

Therefore using the midpoints of the normal ranges, this patient's $PaCO_2$ should be between:

$$(40 - 18·5) \text{ and } (40 - 24·1) = 15·9 - 21·5 \text{ mm Hg.}$$

As this incorporates the level in the arterial blood sample, it is likely that this patient has a single acid–base disturbance which is a metabolic acidaemia.

- Is the PaO_2 uptake abnormal?
  The expected PaO_2 when breathing room air is over 12·0 kPa (over 90 mm Hg). There is, therefore, no evidence of any problem in oxygen uptake in this patient.

Integrate the clinical findings with the data interpretation
The clinical and data analyses tally. This girl has a metabolic acidaemia with respiratory compensation. Your next move would be to determine what is the cause of the acidaemia. This involves carrying out further tests which are selected in the light of the patient's history and physical examination.

ANION GAP

This is defined as the difference in concentration between the plasma cations (i.e. sodium and potassium) and the anions (i.e. bicarbonate and chloride). It is due to the presence of unmeasured anions such as phosphate, sulphate, and albumin, and is normally between 8–16 mmol/l.

$$\text{Anion gap} = ([Na^+] + [K^+]) - ([HCO_3^-] + [Cl^-])$$

In the normal person the anion gap has a range of 6–18 mmol/l. (This will vary as some equations use both sodium and potassium and some do not.) However, it follows from how it is derived that this gap can be altered by changes in the concentration of either the unmeasured anions or unmeasured cations or a combination of the two.

For example, an increase in the anion gap could result from the following.

Increase in the unmeasured anions	Decrease in the *un*measured cations
Metabolic acidosis	Hypokalaemia
Therapy with sodium salt of unmeasured anions (e.g. sodium citrate, lactate or acetate and following excessive doses of penicillins, particularly carbenicillin and ticarcillin)	
Hyperalbuminaemia	Hypocalcaemia
Marked alkalaemia	

Metabolic acidaemia with an increased anion gap

It is important to realise that metabolic acidaemia represents only one of several causes of an increase in anion gap. This finding, therefore, needs to be put into clinical context by reviewing the patient's history and examination findings. By doing this you are less likely to carry out a series of unnecessary investigations whilst trying to find the cause of a condition the patient does not have!

The most likely metabolic acidaemia you will come across is one giving rise to an increase in the anion gap. In these conditions a metabolic acidaemia is produced because the bicarbonate concentration falls:

$$\text{Anion gap} \uparrow = [Na^+] - ([HCO_3^-] \downarrow + [Cl^-])$$

Causes
A metabolic acidaemia with a widened anion gap is common because it is produced by several common clinical conditions. These can be remembered by the mnemonic "mudpiles":

M	Methanol	**P**	Phenformin
U	Uraemia		Paraldehyde
D	Diabetic ketoacidosis	**I**	Isoniazid
			Iron
		L	Lactic acidosis
		E	Ethanol
			Ethylene glycol
		S	Salicylate overdose
			Solvents
			Starvation

The young girl's blood sample was analysed further by measuring the appropriate electrolyte concentrations. In this case these were found to be:

- Na^+ 135 mmol/l
- K^+ 5.0 mmol/l
- HCO_3 10 mmol/l
- Cl^- 95 mmol/l

Using this information it is possible to determine the anion gap:

$$\begin{aligned}
\text{Anion gap} &= [\text{sodium}] - [\text{bicarbonate} + \text{chloride}] \\
&= [135] - [10 + 95] \\
&= 25 \text{ mmol/l}
\end{aligned}$$

Therefore the 17 year old patient has a metabolic acidaemia with a wide anion gap.

SUMMARY

The body's system for removing the carbon dioxide and acid produced by metabolism has both a respiratory and metabolic component. These are linked by the effects of carbonic acid which enables one component to compensate for a defect in the other.

In acute medical emergencies one or both of these systems are often defective. Using a systemic approach to blood gas analysis you can determine where the problem lies. In the common structure of a metabolic acidosis, the use of the anion gap can also be helpful in identifying a specific cause.

The most likely cause of a metabolic acidosis with an increased anion gap in a previously healthy adolescent is an overdose or diabetic ketoacidosis. Consequently the salicylate and blood sugar levels must be checked in this patient.

CHAPTER

23

Dysrhythmia recognition

OBJECTIVES

After reading this chapter you will be able to:

- understand the origin and passage of the electrical activity in the heart
- recognise which patients require this activity to be monitored and how it should be done
- understand the system for analysing electrical activity recorded on a rhythm strip.

CARDIAC ELECTRICAL ACTIVITY: ITS ORIGIN AND ORGANISATION

The sinoatrial node (SAN) is a specialised area of cardiac muscle that generates a continuous sequence of regularly timed waves of electrical activity known as depolarisation. These radiate through both atria, inducing contraction. As the depolarisation spreads through the atria it also gives rise to the "P" wave on the electrocardiogram (ECG). Normally the P wave has a duration of 0·08–0·12 seconds.

Atrial depolarisation normally finishes by converging on a specialised collection of cells called the atrioventricular node (AVN) located at the base of the right atrium. This delays the transmission of the depolarising wave to the ventricles and gives rise to a significant proportion of the PR interval. The latter is measured on the ECG tracing from the start of the P wave to the first deflection of QRS complex (0·12–0·20 seconds).

After the atrioventricular node, the wave of depolarisation is conducted through the fibrous atrioventricular barrier via the bundle of His. At the proximal part of the muscular intraventricular septum this splits into the right and left bundle branches, with the latter subsequently separating into anterior and posterior divisions (fascicles). These, in turn, terminate into small (Purkinje) fibres which transmit the electrical impulse to the non-specialised ventricular myocardium. The passage of the impulse through the specialised ventricular conduction system is rapid compared with the atrioventricular node and is represented by the QRS complex (< 0·12 seconds) on the ECG.

Following stimulation, the myocardial cells recover their normal resting electrical potential in an active biochemical process called repolarisation. The atrial repolarisation wave is usually obscured by the QRS, but the ventricular repolarisation gives rise to the T wave. For most of the period of repolarisation the ventricles remain unresponsive (or "refractory") to further electrical stimulation. A diagrammatical representation of the conducting system and its relationship to the ECG is shown in Figure 23.1.

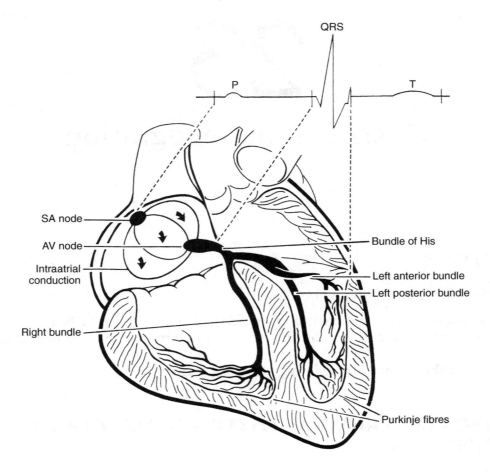

Figure 23.1   The conduction system of the heart and its relationship to the electrocardiogram

The T wave is sometimes followed by a U wave, which is a rounded deflection in the same direction as the T wave. Its exact genesis is unclear but it becomes more prominent in hypokalaemia, hypercalcaemia and inverted in ischaemic heart disease.

The QT interval is measured from the beginning of the QRS complex to the end of the T wave. Consequently it represents the total time for ventricular depolarisation and repolarisation. Nevertheless, prolongation of this interval is mainly associated with clinical conditions that delay ventricular repolarisation. This increases the period of time where the ventricles are susceptible to lethal dysrhythmias (see later).

It is important to realise, however, that the duration of the QT interval is also inversely dependent on the heart rate, and directly dependent on age and gender. The corrected QT interval (QT_c) is the result obtained once the heart rate has been considered (normal range 0·35–0·42 seconds). Fortunately many diagnostic ECG machines do this calculation automatically.

PATHOLOGY OF THE CONDUCTING SYSTEM

The origin and spread of depolarisation through the heart can be affected by ischaemia, drugs, trauma, and abnormal metabolic conditions. This can lead to the depolarisation originating from abnormal areas of the heart and spreading by an atypical route. The ECG can be used in these situations to help locate the affected sites.

All parts of the special conducting system have the ability to initiate a wave of depolarisation but do so at varying frequencies. The eventual heart rate is determined by the part of the conducting system that has the fastest intrinsic rate of depolarisation, normally the sinoatrial node. After the sinoatrial node, the next fastest part is usually the atria. If these are also defective, then the atrioventricular node will take over as the cardiac pacemaker, followed in turn by the bundle of His and the ventricular myocardium.

Occasionally a pathological focus develops in the heart which has a faster intrinsic rate of depolarisation when compared with the sinoatrial node. As a consequence, this focus will replace the sinoatrial node as the cardiac pacemaker.

CAUSES OF DYSRHYTHMIA

Increasing the heart rate

An increase in heart rate occurs normally as a result of emotion, exercise, and fear. The effect is mediated by the sympathetic nervous system which acts on the sinoatrial node to increase its rate of depolarisation. However, an increase in the heart rate can also result from the following pathological reasons:

- automaticity
- reentry
- both.

Automaticity
Automaticity is the ability to depolarise spontaneously. This is a common feature of cells in the conducting system and certain areas of myocardium. As mentioned previously, the sinoatrial node usually has the fastest rate of depolarisation and therefore acts as the dominant pacemaker.

Reentry
Reentry occurs when there is a dual conducting system between the atria and the ventricles. This can be either within the atrioventricular node or bypassing it (e.g. Wolff–Parkinson–White and Lown–Ganong–Levine syndromes). One pathway (**A**) has a unidirectional block (or a longer refractory period) and the other (**B**) has a slow conduction rate (Figure 23.2). In response to a premature beat, the impulse has to go down the slow pathway (**B**). This is because the fast pathway (**A**) has not repolarised from the previous beat and is therefore unable to conduct the electrical impulse. This increase in

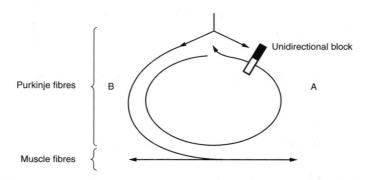

Figure 23.2   The origin of a circus movement

transit time allows **A** to repolarise so that the impulse can be conducted opposite to the normal direction of flow. This gives **B** sufficient time to repolarise and so be able to be stimulated by the retrograde impulse which has travelled along **A**. Consequently a self-sustaining cycle of electrical impulses is created.

Both
Automaticity and reentry can act together.

Slowing of the heart

A reduction in the heart rate is a normal physiological response during sleep, at rest, and in the athletic individual. The heart rate can also fall in certain pathological conditions when the rate of depolarisation of the intrinsic cardiac pacemaker and/or the conducting system has been reduced. Ischaemic heart disease is the most common cause but drugs, trauma, and other diseases can also be responsible.

MONITORING CARDIAC ELECTRICAL ACTIVITY

In the acute situation cardiac electrical activity is usually continuously assessed by an ECG monitor connected to the patient by a standard system of electrical leads (Figure 23.3).

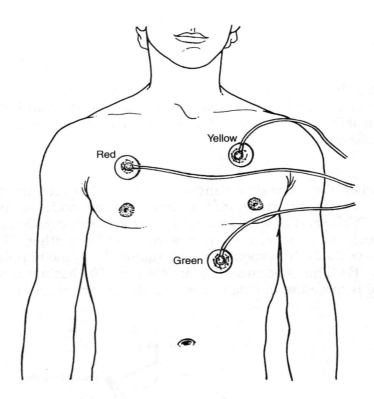

Figure 23.3　Monitoring by the electrocardiogram

Cardiac ECG monitors

Although there are many different types of cardiac monitor, the majority have certain features in common: there is a screen for displaying the cardiac rhythm and a device for obtaining a copy of it. This printout is commonly known as the "rhythm strip". Most models also incorporate a heart rate meter which is triggered by the QRS complexes and a device to automatically store a record of the ECG should the heart rate fall outside certain preset limits. Lights and audible signals may also provide additional indications of the heart rate.

Modern machines tend to convert the electronic signal into digital form. This enables the machine to perform complex functions such as computer aided rhythm analysis, automatic, and semiautomatic defibrillation, and electronic storage of the signal for later playback and analysis.

Leads

Lead I measures the voltage between the right and left shoulder. It gives a good view of the left lateral aspect of the heart and the QRS complex but does not necessarily give a good picture of the P wave (Figure 23.4).

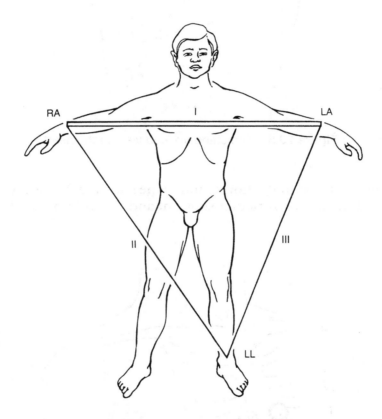

Figure 23.4 The bipolar limb leads

Lead II measures the voltage between the right shoulder and left leg. It is the most commonly used lead for monitoring the cardiac rhythm. As it is in line with the mean frontal cardiac axis, it gives a good view of both the QRS and P wave. It also shows shifts in the direction of the axis (Figure 23.4).

Lead III measures the voltage between the left shoulder and left lower chest (or leg). It is rarely an advantage in dysrhythmia recognition but it does give a good view of the inferior aspect of the heart (Figure 23.4).

The remaining leads are not used during routine monitoring or the initial management of a cardiac arrest. They are, however, required for definitive dysrhythmia analysis and determining the position of the cardiac axis. The MCL1 lead measures the voltage between the right pectoral area (V1 position) and the left shoulder. This gives a good view of the QRS and P wave, but it is not commonly used.

Leads I, II, III, and AVR, AVL, and AVF look at the heart in the vertical plane (Figure 23.5).

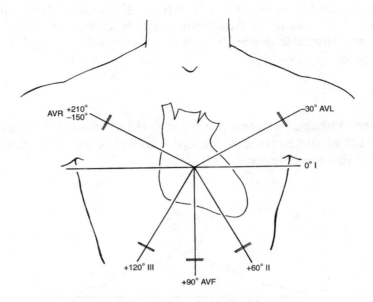

Figure 23.5 The standard lead view of the heart

Leads V1–6 view the heart in the horizontal plane such that V1 and V2 look at the right ventricle, V3 and V4 the interventricular septum, and V5 and V6 mainly the left ventricle (Figure 23.6).

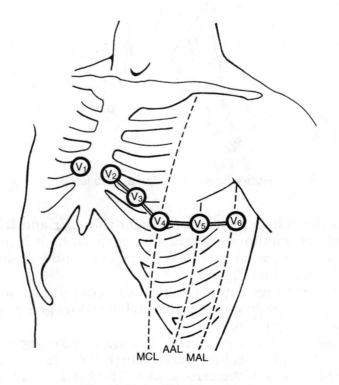

Figure 23.6 The chest leads

Practical points

- The ECG monitor should be used on all patients presenting with chest pain, syncope, dizziness, collapse, hypotension, palpitations, and cardiac arrest.
- ECG machines record at a standard speed of 25 mm/s. Calibrated recording paper is used so that each large square (5 mm) is equivalent to 0·2 s and each small square to 0·04 s. The amplitude of the trace is standardised at 1 mV/cm and most machines have the capability of testing this (Figure 23.7).

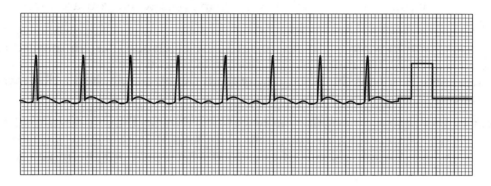

Figure 23.7 Voltage calibration of the electrocardiogram

- To minimise electrical interference the electrodes should be all of the same type, applied over bone rather than muscle and positioned such that they are equidistant from one another. Hair should be removed from the areas where the electrodes are to be attached and the skin cleaned with alcohol to dissolve surface oil. The electrodes should be positioned on the patient's chest so that they will not interfere with any other activities, such as external cardiac massage.
- Adhesive silver/silver chloride electrodes give the best signal and, if readily available, are preferable to defibrillation paddles even for the first "quick look" in cardiac arrest. Another advantage is that paddles will only give a reading when they are in position and, therefore, are not practical for continuously assessing the rhythm. Nevertheless if paddles are used, it is essential that they are placed over gel pads to ensure good electrical contact.
- Ensure that the QRS height is sufficient to stimulate the rate meter by adjusting the gain control. However, this should not be so excessive as to cause artefacts on the monitor.
- Any activity, such as drug use or carotid sinus massage, should be recorded on the rhythm strip as it happens. This helps greatly in the later analysis of the dysrhythmia.
- A common problem is artefact produced by the patient's movements, strenuous respiratory effort or if subjected to external cardiac compression. As the latter is usually sufficient to completely mask the patient's own cardiac rhythm, it must be stopped for the 3–5 s so that the cardiac arrest rhythm can be analysed (see later).
- It is important to realise that the leads used to monitor dysrhythmias are **not** the optimum ones for recording changes in the ST segment and T wave. A "diagnostic" setting may be required to reproduce ST displacement accurately but this produces more baseline wandering.
- If time permits, old notes should be obtained, previous ECGs studied and a full 12 lead ECG should be done as this helps with dysrhythmia analysis.

A SYSTEMATIC APPROACH TO INTERPRETING A RHYTHM STRIP

Avoid the temptation to simply "eye ball" the rhythm strip produced by the ECG monitor. Instead develop a system so that clues and multiple problems are not missed.

Basic principles

It is helpful to remember the following basic principles when you are interpreting the rhythm strip.

- If the depolarisation wave is moving towards the electrode then an upward (positive) deflection is seen on the monitor.
- If the depolarisation wave is moving away from the electrode then a downward (negative) deflection is seen on the monitor.

The next box contains one of the many systems that have been developed to enable health care workers interpret a rhythm strip from lead II in the acute situation. It is an effective system based upon a series of questions which pick out the most life threatening dysrhythmias first.

Systematic approach to interpreting a rhythm strip

How is the patient?

Is there any electrical activity?
  No   Asystole
  Yes   Not asystole
Are there recognisable complexes?
  No   Ventricular fibrillation
  Yes   Not ventricular fibrillation
What is the ventricular rate?
What is the rhythm?
  Regular
  Regular irregularity
  Irregular irregularity
Are the P waves uniform?
  Shape
  Timing – Early or later than normal
Is there atrial flutter?
Are there the same number of P waves as QRS complexes?
  Yes   What is the PR interval?
  No   Is the PR interval constant?
      Is the RR interval constant?
Is the QRS duration normal?
  Yes   Normal ventricular conduction
  No   Abnormal ventricular conduction:
        Shape
        Timing – Early or later than normal
        Frequency
    Ventricular tachycardia:
        Supraventricular tachycardia with aberrant ventricular conduction
        Torsade de pointes
    Idioventricular rhythm:
        Agonal rhythm

---

1. How is the patient?

It is extremely important to see the patient before making a diagnosis and suggesting a treatment from a single rhythm strip. For example, a patient who is not breathing and has no palpable pulse is suffering from a cardiorespiratory arrest irrespective of what the monitor shows. For example, if the arrest occurs despite normal (or near normal) electrical activity then **pulseless electrical activity** (PEA; previously called **electromechanical dissociation**) exists.

2. Is there any electrical activity?
If there is no electrical activity, check:

- connections – to monitor
                – to patient
- QRS gain
- leads I and III.

If there is still no electrical activity diagnose **asystole** (Figure 23.8). However, beware that a completely flat tracing, without any baseline wandering, is usually caused by not connecting the patient's leads.

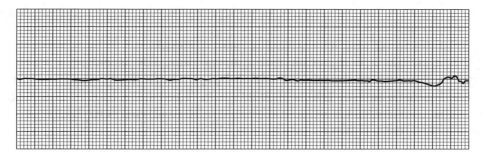

Figure 23.8   Asystole

Occasionally P waves can be detected, indicating that atrial activity is still present. This usually occurs, transiently, shortly after the onset of ventricular asystole and is associated with a better prognosis than when P waves are absent.

3. Are there any recognisable complexes?
If there are no recognisable complexes diagnose **ventricular fibrillation** (VF) (Figure 23.9).

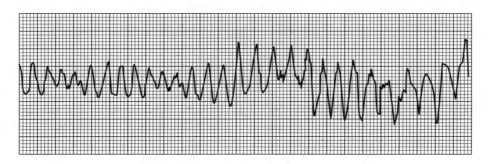

Figure 23.9   Ventricular fibrillation

Ventricular fibrillation is a totally chaotic rhythm because small areas of the myocardium depolarise in a random fashion. Initially, the amplitude of the waveform is large and the dysrhythmia is known as "coarse ventricular fibrillation". Over time "fine ventricular fibrillation" develops because the amplitude diminishes and the tracing becomes flatter. Eventually asystole results.

It is often difficult to determine when the patient has made the transition from fine ventricular fibrillation to asystole. This is made more difficult by the presence of any baseline wandering and electrical interference. In such cases the rhythm should be repeated taking the precautions listed for asystole. In addition all contact with the patient should cease briefly (less than 5 s) so that a reliable tracing can be gained without interference.

Key point

The presence or absence of the commonest cardiac arrest rhythms will have been determined by answering these first three questions. As these require immediate treatment further interpretation of the ECG assumes that these rhythms have been excluded

---

4. What is the ventricular rate?
This can be calculated as follows:

$$\text{ventricular rate} = 300/\text{number of large squares between consecutive R waves}$$

Figure 23.10 demonstrates a ventricular rate of 75/min.

Any rhythm that has a ventricular rate greater than 100 is called a "tachycardia". A common type is a **sinus tachycardia** which has, by definition, one P wave before each QRS and usually has a rate of 100–130 beats/min (Figure 23.11). In contrast, a ventricular rate less than 60/min is called a bradycardia. **Sinus bradycardia** is a common type of bradycardia that has a P wave before each QRS.

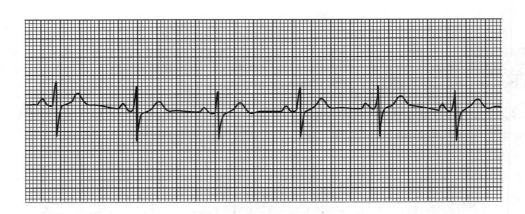

Figure 23.10   Sinus rhythm

Supraventricular tachycardias (SVT) (Figure 23.12) can be divided into two groups depending upon whether it results from reentry or enhanced automaticity. However, in the absence of finding an atrial premature beat (see later) before the tachycardia starts, it is not possible on routine ECG monitoring to distinguish between these two mechanisms.

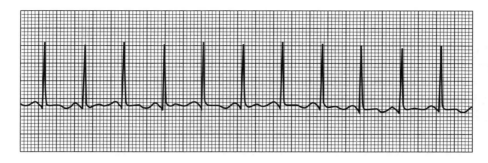

Figure 23.11 Sinus tachycardia

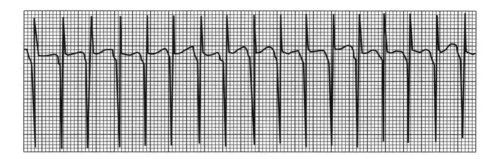

Figure 23.12 Supraventricular tachycardia

In a supraventricular tachycardia the QRS complexes are narrow unless there is an aberrant conduction through the ventricles producing widening of the QRS complex (see later).

5. What is the rhythm?

To answer this question correctly it is important to inspect carefully an adequate length of the rhythm strip tracing. In this way it will be possible to detect subtle variations in rhythm.

Assessment of the regularity of the rhythm is made by comparing the RR intervals of adjacent beats at different places in the tracing. Callipers or dividers are very useful for this but it is also possible to obtain an accurate result by marking the peaks of four adjacent R waves on a piece of paper. This must be done precisely because rhythm irregularity becomes less marked as the heart rate increases. The paper is then moved along the strip to see if the RR gaps correspond. If they do then the rhythm is regular. As interpretation of a fast heart rate can be difficult, a further rhythm strip recorded during carotid sinus massage may help by temporarily slowing the heart rate.

A **sinus rhythm** is diagnosed when:

- the P waves have a normal duration (2–3 small squares)
- the PR interval has a normal and consistent duration (3–5 small squares)
- the heart rate is between 60–100/min
- a P wave precedes each QRS complex.

Usually successive RR intervals are constant but occasionally, in healthy young individuals, the RR interval varies with respiration. Nevertheless the P wave shape and PR interval remain the same. This variation in the RR interval is called **sinus arrhythmia** and results from impairment of the cardioinhibitory centre during inspiration causing the heart rate to increase. The opposite occurs during expiration.

If the RR interval is irregular, it is important to decide whether there is either an "irregular irregularity", with no recognisable pattern, or RR intervals of "regular irregularity", when the variation in the RR intervals repeats in a regular fashion. In the latter case the relationship between the P waves and the QRS waves assumes special importance and will be discussed in greater detail later.

When an irregular irregularity in the RR interval is associated with a constant QRS shape, the likely diagnosis is **atrial fibrillation** (AF) (Figure 23.13). Atrial fibrillation is due to atrial depolarisation in a disorganised fashion at a rate of 350–600/min with conduction through the atrioventricular node occurring at an irregular rate. There are no P waves with AF, but the baseline may vary between fine and course fluctuations in different parts of the strip.

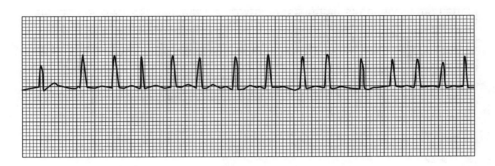

Figure 23.13   Atrial fibrillation

6. Are the P waves uniform?

Normal P waves have a duration of 0·08–0·12 seconds (2–3 small squares) and a vertical deflection of less than 2·5 mm. They can be distinguished from the larger T waves.

It is important to check the whole strip for P waves because they may be hidden in the QRS complex or T wave, producing inconsistent and abnormal "lumps and bumps" (Figure 23.14). Repeating the tracing using a different lead (V1, MCL1 or III) can also help identify apparently missing P waves.

Occasionally, hidden P waves can be revealed in patients with a regular tachycardia by slowing the ventricular rate by either vagal stimulation from carotid sinus massage or drugs (see atrial flutter)

Abnormal shaped P (i.e. "ectopic") waves indicate that the direction of depolarisation through the atria is abnormal and consequently has not been initiated by the sinoatrial node. They have two possible sources.

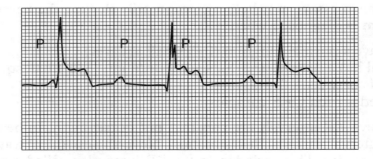

Figure 23.14   P waves hidden in the QRS complex

Premature beats As these usually originate in the atria and, rarely, from the atrio-ventricular junction they are known as **atrial and junctional premature beats**, respectively.

A distinguishing feature of a premature beat is the coupling interval, i.e. the time period between the normal P wave and the abnormal one (P'). This is **shorter** than that between two normal P waves (PP) because the myocardial focus giving rise to the premature atrial beat depolarises before the sinoatrial node (Figure 23.15). The coupling interval is constant if the premature beat is always produced from the same focus.

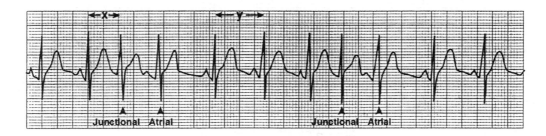

Figure 23.15 Ectopic P waves

The premature P wave (P') (Figure 23.15) blocks the SAN from discharging and so disturbs the subsequent rhythm of P wave production. This can be demonstrated on the rhythm strip by noting the interval between the normal P waves on either side of the ectopic beat. This distance (X) is less than twice the normal PP interval (Y).

The focus may produce single or multiple premature beats. A tachycardia is defined as having three or more such beats occurring in rapid succession. If they occur in discrete self-terminating runs, they are described as being **paroxysmal**. When they occur in longer runs, the abnormal focus may take over completely and not allow any normal (SAN generated) P waves to occur for a prolonged period of time. In these cases it is important to study the whole rhythm strip to determine if a normal PP interval can be found.

Escape beats If the sinoatrial node fails to generate electrical impulse then another part of the conduction system will discharge instead. This gives rise to an escape beat (Figure 23.16). As it occurs later than expected, the coupling interval between the normal and escape P wave is **longer** than the normal (SAN generated) PP interval.

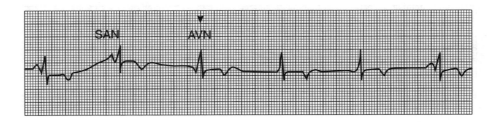

Figure 23.16 Escape P waves

Key point

Premature beat	Reduced coupling interval
Escape beat	Increased coupling interval

7. Is there atrial flutter?

In this condition the atria are depolarising at 250–350 beats/min but in most cases the rate is very close to 300 beats/min (i.e. one per large square). This atrial activity gives rise to regular "F" (flutter) waves which gives the baseline a characteristic "saw-tooth" appearance (Figure 23.17).

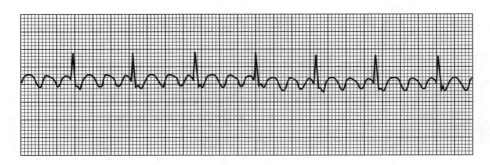

Figure 23.17 Atrial flutter

Only rarely does the atrioventricular node conduct all the atrial impulses to the ventricles. More commonly only one in two or one in four gets through. Nevertheless the QRS complexes which result have a normal shape if the remaining part of the conduction system has not been altered. In cases where the diagnosis is in doubt, carotid sinus massage can be used to increase temporarily the degree of atrioventricular node block so that "F" waves can be seen.

8. Are the number of P and QRS waves the same?

If the number of P and QRS waves are the same, measure the PR interval. In first degree heart block there are the same number of P waves as QRS complexes but the PR interval is constant and longer than 0·2 s (1 large square) (Figure 23.18). This condition is an ECG diagnosis and generally does not progress to more serious forms of heart block. It can, however, result from digoxin and β blockers.

If the number of P waves are greater than the number of QRS complexes then the patient has either second or third degree heart block. To distinguish between them the PR interval must be examined.

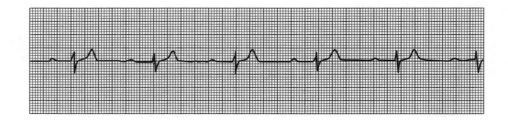

Figure 23.18 First degree block

Second degree heart block – Mobitz type I (Wenckebach) In this condition the PR interval progressively lengthens, until a P wave is not followed by a QRS complex. The atrioventricular node then recovers and the next PR interval reverts to the previous shortest conduction time. This rhythm is therefore distinguished by having **both varying PR and**

RR intervals (Figure 23.19). In some cases this phenomenon is physiological; in others, however, it can be the result of inferior myocardial infarction, digoxin or rheumatic myocarditis.

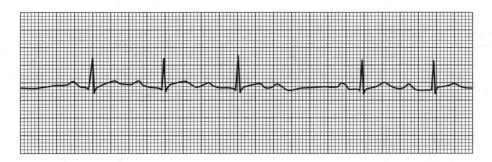

Figure 23.19   Second degree block — Mobitz type I

Second degree heart block – Mobitz type II   In this condition there is an intermittent non-conduction of some P waves but the **PR interval remains constant** (Figure 23.20). However, it may be of a normal or prolonged duration. Mobitz type II is much more likely to progress to third degree heart block than type I and there is a higher chance of developing asystole or ventricular dysrhythmias (see later).

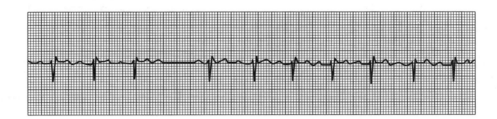

Figure 23.20   Second degree block — Mobitz type II

Third degree (complete heart block)   This results in total dissociation between the depolarisation of the atria and the ventricles with each beating independently (Figure 23.21). As a consequence, there is no consistent relationship between the P waves and the QRS complexes on the ECG trace. The PR interval is, therefore, completely erratic **but the PP and RR intervals are constant**.

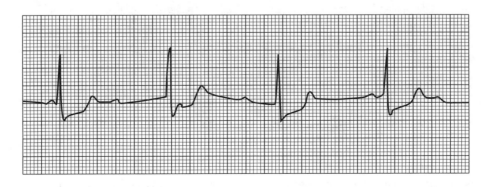

Figure 23.21   Third degree (complete) block

Summary
The different types of heart block are summarised in Table 23.1.

Table 23.1   The different types of heart block

Block	P:QRS	PR interval	RR interval
First degree	Equal	Constant and prolonged	Constant
Second degree, Type I	P > QRS	Variable	Variable
Second degree, Type II	P > QRS	Constant	Variable
Third degree (complete)	P > QRS	Variable	Constant

9. Is the QRS duration normal?
The normal duration for the QRS is 0·10 s (2·5 small squares) or less. This can only occur if the ventricular depolarisation originates from above the bifurcation of the bundle of His. Broader complexes occur as a result of:

- ventricular premature beats
- ventricular escape beats
- bundle branch blocks
- left ventricular hypertrophy
- aberrant conduction.

Ventricular premature beats (VPB) or ectopics   Ventricular premature beats present as bizarre, wide complexes with abnormal ST and T waves (Figure 23.22). Unlike the normal situation, ventricular depolarisation is premature thereby reducing the interval between the normal and abnormal beats (RR').

The QRS complex can be narrow or wide depending on where the source of the ventricular pacemaker is located. An escape focus near the atrioventricular node will result in a rate of around 50/min with narrow complexes as they are conducted via the bundle of His (see later in this chapter). This can result from congenital abnormalities but is also associated with inferior myocardial infarction.

A ventricular focus which is more distal from the atrioventricular node will produce an intrinsic rate of around 30/min (see later in this chapter). However, the QRS complexes will be wide (over 0·10 s) because conduction through the ventricles is not by the normal pathway. This can result from congenital abnormalities as well as from anterior and inferior myocardial infarction. These patients have a worse prognosis than those with a narrow QRS.

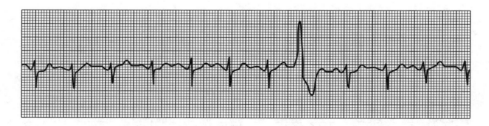

Figure 23.22   Ventricular ectopic

In contrast to atrial premature beats, ventricular premature beats do not alter, or reset, the sinoatrial node. Consequently, the frequency of the P waves will continue undisturbed by the abnormal ventricular activity. There is, therefore, usually a compensatory pause after the ventricular premature beat. As a result the next P wave occurs at the normal time.

A ventricular premature beat discharging during the repolarisation phase of the ventricle runs the risk of precipitating ventricular fibrillation. The chances of this are thought to be higher if the beat occurs close to the T wave. This is known as the **R-on-T phenomenon** (Figure 23.23).

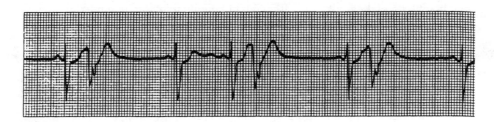

Figure 23.23 R-on-T ectopic

When there is more than one ventricular premature beat, specific terms are used if other features exist.

- Multifocal ventricular ectopics are seen when the ventricular premature beats vary in shape from beat to beat (Figure 23.24). This may or may not represent a number of separate foci but it does indicate a significant increase in ventricular excitability **and a higher chance of deteriorating into ventricular fibrillation**.
- Bigeminy is seen when a normal QRS complex is followed by a ventricular premature beat (Figure 23.25).
- Trigeminy occurs when two normal consecutive QRS complexes are followed by a ventricular premature beat (Figure 23.26).
- A couplet is seen when there are two ventricular ectopic beats in a row (Figure 23.27).

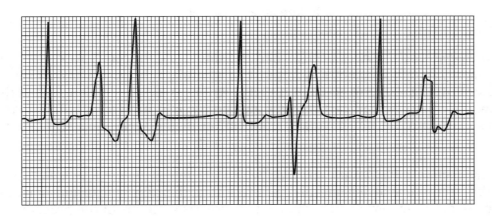

Figure 23.24 Multifocal ventricular ectopics

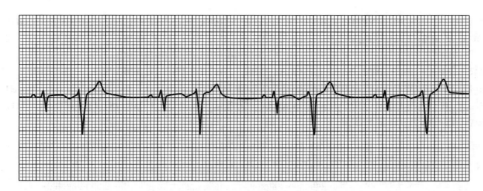

Figure 23.25 Bigeminy

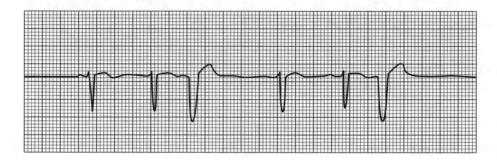

Figure 23.26 Trigeminy

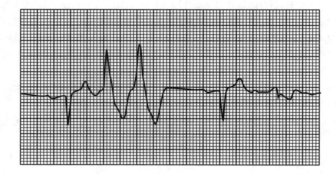

Figure 23.27 Couplets

Ventricular escape beats   These occur when the sinoatrial node and atrioventricular node can no longer generate an electrical impulse or stimulate the ventricles. In such circumstances the ventricles have to rely upon their own intrinsic pacemaker (see earlier in the chapter). Consequently the heart rate is slow and the RR' interval is longer than normal. If P waves exist they do not have any connection to the QRS (see 'third degree heart block').

Aberrant conduction with supraventricular premature stimulation   The QRS is abnormal because the premature atrial impulse gets to either the **atrioventricular node or the ventricles** before they have had a chance to repolarise fully from the preceding stimulation. Consequently, the conduction through the ventricles is abnormal and the resulting QRS complex is broad and abnormal in shape. Occasionally the shape of the QRS varies from beat to beat because the conduction pathway through the ventricles is not consistent. The PR interval is normal or slightly prolonged in this condition.

360

10. Is there ventricular tachycardia?
This occurs when there are three or more consecutive ventricular premature beats, with a rate greater than 140/min. It is said to be sustained if it lasts more than 30 s (Figure 23.28). Ventricular tachycardia produces a regular, or almost regular, rhythm with a constantly abnormally wide QRS complex. The rate usually lies between 140 and 280 beats/min.

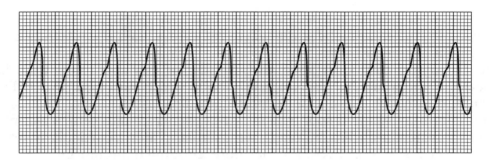

Figure 23.28   Ventricular tachycardia

A regular, broad QRS complex tachycardia can also be due to a supraventricular rhythm with an aberrant conduction. Occasionally the abnormal QRS complexes existed before the supraventricular tachycardia started and the increase in rate simply reflects the increase in rate of stimulation from the atria. However, the complexes may only become abnormal once the supraventricular tachycardia starts. In these circumstances the normal conducting system cannot repolarise quickly enough for the new wave of depolarisation from the atria. As a consequence the ventricular depolarisation takes an abnormal route (usually via an accessory pathway) and this is reflected in the abnormal QRS shape.

Distinguishing between ventricular tachycardia and supraventricular tachycardia with aberrant conduction can be difficult. A search must therefore be made for the following features (Table 23.2).

Table 23.2   Ventricular tachycardia versus supraventricular tachycardia with aberrant conduction

	Ventricular tachycardia	Supraventricular tachycardia and aberrant conduction
Fusion beats	Yes	No
Capture beats	Yes	No
P waves	Absent or not connected with the QRS	Precedes QRS

Fusion beats are produced when the atrial electrical impulse partially depolarises the ventricular muscle which has not been fully depolarised by the ventricular premature beat.

Capture beats occur in the context of atrioventricular dissociation, when the atrial electrical impulse completely depolarises the ventricle before it is depolarised by the ventricular premature beat. The effect is a normal QRS complex in the midst of the sequence of broad QRS complexes.

If the QRS complex was broad before the tachycardia started and its shape does not change during the tachycardia, then the dysrhythmia is likely to be a supraventricular tachycardia with aberrant conduction.

Further clues as to the origin of the broad complex tachycardia come from studying the patient's 12 lead ECG, previous ECG tracings, and medical notes. It is, therefore, essential that attempts are made to obtain these records. However, even after careful ECG evaluation it may still be impossible to distinguish between ventricular tachycardia and a supraventricular tachycardia with an aberrant conduction. In these cases, and especially **after myocardial infarction, it is always safer to assume a ventricular origin for a broad complex tachycardia**.

11. Is there torsade de pointes (polymorphic ventricular tachycardia)?
This is a type of ventricular tachycardia where the cardiac axis is constantly changing in a regular fashion (Figure 23.29).

Torsade de pointes can occur spontaneously, but it can also result from ischaemic heart disease, hypokalaemia, and certain drugs which increase the QT interval. Examples of the latter are tricyclic antidepressants and classes 1a and III antiarrhythmic agents. This condition can end spontaneously or degenerate into ventricular fibrillation. Interestingly, ventricular fibrillation may have a similar pattern, particularly soon after its onset, but this is usually short lived. Furthermore, continued monitoring of the ECG will reveal a far more random appearance and greater variability in QRS morphology in the case of ventricular fibrillation.

Atrial fibrillation in the presence of an anomalous conducting pathway that bypasses the atrioventricular node may permit rapid transmission of atrial impulses to the ventricles. The resulting ventricular rate may be so fast that cardiac output falls dramatically. The ECG appearances are of a very rapid, broad complex tachycardia that may show marked variability in the QRS complexes. However, the QRS complexes do not show the twisting axis characteristic of torsade de pointes. Furthermore, it is often impossible to recognise occasional fusion beats in cases of atrial fibrillation. The rhythm overall is also more organised than ventricular fibrillation and lacks the random change in amplitude.

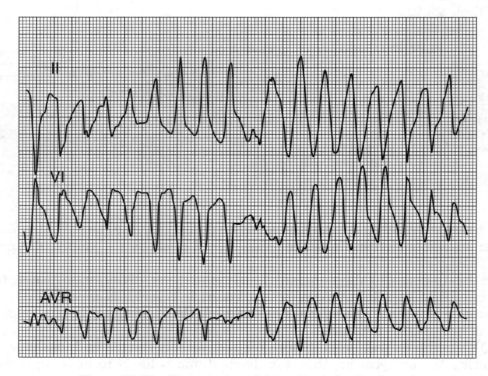

Figure 23.29   Torsade de pointes, showing axis change

12. Is there an idioventricular rhythm (IVR)?
This occurs when the ventricles have taken over as the cardiac pacemaker due to failure of the sinoatrial node, atria or atrioventricular node. In view of the ventricles' slow intrinsic rate of depolarisation the heart rate is usually slow (< 40 beats/min). However, it can be accelerated and produce rates up to 120 beats/min.

Acute idioventricular rhythm commonly occurs after a myocardial infarction.

An **agonal rhythm** is characterised by the presence of slow, irregular, wide ventricular complexes of varying morphology. This rhythm is usually seen during the latter stages of unsuccessful resuscitation attempts. The complexes gradually slow and often become progressively broader before all recognisable electrical activity is lost.

SUMMARY

The electrical activity of the heart is highly organised and monitoring of this activity should be carried out in a particular way to minimise the chances of artefacts. By using a systematic approach it is possible to interpret ECG rhythm strips effectively. **It is important to remember to treat the patient and not the monitor.**

CHAPTER

24

Chest X-ray interpretation

OBJECTIVES

After reading this chapter you will be able to:

- describe an effective system for non-radiologists to interpret chest X-rays.

INTRODUCTION

To aid understanding, the chapter will begin by reviewing important anatomical features and considering how each particular area can be affected.

It is important that a systematic method is followed when studying any X-ray, so that subtle and multiple pathologies are not missed. Once the patient's details have been checked use the system recommended for chest X-ray interpretation shown in the box.

The 'AABCS' approach to radiographic interpretation

- **A** – **A**dequacy
- **A** – **A**lignment
- **B** – **B**ones
- **C** – **C**artilage and joints
- **S** – **S**oft tissue

Most patients require only one good quality film and the ideal is a posteroanterior view (PA) taken in the X-ray department. The clinical condition of acutely ill patients usually prohibits this. Thus an anteroposterior (AP) view is taken in the resuscitation room or on the ward. This enables monitoring and treatment to be continued because the film cartridge is placed behind the patient lying on the trolley or bed. However, the apparent dimensions of the heart shadow are altered as a result of this projection.

INTERPRETATION OF FRONTAL CHEST RADIOGRAPHS

Adequacy

Having made sure it is the correct radiograph, check the side marker and look for any details written or stamped on the film. This will tell you if the film is posteroanterior or anteroposterior. Assess the exposure, by looking at the midthoracic intervertebral discs and noting if they are just visible through the mediastinal density. In overexposed films all the intervertebral discs are seen and the radiograph appears generally blacker. In contrast underexposure gives rise to poor definition of structures and boundaries.

The film should show the lung apices and bases including the costophrenic recesses, the lateral borders of the ribs, and peripheral soft tissues. The right hemidiaphragm should reach the anterior end of the right sixth/seventh rib or the ninth/tenth rib posteriorly on full inspiration. Poor inspiration (diaphragm higher than anterior fifth rib) affects the lower zone vessels such that they are compressed and appear more prominent. This in turn leads to vague lower zone shadowing. In addition, the heart appears enlarged because the diaphragms are high and the heart lies more horizontally.

Alignment

This is determined by looking at the relationship between the spinous processes of the upper thoracic vertebrae and the medial aspects of the clavicles. The ends of both clavicles should be equidistant from the central spinous process.

As with adequacy, alignment of the patient to the X-ray can significantly alter the size and shape of the chest contents on the radiograph. For example, if the patient is rotated there is distortion of the mediastinal contours as well as inequality in the transradiancy of the hemithoraces.

In addition to postural and rotational artefacts, remember the configuration of the patient's chest wall can also give rise to abnormal appearances. For example, pectus excavatum can alter the size, shape, and position of the mediastinum, as well as producing inequality in the transradiancy of the lungs.

Bones

The posterior, lateral, and anterior aspects of each rib must be examined in detail. This can be done by tracing out the upper and lower borders of the ribs from the posterior costochondral joint to where they join the anterior costal cartilage at the midclavicular line. The internal trabecula pattern can then be assessed.

Finish assessing the bones by inspecting the visible vertebrae, the clavicles, scapulae and proximal humeri. However, for full assessment specific views must be obtained.

Cartilage and joints

Calcification in the costal cartilage is common in the elderly – similarly in the larynx. Occasionally the glenohumeral joints are seen on the chest X-ray. They may show either degenerative or inflammatory changes.

Soft tissue

The soft tissue can be considered in three parts.

- Mediastinum
- Lungs and diaphragm
- Extrathoracic soft tissues.

Mediastinum

The mediastinum normally occupies the centre of the chest radiograph and has a well defined margin. You should consider the upper, middle (hila), and lower (heart) parts of the mediastinum.

Upper mediastinum

Check the position of the trachea. This should be central.

The upper left mediastinal shadow is formed by the left subclavian artery. This normally gives rise to a curved border which fades out where the vessels enter the neck. The left outer wall of the trachea is not visible in this area because the subclavian vessels separate the trachea from the aerated lung. Inferiorly, the left paratracheal region is interrupted by both the aortic knuckle and the main pulmonary artery with the space between the two being known as the 'aortopulmonary window'. The aortic knuckle should be well defined.

Middle mediastinum

The hila shadows are produced mainly by the pulmonary arteries and veins. The major bronchi can be identified as air containing structures but the bronchial walls are commonly only visible when seen end on. Though a contribution is made to these shadows by the hilar lymph nodes, they cannot be identified separately from the vascular shadows. The left hilum is usually higher than the right.

Any lobulation of the hilar shadow, local expansion or increase in density compared with the opposite side indicates a central mass lesion. Central enlargement of the pulmonary arteries may mimic mass lesions but the vascular enlargement is usually bilateral, accompanied by cardiomegaly and forms a branching shadow.

Lower mediastinum

The overall position, size, and shape of the heart should be noted first. Normally the cardiac shadow can have a transverse diameter which is up to 50% of the transverse diameter of the chest on a posteroanterior film. Cardiomyopathy or pericardial effusion can both give rise to a globular heart shadow but further diagnostic clues are usually available from the clinical history and examination.

The heart borders can then be assessed. The heart silhouette should be sharp and single with loss of a clear border indicating neighbouring lung pathology. A double outline suggests a pneumomediastinum/pneumopericardium. With a pneumomediastinum a translucent line can usually be seen to extend up into the neck and be accompanied by subcutaneous emphysema.

Inspection of the heart is completed by checking for calcification (valves and pericardium) and retrocardiac abnormalities, e.g. hiatus herniae, increased density or the presence of foreign bodies.

Lungs and diaphragm

Lungs

These are best assessed initially by standing back from the radiograph so that you can compare the overall size and transradiancy of both hemithoraces. A number of changes may be seen.

Reduced volume The commonest cause of lung volume loss is lobar collapse. When complete, these give rise to dense white shadows in specific locations and are usually accompanied by hilar displacement, increased radiolucency in the remaining lobes and reduction in the vascular pattern due to compensatory emphysema. When the collapse is incomplete, consolidation in the remaining part of the lobe is evident.

Reduced density   The transradiancy of both lungs should be equal and their outer edges should extend out to the ribs laterally and the diaphragm below. Any separation indicates that there is a pneumothorax. Within the normal lungs the only identifiable structures are blood vessels, end on bronchi and the interlobar fissures. Air trapping gives rise to increased translucency and flattening of the dome of the diaphragm. In extreme cases the mediastinum may be displaced to the contralateral side.

Increased density   There are several causes for an increase in pulmonary density. In consolidation the density is restricted to either part or all of a pulmonary lobe as a result of the air being replaced with fluid. With segmental consolidation the density is rounded and the edges blurred. When the whole of the lobe is involved the interface with neighbouring soft tissues is lost. This can lead to alteration in the outline of the heart and diaphragm depending upon the location of the lobe (see earlier).

Pleural fluid is seen initially as blunting of the costophrenic angle. As more accumulates the fluid level is easier to make out. However, if the patient is supine the fluid collects posteriorly and gives rise to a general ground-glass appearance on the affected side. Consequently, an effusion may be missed until it is large or the frontal and erect chest radiograph is carried out.

Pulmonary oedema presents as generalised fluffy air space shadowing which can be accompanied by Kerley B lines due to interstitial lymphatic congestion.

The position, configuration, and thickness of the fissures should also be checked – anything more than a hairline thickness should be considered abnormal. To visualise a fissure the X-ray beam needs to be tangential; therefore, only the horizontal fissure is evident on the frontal film, and then only in 50% of the population. It runs from the right hilium to the sixth rib in the axilla. The azygos fissure is seen in approximately 1% of the population. The oblique fissures are only identified on the lateral view.

Diaphragm

The diaphragm must be checked for position, shape, and clarity of the cardiophrenic and costophrenic angles. The outline of the diaphragm is normally smoothly arcuate with the highest point medial to the midline of the hemithorax. Lateral peaking, particularly on the right, suggests a subpulmonary effusion or a haemothorax in the appropriate clinical setting.

In the vast majority of patients the right diaphragm is higher than the left. However, elevation of either side can result from pathology in the abdomen or damage to the phrenic nerve. In this situation the patient's history will be very helpful in distinguishing between these possible causes.

The upper surface of the diaphragm is normally clearly outlined by air in the lung except where it is in contact with the heart and pericardial fat. Loss of clarity may indicate collapse or consolidation of the lower lobe. It could also indicate diaphragmatic rupture.

Extrathoracic soft tissue

Start at the top with the neck and supraclavicular area, and continue down the lateral wall of the chest on each side. Note any foreign bodies and subcutaneous emphysema. The latter is often seen in the cervical region and appears as linear transradiancies along tissue planes. When gross it may interfere with the assessment of the underlying lung. Finally, check under the diaphragm for abnormal structures or free gas.

Presence and position of any medical equipment

The position and presence of any invasive medical equipment must be assessed while the radiograph is examined so that potential complications can be identified. A further chest X-ray should be performed after the placement of any of these devices in order to exclude or detect the above complications.

Reassess commonly missed areas

Once the system described above has been completed, it is important to reevaluate those areas where pathology is often overlooked. These include:

- the lung apices
- behind the heart shadow
- under the diaphragm
- peripheral soft tissues.

Summary of the system for assessing frontal chest radiographs

- **Assess the adequacy of the film**
  - Patient's personal details
  - Projection of the X-ray beam
  - Exposure of the film
  - Area of the chest on the film
  - Degree of inspiration
- **Assess the alignment of the film**
- **Assess the bones**

Extrathoracic	Spine
	Shoulder
	Foreign bodies
	Air
	Under the diaphragm

- **Assess the cartilage and joints**
- **Assess the soft tissue**

Mediastinum	Upper
	Middle (hila)
	Lower (heart)
Lungs and diaphragm	Lungs
	Size
	Density
	Fissures
	Nodules and opacifications
	Diaphragm
	Position
	Shape
	Clarity of the angles
	Foreign bodies
	Air
	Under the diaphragm

- **Reassess commonly missed areas of the film**
  - Apices
  - Behind the heart
  - Under the diaphragm
  - Peripheral soft tissues

CHAPTER

25

Haematological investigations

OBJECTIVES

After reading this chapter you will be able to:

- identify which haematological tests are useful in the acute medical patient
- describe the rational use of such tests
- use test results to aid further clinical management.

INTRODUCTION

A full blood count is probably the commonest laboratory investigation that is requested because it is a "routine test". There is, however, no such commodity as a routine test and you should be able to justify requesting any investigation. A similar situation, though much less common, exists when requesting assessment of the components of the clotting cascade. It is, therefore, important that you critically appraise your requests and also interpret all the available information provided by, for example, a full blood count, and not just the haemoglobin, as often occurs.

RULES

When interpreting haematological results:

- Always request investigations and interpret results in light of clinical findings.
- Beware:
  - the isolated abnormality
  - bizarre results
  - results that do not fit with the clinical picture.
- If in doubt repeat the test.
- Always seek corroborative evidence from:
  - clinical findings
  - other test results.
- Always observe serial results for trends.

371

REVISION

Many haematological disorders are identified by, or suggested by, an abnormality in the full blood count. The result usually relates to three major cell lines in peripheral blood: erythrocytes, leucocytes, and platelets. In addition there is a wealth of numerical information describing these cell lines that is often ignored – at the clinician's peril. This information, generated by automatic haematology counters, should be used to the clinician's advantage – hence the need for revision of some of the key cell count components.

HAEMOGLOBIN LEVEL

The normal levels of haemoglobin are 15 ± 2 g/dl (150 ± 20 g/l) for men and 14 ± 2 g/dl (140 ± 20 g/l) for women. In the acute medical patient a raised haemoglobin often indicates polycythaemia. This is commonly associated with chronic respiratory disease rather than the rare polycythaemia rubra vera. In contrast, the haemoglobin level may be low indicating anaemia. However, remember that in patients with acute blood loss the haemoglobin level may be normal initially, until either compensatory measures fail or haemodilution occurs.

The red cell count is quoted by some laboratories, but this has little diagnostic value in the acute medical patient. However, the combination of haemoglobin and red cell count can be used to derive the mean cell haemoglobin (MCH). This gives a reliable indication of the amount of haemoglobin per red cell and is measured in picograms (normal range $29.5 \pm 2 \cdot 5$ pg). The mean cell haemoglobin concentration (MCHC) represents the concentration of haemoglobin in grams per decilitre (100 ml) of erythrocytes (normal range $33 \pm 1 \cdot 5$ g/dl). This is obtained by dividing the haemoglobin concentration by the packed cell volume. A low mean cell haemoglobin concentration is due to a low haemoglobin content in the red cell mass and indicates deficient haemoglobin synthesis. Thus the red cells will appear pale (hypochromic). Remember that high mean cell haemoglobin concentrations do not occur in red cell disorders because the haemoglobin concentration is already near saturation point in normal red cells. The mean cell haemoglobin concentration, unlike the mean cell haemoglobin, assesses the degree of haemoglobinisation of the red cells irrespective of their size and is useful in assessing the extent of under-haemoglobinisation. The packed cell volume (PCV or haematocrit) represents a proportion (by volume) of whole blood occupied by the red cells and is expressed as a percentage (normal range for men 47 ± 7, women $42 \pm 5\%$). The packed cell volume or haematocrit is always elevated in polycythaemia irrespective of cause. However, this may only be relative when haemoconcentration occurs as a result of fluid loss producing a decrease in plasma volume. The packed cell volume is therefore reduced in the presence of excess extracellular fluid and raised in fluid depletion. The mean cell value (MCV) measured in femtolitres (normal range 85 ± 10 fl) indicates erythrocyte size. Thus, it is increased in patients with macrocytic disorders (e.g. vitamin B12/folate deficiency) and reduced in the presence of microcytes (e.g. iron deficiency anaemia).

It is important to realise that red cell indices indicate the average size and degree of haemoglobinisation of red cells. They are, therefore, only of value if combined with a blood film examination that will augment the information about the relative uniformity of changes in either cell size or haemoglobin concentration.

THE BLOOD FILM

The benefits of the blood film have already been described. Some of the common terms used to describe cell morphology are listed in the box.

Morphological terms on blood cell reports		
Red cells	Pale cells	Hypochromia indicating defective haemoglobinisation or haemoglobin synthesis
	Macrocytes	Large cells, abnormal red cell production, premature release, megaloblastic erythropoiesis, haemolysis
	Anisocytes	Variation in cell size
	Poikilocytes	Variation in cell shape
		Schistocytes
		Burr cells
		Fragmented forms, usually indicate red cell trauma
	Sickle cells	Sickling disorders
White cells	Hypersegmented neutrophils	Usually indicates vitamin B12 or folate deficiency
	Left shift neutrophils	Indicate that neutrophils are being prematurely released
	Toxic granulation	Increased neutrophils
		Cytoplasmic granularity
		Usually associated with underlying infection
	Atypical lymphocytes	Likely viral infection
	Blast cells	Usually indicate leukaemia
Platelets	Clumping	Often causing an artificially low platelet count

RED CELL ABNORMALITIES

Red cell abnormalities can be classified as alterations in either number or morphology.

Alteration in number

An increase in red cells is described as polycythaemia (see earlier). In contrast anaemia is described as diminished oxygen carrying capacity of the blood due to either a reduction in the number of red cells or in the content of haemoglobin or both. This may be due to deficient red cell production and/or excessive loss. Although there is some overlap between these conditions this classification does provide a convenient way of considering this condition (see the next box).

Deficient red cell production

Iron deficiency anaemia secondary to:
- poor dietary intake
- malabsorption
- chronic blood loss

Vitamin B12 or folic acid deficiency secondary to:
- pernicious anaemic
- malabsorption of vitamin B12 or folic acid
- pregnancy
- hypothyroidism
- vitamin C deficiency
- drug use including alcohol
- aplasia
- invasion of bone marrow by, e.g. leukaemia, Hodgkin's lymphoma, myeloma
- toxic effects on erythroblasts, e.g. uraemia, chronic infections, and malignant disease

---

> **Excessive loss of red blood cells**
>
> - Haemorrhage
> - Abnormal haemolysis
> - Hypersplenism
> - Drugs

An anaemia with a coexistent reduction in both white cells and platelets is referred to as pancytopenia.

Alteration in morphology

An anaemia with reduced mean cell volume, mean cell haemoglobin, and mean cell haemoglobin concentration, i.e. microcytic hypochromic anaemia, is highly suggestive of iron deficiency. Therefore a serum ferritin should be requested before treatment with iron is started. However, if there is coexistent thrombocytosis then this type of anaemia could indicate ongoing blood loss or inflammation. If none of these conditions are evident then it is possible that the microcytic hypochromic picture is a manifestation of thalassaemia, which is rare in the United Kingdom. In contrast an anaemia with raised mean cell volume and mean cell haemoglobin is suggestive of a variety of conditions including a deficiency in vitamin B12 and/or folic acid, hypothyroidism, and alcohol use. An anaemia with normal mean cell volume, mean cell haemoglobin and mean cell haemoglobin concentration, i.e. a normochromic normocytic anaemia, can reflect chronic disease (e.g. inflammation, myeloma), acute blood loss or haemolysis.

Haemolysis is usually associated with a normochromic normocytic anaemia although some of the red cells can be large due to the release of a large number of immature red cells, i.e. reticulocytes. The latter can also occur following haemorrhage or in response to treatment with iron, folic acid, and vitamin B12. The comment polychromasia (grey/blue tint to cells) is often recorded on the full blood count indicating a reticulocyte response. A formal count of these cells can also be done.

Haemolytic anaemia is a term that describes a group of anaemias of differing cause, which are all characterised by abnormal destruction of red cells. The questions asked to identify the cause of haemolysis are shown in the box.

> **Three key questions in the diagnosis of haemolytic anaemia**
>
> - Is it an inherited or acquired disorder?
> - Is the location of the abnormality within the red cells (intrinsic) or outside (extrinsic)?
> - Are the red cells prematurely destroyed in the blood stream (intravascular) or outside in the spleen and liver (extravascular)?

These questions can be used to produce a "user frendly" classification of haemolytic anaemia as shown in the box.

Classification of haemolytic anaemias

- Inherited disorders
Red cell membrane	hereditary spherocytosis
	hereditary elliptocytosis
Haemoglobin	thalassaemia syndromes
	sickle cell disorders
Metabolic pathways	glucose 6 phosphate dehydrogenase deficiency
	pyruvate kinase deficiency
- Acquired disorders
Immune	warm and cold autoimmune haemolytic anaemia
Isoimmune	rhesus or ABO incompatibility
Non-immune and trauma	valve prosthesis, microangiopathy, drugs,
	infection, chemicals, hypersplenism

LABORATORY DIAGNOSIS OF HAEMOLYTIC ANAEMIA

The most likely clue is a normochromic normocytic anaemia with prominent reticulocytes. Other laboratory results include:

- unconjugated hyperbilirubinanaemia (thus a lack of bilirubin in the urine).
- low haptoglobin (a glycoprotein that binds to free haemoglobin and is thus depleted in haemolysis).
- Haemoglobin and haemosiderin can be detected in the urine with intravascular haemolysis.

Inherited disorders

More specific tests will be requested after taking a comprehensive history as this is likely to provide clues to underlying inherited disorders. The presence of hereditary spherocytosis or elliptocytosis will be seen on the blood film.

The thalassaemias are a heterogeneous group of disorders affecting haemoglobin synthesis; they will be diagnosed from the medical history, clinical examination, blood film, and haemoglobin electrophoresis to identify structural haemoglobin variants. In addition, the presence of sickle cell syndromes will be diagnosed from the clinical history, in particular that of the family, and the presentation with haemolysis, vascular occlusive crises, and sequestration crises. Under these circumstances the blood film is likely to show the presence of sickle shaped cells. Haemoglobin electrophoresis may reveal an abnormal haemoglobin such as Hbss in sickle cell anaemia with no detectable haemoglobin A.

The two common abnormalities of red cell metabolism resulting in haemolysis are glucose 6 phosphate dehydrogenase deficiency and pyruvate kinase deficiency. As well as the features of intravascular haemolysis described earlier, specific enzyme levels can also be measured to produce a definitive diagnosis.

Acquired disorders

Autoimmune haemolytic anaemia is a form of acquired haemolysis with a defect outside the red cell. The bone marrow produces structurally normal red cells. These are prematurely destroyed by the production of an aberrant antibody targeted against one or more antigens on the red cell membrane. Once the autoantibody has bound with the antigen on the red cell the exact type of haemolysis is determined by the class of antibody as well as the surface antigen. A simple classification of these conditions is either warm and cold depending on whether the antibody reacts better with red cells at 37°C or 4°C respectively.

Classification of autoimmune haemolytic anaemia

- Warm (usually IgG mediated)

Primary
    idiopathic
Secondary
    lymphoproliferative disorders
    other neoplasms
    drugs
    infections
    connective tissue disorders

- Cold (usually IgM mediated)

Primary
    cold haemagglutinin disease
Secondary
    lymphoprolific disorders
    infections, e.g. mycoplasma
    paroxysmal nocturnal haemoglobinuria
    cold haemoglobinuria

Warm autoimmune haemolytic anaemia

This is the commonest form of haemolytic anaemia. The erythrocytes are coated with either IgG alone or IgG and complement or complement alone. Premature destruction of red cells usually occurs in the liver and spleen. The most characteristic laboratory abnormality in warm autoimmune haemolytic anaemia is a positive direct antiglobulin test (DAT or Coombs test). As a reminder the DAT is where red cells are already sensitised and have immunoglobulin bound to their surface antigens. Addition of extrinsic antihuman globulin results in haemolysis, i.e. a positive direct Coombs test. In contrast, the indirect test is where normal red cells have to be sensitised *in vitro* by the addition of the test serum containing red cell antibodies. Finally antihuman globulin is added. Agglutination indicates the presence of red cell antibodies, as used in red cell typing.

Cold autoimmune haemolytic anaemia

This is generally associated with an IgM antibody. Isoimmune haemolytic anaemia may occur with rhesus or ABO incompatibility, and in the context of adult medicine this may follow a blood transfusion reaction.

Non-immune and traumatic autoimmune haemolytic anaemia is most frequently manifested by a microangiopathic picture. This is one of the most frequent causes of haemolysis and describes intravascular destruction of red cells in the presence of an abnormal microcirculation. Causes of microangiopathic haemolytic anaemia are listed in the box.

Causes of microangiopathic haemolytic anaemia

- Disseminated intravascular coagulation (DIC)
- Valve prosthesis
- Malignancy
- Severe infections
- Glomerulonephritis
- Vasculitis
- Accelerated (malignant) hypertension

TOTAL AND DIFFERENTIAL LEUCOCYTE COUNT

The total white count varies markedly as there is a diurnal rhythm with minimal counts occurring in the morning. This may rise during the rest of the day or following stress, eating or during the menstrual cycle. The total leucocyte count is $7 \pm 3 \times 10^9/l$. This comprises:

- neutrophils $2–7 \times 10^9/l$ (40–80% of total count)
- lymphocytes $1–3 \times 10^9/l$ (20–40% of total count)
- monocytes $0·2–1 \times 10^9/l$ (2–10% of total count)
- eosinophils $0·04–0·4 \times 10^9/l$ (1–6% of total count)
- basophils $0·02–0·1 \times 10^9/l$ (< 2% of total count).

DISORDERS OF LEUCOCYTES

There are many conditions that will affect both the total and differential white cell count. Common disorders are listed in the next four tables.

Disorders of neutrophils

Raised number	Bacterial infection
	Myeloproliferative disease
	Tissue damage
	Malignancy
	Drugs
Reduced numbers	Drugs
(production failure)	Chemicals
	Severe infection
	Marrow infiltration by malignant tumour or marrow fibrosis
	Specific deficiencies of vitamin B12 and folic acid
Idiopathic	Peripheral sequestration/hypersplenism
	Shock
	Severe infection

Disorders of lymphocytes	
Raised numbers (lymphocytosis, i.e. > 4 × 10⁹/l)	Viral infection, especially glandular fever*
	Chronic lymphatic leukaemia
	Typhoid fever
	Brucellosis
Reduced numbers (lymphopenia)	Corticosteroids
	Viral infections*
	Cytotoxic drugs
	Ionising radiation

* In suspected viral infections a blood film may show changes in lymphocyte numbers and morphology.

Disorders of monocytes	
Raised numbers	Infective endocarditis
	Typhus fever
	Malaria
	Kala-azar
	Systemic lupus erythematosus
	Certain clinical poisonings, e.g. trichloroethylene

Disorders of eosinophils	
Raised numbers	Parasitic infections
	Atopy including asthma and drugs insensitivity
	Chronic eczema
	Malignant tumours, e.g. Hodgkin's disease

Basophils rarely have any significance in the acute medical setting.

THE PLATELET COUNT

There is a marked variation in the normal platelet count ranging from 150 to 400 × 10⁹/l. Common platelet disorders are listed in the next box.

Disorders of platelets

Raised number (thrombocytosis)	Inflammation, e.g. Crohn's disease
	Haemorrhage
	Essential thrombocytosis (rare)
	Polycythaemia rubra vera (rare)
Reduced number (thrombocytopenia)	Deficient production, e.g. hypoplasia replacement with leukaemic cells or fibrosis
	Dyshaemopoiesis secondary to vitamin B12 deficiency
	Increased destruction of platelets, e.g. drugs or autoimmune
	Sequestrated in the spleen
	Increased consumption (disseminated intravascular coagulation)

Thrombocytopenia is a common finding. The risk of spontaneous haemorrhage is unusual unless the platelet count falls below $20 \times 10^9/l$.

COAGULATION

The physiological pathway of blood coagulation is an interlinked cascade of factors which most doctors learn for examinations. The basic principles are three activation pathways: intrinsic, extrinsic, and alternative, which have a final common pathway. Individual components of these pathways are shown in Figures 25.1 and 25.2.

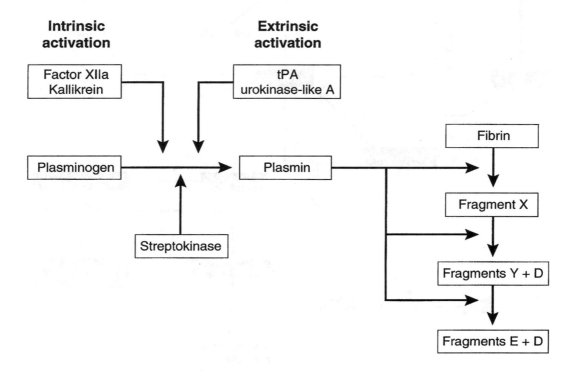

Figure 25.1 Clotting pathways

Blood clotting is a vital defence mechanism that is regulated to ensure adequate and appropriate activation.

The major inhibitors of coagulation circulating in the plasma are:

- Antithrombin III. This is the most potent inhibitor of the terminal proteins of the cascade, particularly factor X and thrombin. Its activity is greatly increased by interaction with heparin.
- Protein C is a vitamin K dependent plasma protein which inactivates cofactors Va and VIIIa as well as stimulating fibrinolysis. Protein C is converted to an active enzyme from interaction with thrombin. Protein S is a cofactor for protein C.
- Fibrinolytic systems. This is the endogenous system for fibrin digestion and is shown in Figure 25.2. Fibrin clots are broken down by plasmin that is produced from plas-

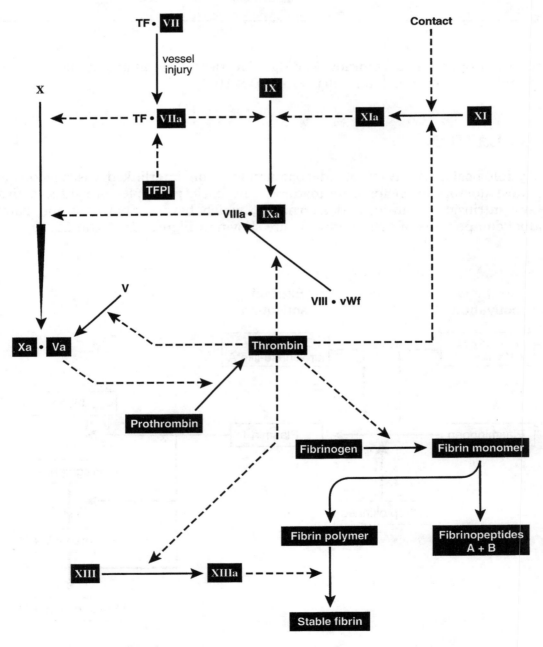

Figure 25.2 The endogenous system for fibrin digestion.

minogen by "activator enzymes". Plasmin also inhibits thrombin generation, thus reacting as an anticoagulant. In addition, fibrin degradation products have a similar effect. Fibrinolysis is also under strict control. Circulating plasmin is inactivated by the protease inhibitor α2 antiplasmin.

Tests for the assessment of coagulation

In most acute medical situations, an assessment of the coagulation cascade only requires:

- prothrombin time – a measure of the function of the extrinsic pathway
- activated partial thromboplastin time – assesses the intrinsic pathway
- assessments of fibrinolysis, e.g. fibrinogen level, fibrin degradation product level or D-dimer quantitation – are often used as markers of disseminated intravascular coagulation.

The common causes of prolonged prothrombin and activated partial thromboplastin times are listed in the box.

Common causes of prolonged prothrombin and activated partial thromboplastin times

Prothrombin times	Activated partial thromboplastin times
Warfarin	Heparin
Liver disease	Haemophilia
Vitamin K deficiency	von Willebrand's disease
Disseminated intravascular coagulation	Liver disease
	Lupus anticoagulant syndrome

SUMMARY

A limited number of haematological investigations are required in the acutely ill medical patient. Much of the information available is often underused; therefore a thorough understanding of the morphology and normal values of, in particular, red cells is extremely useful. A blood film is an underused investigation that can yield significant relevant information in the acute medical setting. These initial investigations, combined with a phased history, will influence the selection of subsequent haematological tests.

CHAPTER

26

Biochemical investigations

OBJECTIVES

After reading this chapter you will be able to:

- understand the importance of interpreting urea, electrolyte, and creatinine results in light of clinical findings
- systematically assess urea, electrolyte, and creatinine results
- use these results to aid your clinical management.

INTRODUCTION

Urea, electrolytes, and creatinine are commonly requested laboratory investigations. All too often there is little thought about why these investigations have been requested and what the abnormalities, in particular of the electrolytes, may indicate. This chapter will provide a systematic approach to the assessment of such investigations, but before this is described there are certain rules which have to be obeyed.

RULES FOR THE INTERPRETATION OF UREA, ELECTROLYTES AND CREATININE

- Always interpret the results in the light of clinical findings
- Beware – the isolated abnormality
           – bizarre results
           – results that do not fit the clinical picture
- If in doubt, repeat the test
- Always seek corroborative evidence from   – clinical findings
                                             – other test results
- Always observe serial results for trends

GUIDELINES FOR INTERPRETATION OF UREA, ELECTROLYTES AND CREATININE

A review of essential facts.

Urea

Blood urea provides an assessment of glomerular function. However, it can be influenced by many exogenous factors including food intake, fluid balance, gastrointestinal haemorrhage, drugs, and liver function. Normal plasma urea is 4·6–6·0 mmol/l.

Creatinine

This provides a better indication of renal function. Plasma creatinine levels are proportional to muscle mass. Creatinine gives a reasonable indication of changes in glomerular filtration providing the body weight remains stable. Normal plasma creatinine is 60–125 micromol/l.

Potassium

This is the most important intracellular cation and only approximately 2% of the total body potassium is found in the extracellular fluid. Normal plasma potassium is 3·5–5·0 mmol/l.

Bicarbonate

Bicarbonate is an important anion. Normal plasma bicarbonate is 24–28 mmol/l. In a venous blood sample the bicarbonate provides a useful, but crude, indication of the acid–base status.

Sodium

Sodium is the major extracellular cation and is intimately related to water balance. The normal plasma sodium is 135–145 mmol/l.

A SYSTEMATIC EXAMINATION OF UREA, ELECTROLYTES AND CREATININE

It is impossible to provide an accurate diagnosis purely by assessing a patient's urea, creatinine, and electrolytes. However, this system, especially when viewed with a patient's clinical picture, will help to discriminate between many of the common conditions.

A systematic approach comprises:

1. assessment of the patient's urea and creatinine
2. the relationship between the urea and creatinine
3. assessment of potassium, bicarbonate, and sodium.

Examine the urea and creatinine; five patterns are seen, as described below.

Diagnosis		
↑↑ Urea	↑↑ Creatinine	Renal failure
↓ Urea	↓ Creatinine	Fluid overload
Urea < creatinine		Low protein diet
		Liver failure
		Dialysis
Urea > creatinine		Fluid depletion, e.g. dehydration, fever, trauma
		Drugs, e.g. diuretics
		Elevated protein, e.g. diet, gastrointestinal bleed, catabolism
Urea normal	Creatinine normal	Check for any electrolyte abnormality

All results will fall into one of these five broad categories and each will be examined.

Urea raised and creatinine raised

The most common diagnosis would be renal failure. Therefore confirmatory evidence should be sought.

- Check plasma potassium – this will remain normal until the glomerular rate has fallen below 10 ml/min. Hyperkalaemia is common, but can be secondary to a metabolic acidosis, catabolism or haemolysis.
- Check bicarbonate – this is often reduced reflecting the acidosis associated with uraemia or a failure of bicarbonate secretion.
- Check serum sodium – this may be normal but is often low due to overhydration and dilution. To provide further information, plasma osmolality along with urine, sodium, osmolality, and urea should be measured to distinguish between acute and established renal failure.

Urea low and creatinine low

This commonly results from fluid overload.

- Check potassium, bicarbonate and sodium. Low values would be expected.

The basic problem is that sodium is retained but to a significantly lesser extent than the degree of water retention. This commonly results from two mechanisms.

- Increased water intake, e.g. excess intravenous fluids, excess drinking (both pathological and psychological polydipsia) and water absorption during bladder irrigation.
- Inability to excrete water, e.g. SIADH, adrenocortical insufficiency, hypothyroidism, and drugs that reduce renal diluting capacity, e.g. diuretics. Under these circumstances there is water retention but body sodium is normal with possibly only small increase in extracellular fluid volume which will be undetected clinically. In contrast if both extracellular fluid sodium and water are increased, but more water is retained than sodium, hyponatraemia will result with expansion of the extracellular fluid volume producing oedema. Note that the discriminating factor between these conditions is based on the clinical presence of oedema.

The first group of conditions with water retention and a normal serum sodium is often referred to as hyponatraemia with clinically normal extracellular fluid volume. In contrast hyponatraemia with expansion of the extracellular volume occurs with cardiac, renal, and liver failure. The urine sodium can provide further clues, in particular, in the patient who is hyponatraemic with an increased extracellular volume where the urine sodium is usually less than 10 mmol/l (except in renal failure).

An interesting variant is beer drinker's hyponatraemia. Beer has a low sodium content. If in excess of five litres is consumed daily then hyponatraemia may result, usually with a clinically normal extracellular volume.

Urea less than creatinine

Low urea in relation to the creatinine usually indicates low protein diet or rarely liver failure or post dialysis. Low urea in liver disease is usually attributed to reduced synthesis.

● Check potassium
   - normal with low protein diet and post dialysis
   - normal in liver disease unless diuretics are used
   - low in liver disease with diuretic use.

Urea greater than creatinine

These results suggest fluid depletion, e.g. associated with dehydration, fever, infection or trauma. Drugs, in particular diuretics, can induce a similar problem. An alternative explanation is increased protein which may be from a dietary source, following a gastro-intestinal haemorrhage, or secondary to catabolism.

● Check potassium
   - low values would suggest gastrointestinal fluid loss
   - high values are likely to indicate incipient renal failure or potassium sparing diuretic
● Check sodium
   - low values indicate hyponatraemia with reduced extracellular fluid volume reflecting reduced intake (rare), usually attributed to inappropriate replacement of gastro-intestinal fluid loss with 5% dextrose only

The major cause is excessive sodium loss which is usually:

● from the gastrointestinal tract secondary to vomiting, diarrhoea, fistulae or intestinal obstruction
● from the kidney, for example, during the diuretic phase of acute tubular necrosis
● due to excess diuretic therapy (including mannitol or the osmotic effect of hypoglycaemia)
● due to postobstructive diuresis
● due to adrenocortical insufficiency or severe alkalosis where increased urinary loss of bicarbonate necessitates an accompanying cation, usually sodium.

In addition, salt may be lost:

● from the skin in severe sweating, burns or erythroderma
● in association with inflammation of the peritoneum or pancreas
● following the removal of serous effusions, for example, ascites.

The key feature to remember is that salt loss is always associated with loss of water and other ions, in particular, potassium. However, it is often easy to underestimate the loss of salt if another solute such as glucose is present in excess, i.e. hyperglycaemia. This will tend to retain fluid within the extracellular fluid and the severity of the situation will be only unmasked when the hyperglycaemia is treated. The urine sodium again will provide a good indicator in that it will be less than 10 mmol/l in all conditions, unless there is an intrinsic salt losing problem with the kidneys.

Urea normal and creatinine normal

Therefore exclude any electrolyte abnormality.

- Check potassium – high; secondary to haemolysis, increased intake (usually iatrogenic) or redistribution, e.g. with acidosis or muscle injury

Under these situations the serum sodium is normal. Hyperkalaemia may also be present because of reduced excretion, for example, with acute renal failure or the use of potassium sparing diuretics. Again the sodium is usually normal although it can be reduced in the former because of dilution.

An elevated potassium in the presence of reduced sodium is suggestive of adrenal insufficiency.

- Check potassium – if low the commonest cause is a metabolic alkalosis; therefore check the bicarbonate level

Potassium may be lost from the gastrointestinal tract, for example, with diarrhoea or malabsorption. Under these circumstances the serum sodium is usually normal. In contrast, renal loss, associated with either diuretic therapy or cardiac or liver failure, is accompanied by hyponatraemia. A normal urea and creatinine with low potassium and high sodium combined means that excess of glucocorticoid and mineral corticoid hormones has to be excluded.

- Check bicarbonate – high, when associated with metabolic alkalosis and hypokalaemia.
- Check sodium – hyponatraemia in the context of normal urea, creatinine, and potassium is related to the extracellular fluid volume (see earlier).

Pseudohyponatraemia is a trap for the unwary. Sodium is present only in the aqueous phase of plasma. If there is an associated abnormal amount of lipid the water volume will be reduced and the measured sodium will be low. This result will be spurious because of the high proportion of lipid. In nephrotic syndrome or diabetes mellitus, for example, one litre of plasma may comprise 600 ml of water and 400 ml of lipid with a measured sodium of 120 mmol/l. The true calculated value of sodium, however, when expressed according to the volume of water, is 120 mmol/l of sodium in 600 ml of water – 200 mmol/l. Although this is an extreme example, it indicates that if such problems are not identified inappropriate treatment may occur. A way to clarify this situation is to measure urine sodium and chloride which are low in true hyponatraemia.

SUMMARY

These guidelines must be interpreted in the light of clinical findings. They will, however, facilitate the diagnosis of common conditions.

CHAPTER

27

Practical procedures: airway and breathing

PROCEDURES

- Oropharyngeal airway insertion
- Nasopharyngeal airway insertion
- Ventilation via a Laerdal pocket mask
- Orotracheal intubation
- Insertion of a laryngeal mask airway
- Insertion of a Combitube
- Surgical airway:
    needle cricothyroidotomy
    surgical cricothyroidotomy
- Needle thoracocentesis
- Aspiration of pneumothorax
- Aspiration of pleural fluid
- Chest drain insertion

OROPHARYNGEAL AIRWAY

Equipment

- A series of oropharyngeal (Guedel) airways
- Tongue depressor
- Laryngoscope

Procedure

The correct size of airway is selected by comparing it with the vertical distance from the angle of the mandible to the centre of the incisors. The airway is inserted in adults and older children as follows.

1. Open the patient's mouth and check for debris. This may be inadvertently pushed into the larynx as the airway is inserted
2. Insert the airway into the mouth either (i) "upside down" (concave uppermost) as far as the junction between the hard and soft palates and rotate through 180° or (ii) use

391

a tongue depressor or the tip of a laryngoscope blade to aid insertion of the airway "the right way up" under direct vision.

3. Insert so that the flange lies in front of the upper and lower incisors or gums in the edentulous patient (Figure 27.1) .
4. Check the patency of the airway and ventilation by "looking, listening, and feeling".

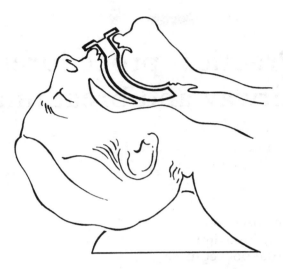

Figure 27.1   Oropharyngeal airway *in situ*

Complications

- Trauma resulting in bleeding
- Vomiting or laryngospasm: if the patient is not deeply unconscious

Key point
Use the oropharyngeal airway with caution in patients with a suspected base of skull fracture

NASOPHARYNGEAL AIRWAY

Equipment

- A series of nasopharyngeal airways
- Lubricant
- Safety pin

Procedure

Choose an airway approximately the same size as the patient's little finger or similar in diameter to the nares. Nasopharyngeal airways are designed to be inserted with the bevel facing medially. Consequently, the right nostril is usually tried first, using the following technique.

1. Lubricate the airway thoroughly.
2. Check the patency of right nostril.

3. Insert the airway bevel end first, along the floor of the nose (i.e. vertically in a supine patient) with a gentle twisting action.
4. When fully inserted, the flange should lie at the nares (Figure 27.2).
5. Once in place insert a safety pin through the flange to prevent the airway being inhaled.
6. If the right nostril is occluded or insertion is difficult, use the left nostril.
7. Check the patency of the airway and ventilation by "looking, listening, and feeling".

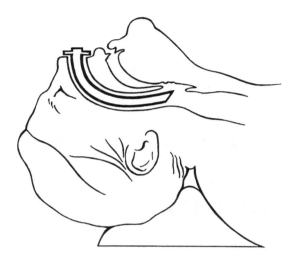

Figure 27.2   Nasopharyngeal airway *in situ*

Complications

- Bleeding
- Vomiting and laryngospasm if the patient not deeply unconscious

LAERDAL POCKET MASK

Equipment

Laerdal pocket mask
Airway mannikin

Procedure

The technique for using the mask is as follows.

1. With the patient supine, apply the mask to the patient's face using the thumbs and index fingers of both hands.
2. The remaining fingers are used to exert pressure behind the angles of the jaw (as for the jaw thrust) at the same time as the mask is pressed on to the face to make a tight seal (Figure 27.3).
3. Blow through the inspiratory valve for 1–2 s, at the same time looking to ensure that the chest rises and then falls.
4. If oxygen is available, add via the nipple at 12–15 l/min.

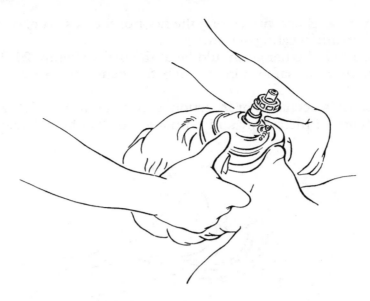

Figure 27.3   Haerdal pocket mask

OROTRACHEAL INTUBATION

Equipment

- Laryngoscope: most commonly with a curved (Macintosh) blade
- Tracheal tubes:
    females 7·5–8·0 mm internal diameter, 21 cm long
    males 8·0–9·0 mm internal diameter, 23 cm long
- Syringe, to inflate the cuff
- Catheter mount, to attach to ventilating device
- Lubricant for tube, water soluble, preferably sterile
- Magill forceps
- Introducers, malleable and gum elastic, for difficult cases
- Adhesive tapes or bandages for securing tube
- Ventilator
- Suction
- Stethoscope

Procedure

1. Whenever possible, ventilate the patient with 100% oxygen, using a bag–valve–mask device before intubation. During this time, check the equipment and ensure that all components are complete and functioning, particularly the laryngoscope, suction, and ventilating device.
2. Choose a tracheal tube of the appropriate length and diameter, and check the integrity of the cuff.
3. Position the patient's head to facilitate intubation; flex the neck and extend the head at the atlantooccipital joint ("sniffing the morning air" position), providing there are no contraindications. This is often made easier by having a small pillow under the patient's head.
4. Hold the laryngoscope in your left hand, open the patient's mouth and introduce the blade into the right-hand side of the mouth, displacing the tongue to the left.

5. Pass the blade along the edge of the tongue. The tip of the epiglottis should be seen emerging at the base of the tongue.
6. Advance the tip of the blade between the base of the tongue and the anterior surface of the epiglottis (vallecula).
7. The tongue and epiglottis are then **lifted** to reveal the vocal cords; **note that the laryngoscope must be lifted in the direction that the handle is pointing and not levered** by movement of the wrist, as this might damage the teeth and will not provide as good a view (Figure 27.4).

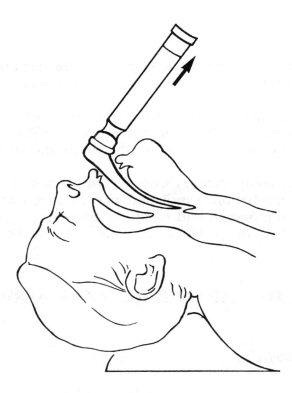

Figure 27.4 Laryngoscopy

8. Introduce the tracheal tube from the right-hand side of the mouth and insert it between the vocal cords into the larynx under direct vision, until the cuff just passes the cords.
9. Once the tube is in place, inflate the cuff sufficiently to provide an air-tight seal between the tube and the trachea. (As an initial approximation, the same number of millilitres of air can be used as the diameter of the tube in millimetres, and adjusted later.)
10. Attach a catheter mount to the tube and ventilate. Ensure that the tube is in the correct position and confirm ventilation of both lungs, by:
    - looking for bilateral chest movement with ventilation
    - listening for breath sounds bilaterally in the midaxillary line
    - listening for gurgling sounds over the epigastrium, which may indicate inadvertent oesophageal intubation
    - measuring the carbon dioxide in the expired gas. This will be greater than 0·2% in gas leaving the lungs providing there is a spontaneous circulation or good quality cardiopulmonary resuscitation in progress. Less than 0·2% indicates oesophageal placement of the tube.

Manoeuvres to assist with intubation

Occasionally, when the larynx is very anterior, direct pressure on the thyroid cartilage by an assistant may aid visualisation of the cords (not to be confused with cricoid pressure). However, despite this manoeuvre, in a small percentage of patients only the very posterior part of the cords (or none) can be seen and passage of the tracheal tube becomes difficult. In these cases, a gum elastic introducer can often be inserted into the larynx initially and then the tracheal tube slid over the introducer into the larynx. However, remember that the patient must be oxygenated between attempts at intubation.

Complications

- All the structures encountered from the lips to the trachea may be traumatised.
- When the degree of unconsciousness has been misjudged, vomiting may be stimulated
- A tube that is too long may pass into a main bronchus (usually the right), causing the opposite lung to collapse, thereby severely impairing the efficiency of ventilation. This is usually identified by the absence of breath sounds and reduced movement on the unventilated side.
- The most dangerous complication associated with tracheal intubation is **unrecognised** oesophageal intubation. Ventilation may appear adequate, but in fact the patient is not receiving oxygen and is rapidly becoming hypoxaemic. **If in doubt, take it out** and ventilate the patient using a bag–valve–mask.

INSERTION OF THE LARYNGEAL MASK AIRWAY (LMA)

Equipment

- Laryngeal mask airway, size   cuff volume
  5   large adult   40 ml
  4   adult male   30 ml
  3   adult female, child 30–35 kg   20 ml
- Lubricant
- Syringe to inflate cuff
- Adhesive tape to secure laryngeal mask airway
- Suction
- Ventilating device

Procedure

1. Whenever possible, ventilate the patient with 100% oxygen using a bag–valve–mask device before inserting the laryngeal mask airway. During this time, check that all the equipment is present and working, particularly the integrity of the cuff.
2. Deflate the cuff and lightly lubricate the back and sides of the mask.
3. Tilt the patient's head (if safe to do so), open the mouth fully, and insert the tip of the mask along the hard palate with the open side facing, but not touching the tongue (Figure 27.5a).
4. Insert the mask further, along the posterior pharyngeal wall, with your index finger initially providing support for the tube (Figure 27.5b). Eventually resistance is felt as the tip of the laryngeal mask airway lies at the upper end of the oesophagus (Figure 27.5c).

5. Fully inflate the cuff using the air filled syringe attached to the valve at the end of the pilot tube using the volume of air shown in the earlier box (Figure 27.5d).
6. Secure the laryngeal mask airway with adhesive tape and check its position during ventilation as for a tracheal tube.
7. If insertion is not accomplished in less than 30 seconds, reestablish ventilation using a bag–valve–mask.

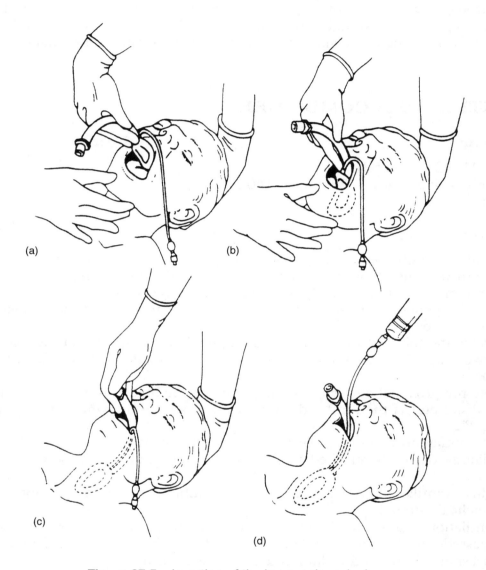

Figure 27.5   Insertion of the laryngeal mask airway

Complications

*   Incorrect placement is usually due to the tip of the cuff folding over during insertion. The laryngeal mask airway should be withdrawn and reinserted.
*   Inability to ventilate the patient, because the epiglottis has been displaced over the larynx. Withdraw the laryngeal mask airway and reinsert ensuring that it closely follows the hard palate. This may be facilitated by the operator or an assistant lifting the jaw upwards. Occasionally rotation of the laryngeal mask airway may prevent its insertion. Check that the line along the tube is aligned with the patient's nasal septum; if not, reinsert.

- Coughing or laryngeal spasm is usually due to attempts to insert the laryngeal mask airway into a patient whose laryngeal reflexes are still present.

Intubation via the laryngeal mask airway

Insert an introducer through the laryngeal mask airway into the trachea, remove the laryngeal mask airway and then pass the tracheal tube over the introducer into the trachea. Alternatively, a small diameter cuffed tracheal tube (6·0 mm) may be passed directly through a size 4 laryngeal mask airway into the trachea. A laryngeal mask airway is currently being designed to allow intubation through it with a larger diameter tracheal tube.

INSERTION OF A COMBITUBE

Equipment

- 37 or 41 FG Combitube
- Accompanying syringes: 20 ml and 140 ml
- Lubricant
- Suction
- Ventilating device

1. Whenever possible ventilate the patient with 100% oxygen, using a bag–valve–mask device before inserting the Combitube. During this time, check the equipment is present and working, particularly the integrity of the cuffs.
2. Grasp the patient's jaw and tongue between your thumb and index finger and lift them forwards.
3. Advance the tube with the curve pointing towards the larynx, in the midline, until the two black lines are positioned between the patient's teeth or gums (if edentulous).
4. Inflate the proximal cuff with 100 ml of air via the blue pilot tube marked "No. 1". The distal cuff is then inflated with 15 ml of air via the white pilot tube marked "No. 2".
5. Start ventilation assuming oesophageal placement as this commonly occurs. The ventilating device is attached to the No. 1 (blue) end of the Combitube (Figure 27.6a).
6. Confirm ventilation is successful (i.e. the Combitube lies in the oesophagus) as for orotracheal intubation.
7. If ventilation is unsuccessful and accompanied by gastric inflation, the Combitube has passed into the trachea. The ventilating device should be connected to the No. 2 (clear, shorter) end of the Combitube (Figure 27.6b).
8. Confirm satisfactory ventilation as previously described.

In the oesophageal position, regurgitation and aspiration are prevented by the distal cuff sealing the oesophagus. In the tracheal position aspiration of regurgitated contents is prevented by the distal cuff sealing the airway as with a conventional tracheal tube.

Complications

- Damage to the cuffs by the patient's teeth during insertion.
- Unable to insert due to limited mouth opening.
- Trauma to the oesophagus or trachea due to poor technique of insertion or wrong size used.
- Failure to achieve ventilation as a result of using the wrong lumen.

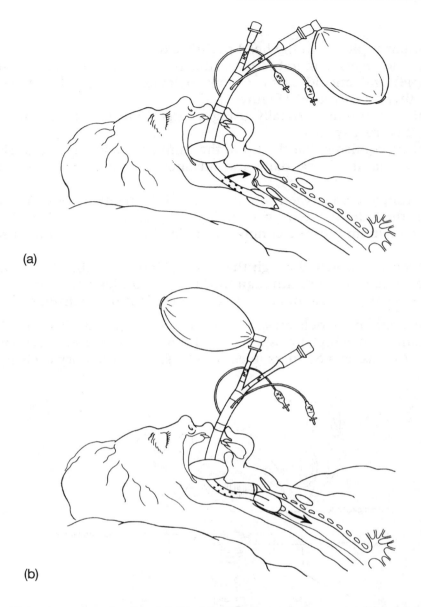

(a)

(b)

Figure 27.6 Insertion of a Combitube (a) oesophageal placement (b) tracheal placement

THE SURGICAL AIRWAY

It is important to realise that these techniques are temporising measures, while preparing for a definitive airway.

Needle cricothyroidotomy

Equipment

- Venflons 12–14 gauge
- Jet insufflation equipment
- Oxygen tubing with either a threeway tap or a hole cut in the side
- 20 ml syringe
- Mannikin/sheep's larynx

Procedure

1. Place the patient supine with the head slightly extended.
2. Identify the cricothyroid membrane as the recess between the thyroid cartilage (Adam's apple) and cricoid cartilage (approximately 2 cm below the "V" shaped notch of the thyroid cartilage) (Figure 27.7).
3. Puncture this membrane vertically using a large bore (12–14 gauge) intravenous cannula attached to a syringe
4. Aspiration of air confirms that the tip of the cannula lies within the tracheal lumen.
5. Angle the cannula at 45° caudally and advance over the needle into the trachea (Figure 27.8).
6. Attach the cannula to an oxygen supply at 12–15 l/min either via a "Y" connector or a hole cut in the side of the oxygen tubing. Oxygen is delivered to the patient by occluding the open limb of the connector or side hole for 1 s and then releasing for 4 s.
7. Expiration occurs passively through the larynx. Watch the chest for movement and auscultate for breath sounds, although the latter are difficult to hear.
8. If satisfactory, secure the cannula in place to prevent it being dislodged.

An alternative method of delivering oxygen is to use jet ventilation. This involves connecting the cannula to a high pressure oxygen source (4 bar, 400 kPa, 60 psi) via luer-lock connectors or by using a Sanders injector. The same ventilatory cycle is used.

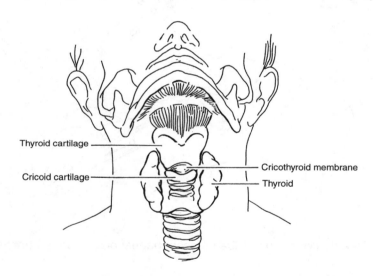

Figure 27.7   Cricothyroidotomy: relevant anatomy

Complications

- Asphyxia
- Pulmonary barotrauma
- Bleeding
- Oesophageal perforation
- Kinking of the cannula
- Subcutaneous and mediastinal emphysema
- Aspiration

Occasionally, this method of oxygenation will disimpact a foreign body from the larynx, allowing more acceptable methods of ventilation to be used.

Key point
There are two important facts to remember about transtracheal insufflation of oxygen. Firstly, it is not possible to deliver oxygen via a needle cricothyroidotomy using a self-inflating bag and valve. This is because these devices do not generate sufficient pressure to drive adequate volumes of gas through a narrow cannula. In comparison, the wall oxygen supply will provide a pressure of 400 kPa (4000 cm H_2O), which overcomes the resistance of the cannula.

Secondly, expiration cannot occur through the cannula or through a separate cannula inserted through the cricothyroid membrane. The pressure generated during expiration is generally less than 3 kPa (30 cm H_2O), which is clearly much less than the pressure required to drive gas in initially. Expiration must occur through the upper airway, even when partially obstructed. If the obstruction is complete, then the oxygen flow must be reduced to 2–4 l/min to avoid the risk of barotrauma, in particular the creation of a tension pneumothorax

Surgical cricothyroidotomy

Equipment

- Antiseptic solution
- Swab
- Syringe, needle, and local anaesthetic
- Scalpel
- Two arterial clips
- Endotracheal tube or size 5 tracheotomy tubes
- Tape
- Gloves
- Mannikin/sheep's larynx

Procedure

1. Place the patient supine if possible with the head extended.
2. Identify the cricothyroid membrane as described earlier (Figure 27.8).
3. Stabilise the thyroid cartilage using the thumb, index, and middle fingers of the left hand.
4. If the patient is conscious, consider infiltrating with local anaesthetic containing adrenaline (lignocaine 1% with adrenaline 1:200 000).
5. Make a longitudinal incision down to the membrane, pressing the lateral edges of the skin outwards to reduce bleeding.
6. Incise the membrane transversely and dilate the channel with the scalpel handle to accept a small (4·0–7·0 mm) cuffed tracheostomy tube. If one of these is not immediately available, a similarly sized tracheal tube can be used.
7. Ensure that the tube enters the tracheal lumen, rather than just running anteriorly in the soft tissues.
8. Inflate the cuff and commence ventilation.
9. Check the adequacy of ventilation as described earlier and, if satisfactory, the tube can be secured.
10. Suction the upper airway via the tube to remove any inhaled blood or vomit.

An alternative technique in these circumstances is the "Mini-Trach" (Portex). This was originally designed to facilitate the removal of secretions from the chest. The "kit" contains everything required to create an emergency surgical airway.

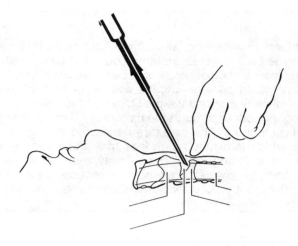

Figure 27.8 Needle cricothyroidotomy

1. Use a guarded scalpel to puncture the cricothyroid membrane percutaneously, to the correct depth.
2. Pass the rigid, curved introducer through the puncture site into the trachea.
3. Pass the 4·0 mm PVC flanged tracheal cannula (with a standard 15 mm connector attached) over the introducer into the trachea.
4. Remove the introducer and secure the cannula via the flanges with tapes. Ventilate the patient using the devices already described.

Complications

-   Similar to needle cricothyroidotomy, except that bleeding is more profuse due to the larger incision
-   Vocal cord damage may result in hoarseness
-   Cricoid cartilage damage may cause laryngeal stenosis

NEEDLE THORACOCENTESIS

Equipment

-   Alcohol swab
-   Intravenous cannula (16 gauge minimum)
-   20 ml syringe

Procedure

1. Identify the second intercostal space in the midclavicular line on the side of the pneumothorax (the opposite side to the direction of tracheal deviation).
2. Swab the chest wall with surgical preparation or an alcohol swab.
3. Attach the syringe to the cannula.
4. Insert the cannula into the chest wall, just over the rib, aspirating all the time.
5. If air is aspirated, remove the needle, leaving the plastic cannula in place.
6. Tape the cannula in place and proceed to chest drain insertion (see later) as soon as possible.

> **Key point**
> If needle thoracocentesis is attempted, and the patient does not have a tension pneumothorax, the chance of causing a pneumothorax is 10–20%. Patients must have a chest X-ray, and will require chest drainage if ventilated

Complications

- Local haematoma
- Lung laceration

ASPIRATION OF PNEUMOTHORAX

Equipment

- Alcohol swab
- Intravenous cannula (minimum 16 gauge)
- 20 ml syringe
- Threeway tap

Procedure

The equipment is the same as for needle thoracocentesis, plus threeway tape.

1. Explain to the patient the nature of the procedure.
2. Use appropriate aseptic techniques.
3. Identify the second intercostal space in the midclavicular line.
4. After appropriate skin preparation, infiltrate the area with 1% lignocaine.
5. Insert a large (14 or 16 gauge) cannula, remove the central trochar, and attach a threeway tap and 50 ml syringe.
6. Continue to aspirate until resistance is encountered or the patient experiences discomfort or coughing.

> **Key point**
> Aspiration of 2 litres of air may suggest a persistent air leak; the procedure should be abandoned and a formal chest drain insertion considered

Complications

- As for needle thoracocentesis

ASPIRATION OF PLEURAL FLUID

Equipment

Skin preparation:
    local anaesthetic
    5 ml syringe with orange, blue, and green hubbed needles
    50 ml syringe with threeway tap
    16 gauge cannula

Procedure

1. Explain to the patient the nature of the procedure.
2. Identify the appropriate side for aspiration of pleural fluid and recheck the X-ray.
3. Clean the skin.
4. After raising the skin bleb, the local anaesthetic is injected via the orange hubbed needle. Introduce the larger blue hubbed needle over the superior aspect of the rib through the intercostal tissues down to the pleura.
5. Always aspirate before injecting to ensure that a blood vessel has not been traumatised.
6. For a diagnostic aspiration a green hubbed 21 gauge needle can be inserted through this anaesthetised area into the pleural space, and fluid aspirated into a 30 ml syringe.
7. In contrast, fluid can be aspirated after insertion of a large cannula through this area and attaching the syringe to the cannula via a threeway tap.

Failure of aspiration

- Attempted aspiration too high
- Thickened pleura
- Pleural tumour
- Viscid empyema fibrinous exudate
- Complication – dry tap for reasons described above
- Haematoma
- Bleeding
- Pneumothorax

Complications

- As for needle thoracocentesis

CHEST DRAIN INSERTION

Equipment

Skin preparation and surgical drapes
Local anaesthetic
Scalpel
Scissors
Large clamps × 2
Chest drain tube without trochar
Suture
Underwater seal
10 ml syringe with orange, blue and green needles

Procedure

1. Identify relevant landmarks (usually the fifth intercostal space anterior to the midaxillary line) on the side with the pneumothorax.
2. Swab the chest wall with surgical preparation or an alcohol swab.
3. Use local anaesthetic if necessary.

4. Make a 2–3 cm transverse skin incision along the line of the intercostal space, towards the superior edge of the sixth rib (thereby avoiding the neurovascular bundle).
5. Bluntly dissect through the subcutaneous tissues just over the top of the rib, and puncture the parietal pleura with the tip of the clamp.
6. Put a gloved finger into the incision and clear the path into the pleura.
7. Advance the chest drain tube into the pleural space **without** the trochar.
8. Ensure that the tube is in the pleural space by listening for air movement, and by looking for fogging of the tube during expiration.
9. Connect the chest drain tube to an underwater seal.
10. Suture the drain in place, and secure with tape.
11. Obtain a chest X-ray.

Complications

- Damage to intercostal nerve, artery or vein
- Introduction of infection
- Tube kinking, dislodging or blocking
- Subcutaneous emphysema
- Persistent pneumothorax due to faulty tube insertion, leaking around chest drain, leaking underwater seal, bronchopleural fistula
- Failure of lung to expand due to blocked bronchus
- Anaphylactic or allergic reaction to skin preparation

CHAPTER

28

Practical procedures: circulation

PROCEDURES

- Peripheral venous cannulation
- Central venous cannulation:
  - internal jugular vein
  - subclavian vein
  - femoral vein
  - Seldinger technique

VENOUS ACCESS

Venous access is an essential part of resuscitation. It is an invasive procedure that must not be treated with complacency.

Vascular access can be achieved via several routes:

- percutaneous cannulation of a peripheral vein
- following surgical exposure of a vein in the "cutdown" technique
- percutaneous cannulation of a central vein
- intraosseous route.

Success is optimised and complications minimised when the operator understands the:

- local anatomy
- equipment
- technique
- complications.

PERIPHERAL VENOUS CANNULATION

The antecubital fossa is the commonest site for peripheral venous cannulation.

The cephalic vein passes through the antecubital fossa on the lateral side and the basilic vein enters very medially just in front of the medial epicondyle of the elbow. These two large veins are joined by the **median cubital or antecubital vein**. The median vein of the forearm also drains into the basilic vein (Figure 28.1).

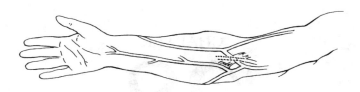

Figure 28.1   Veins of the forearm and antecubital fossa

Although the veins in this area are prominent and easily cannulated, there are many other adjacent vital structures which can be easily damaged.

The most popular device for peripheral intravenous access is the cannula over needle, available in a wide variety of sizes, 12–27 gauge (g). It consists of a plastic (PTFE or similar material) cannula which is mounted on a smaller diameter metal needle, the bevel of which protrudes from the cannula. The other end of the needle is attached to a transparent "flashback chamber", which fills with blood indicating that the **needle** bevel lies within the vein. Some devices have flanges or "wings" to facilitate attachment to the skin. All cannulae have a standard luer-lock fitting to attach a giving set and some have a valved injection port attached through which drugs can be given.

Equipment

Alcohol swab
Intravenous cannulae
Tourniquet
Tape

Procedure

1. Choose a vein capable of accommodating a large cannula, preferably one that is both visible and palpable. The junction of two veins is often a good site as the "target" is relatively larger and more stable.
2. Encourage the vein to dilate as this increases the success rate of cannulation. In the limb veins use a tourniquet that stops venous return but permits arterial flow. Further dilatation can be encouraged by gently tapping the skin over the vein. If the patient is cold and vasoconstricted, if time permits, topical application of heat from a towel soaked in warm water can cause vasodilatation.
3. If time permits, the skin over the vein should be cleaned. Ensure there is no risk of allergy if iodine based agents are used. If alcohol based agents are used, they must be given time to work (2–3 min), ensuring that the skin is dry before proceeding further.
4. In the conscious patient, consider infiltrating a small amount of local anaesthetic into the skin at the point chosen using a 22–25 gauge needle, particularly if a large (>1·2 mm, 18-gauge) cannula is to be used. This reduces the pain of cannulation, therefore making the patient less likely to move and less resistant to further attempts if the first is unsuccessful!
5. If a large cannula is used, insertion through the skin may be facilitated by first making a small incision with either a 19 gauge needle or a scalpel blade, taking care not to puncture the vein.
6. Immobilise the vein to prevent displacement by the advancing cannula. Pull the skin over the vein tight, with your spare hand (Figure 28.2).

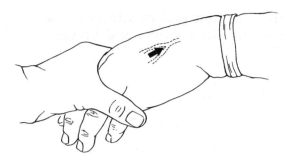

Figure 28.2   Vein immobilised

7.   Hold the cannula firmly, at an angle of 10–15° to the skin and advance through the skin and then into the vein. Often a slight loss of resistance is felt as the vein is entered. This should be accompanied by the appearance of blood in the flashback chamber of the cannula (Figure 28.3). However, the appearance of blood only indicates that the tip of the needle is within the vein, not necessarily any of the cannula.

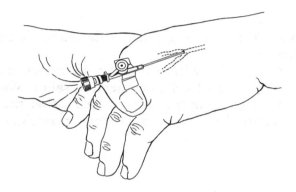

Figure 28.3   Cannula inserted (note the flashback of blood)

8.   Whilst keeping the skin taut, the next step is to reduce the angle of the cannula slightly and advance it a further 2–3 mm into the vein. This is to ensure that the first part of the plastic cannula lies within the vein. Care must be taken at this point not to push the needle out of the back of the vein.

9.   Withdraw the needle 5–10 mm into the cannula so that the point no longer protrudes from the end. Often as this is done, blood will flow between the needle body and the cannula, confirming that the tip of the cannula is within the vein (Figure 28.4).

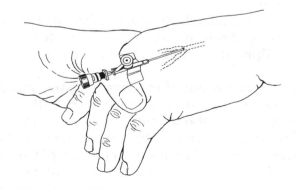

Figure 28.4   Cannula with needle slightly withdrawn

10. Advance the combined cannula and needle along the vein. The needle is retained within the cannula to provide support and prevent kinking at the point of skin puncture (Figure 28.5).

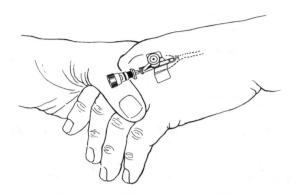

Figure 28.5   Cannula fully inserted

11. Insert the cannula as far as the hub, release the tourniquet and remove the needle and place in a sharps bin.
12. Confirm that the cannula lies within the vein by either attaching an intravenous infusion, ensuring that it runs freely, or injecting saline. Watch the tissues around the site for any signs of swelling that may indicate that the cannula is incorrectly positioned. Finally secure the cannula in an appropriate manner.

Complications

- Failed cannulation is the most common, usually as a result of pushing the needle completely through the vein. It is inversely related to experience.
- Haematomata are usually secondary to the above with inadequate pressure applied to prevent blood leaking from the vein after the cannula is removed. They are made worse by forgetting to remove the tourniquet!
- Extravasation of fluid or drugs is commonly a result of failing to recognise that the cannula is not in the vein before use. Placing a cannula over a joint or prolonged use to infuse fluids under pressure also predisposes to leakage. The faulty cannula must be removed. Damage to the surrounding tissues will depend primarily on the nature of the extravasated fluid.
- Damage to other local structures is secondary to poor technique and lack of knowledge of the local anatomy.
- The plastic cannula can be sheared, allowing fragments to enter the circulation. This is usually a result of trying to reintroduce the needle after it has been withdrawn. The safest action is to withdraw the whole cannula and attempt cannulation at another site with a new cannula.
- The needle may fracture as a result of careless excessive manipulation with the finer cannulae. The fragment will have to be removed surgically.
- Inflammation of the vein (thrombophlebitis) is related to the length of time the vein is cannulated and the irritation caused by the substances flowing through it. High concentrations of drugs and fluids with extremes of pH or high osmolality are the main causes. Once a vein shows signs of thrombophlebitis, i.e., tender, red, and the flow rate is deteriorating, the cannula must be removed to prevent subsequent infection or thrombosis which may spread proximally.

CENTRAL VENOUS CANNULATION

Catheterisation of a central vein is relatively easy. However, at a cardiac arrest, it may be necessary for someone to catheterise a central vein safely and quickly but without the benefit of a great deal of experience. Therefore an easy technique is required that has a high success rate with few complications. Central venous cannulation is a common technique in acutely ill patients for:

- drug delivery
- central pressure monitoring
- pacing
- inserting a pulmonary artery flotation catheter
- parenteral nutrition.

Equipment

Skin preparation
Local anaesthetic
10 ml syringe with blue and green needles
Appropriate catheter for central venous cannulation (see Seldinger technique)
Suture
Tape

Procedure

Whenever possible place the patient in a head-down position to dilate the vein and reduce the risk of air embolus. Many approaches and different types of equipment have been described to secure central venous access. This chapter describes three approaches (internal jugular, subclavian and femoral) using a single standard technique. This has been found to be successful in both experienced and inexperienced hands. No further justification of the choice is offered. For those already skilled at central venous cannulation using a different technique (**with an acceptable rate of complications**), carry on!

The internal jugular vein – paracarotid approach (Figure 28.6)

At the level of the thyroid cartilage, the internal jugular vein runs parallel to the carotid artery in the carotid sheath and therefore rotation of the head, obesity and individual variations in anatomy have less effect on the location of the vein.

1. Place the patient in the supine position, arms at their side and the head in a neutral position.
2. Standing at the head of the patient identify the thyroid cartilage and use the fingers of the left hand to palpate the carotid pulse. The right internal jugular vein is the one most commonly used initially.
3. Identify the apex of a triangle formed by the two heads of sternoclavicular muscle (the base is the clavicle).
4. Under sterile conditions, infiltrate with 1% lignocaine.
5. With the fingers of the left hand "guarding" the carotid artery, insert a needle 0·5 cm lateral to the artery. Inject 0·5–1 ml of air to expel any skin plug in the needle tip.
6. Advance the needle slowly caudally, parallel to the sagittal plane at an angle of 45° to the skin, aspirating at all times.

411

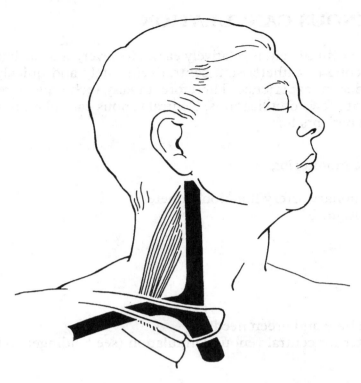

Figure 28.6   The course of the central veins of the neck

7. Confirm entry into the vein by blood entering the syringe. Introduce the catheter via a guide wire as described later.
8. If the vein is not entered at the first attempt, then subsequent punctures should be directed slightly more laterally (never medially towards the artery).

   Although a chest X-ray should be taken it is less urgent than when using the subclavian vein, as the catheter is more likely to be correctly positioned and the incidence of pneumothorax is much lower with this approach.

The subclavian vein – infraclavicular approach

1. Place the patient in supine position, with arms at their side and head turned away from the side of the puncture. Occasionally it may be advantageous to place a small support (a 500 ml bag of fluid!) under the scapula of the side of approach, to raise the clavicle above the shoulder.
2. Standing on the same side as that to be punctured (usually the right), identify the midclavicular point and the suprasternal notch.
3. Under sterile conditions infiltrate with 1% lignocaine.
4. Insert the needle 1 cm below the midclavicular point and inject 0·5–1 ml of air to expel any skin plug in the needle tip. Advance the needle posterior to the clavicle towards a finger in the suprasternal notch. Keep the syringe and needle horizontal during advancement. Aspirate at all times.
5. Blood entering the syringe will confirm entry into the vein. Introduce the catheter via a guide wire as already described.
6. A chest X-ray should be taken as soon as possible to exclude a pneumothorax and confirm the correct position of the catheter.

The femoral vein

1. Place the patient in a supine position.
2. Under sterile conditions, palpate the femoral artery (midinguinal point). The femoral vein lies directly medial to the femoral artery (remember lateral to medial structures are femoral nerve, artery, vein, space).
3. Infiltrate the puncture site with local anaesthetic.
4. While palpating the femoral artery insert the needle over the femoral vein parallel to the sagittal plane at an angle of 45° to the skin, aspirating at all times. A free flow of blood entering the syringe will confirm entry into the vein.
5. Advance the guide wire through the needle as described below.

Complications

- Venous thrombosis
- Injury to artery or nerve
- Infection
- Arteriovenous fistula
- Air embolism

In addition, attempts at internal jugular or subclavian vein access may cause pneumothorax, haemothorax, and chylothorax.

Seldinger technique

Equipment

Skin cleaning swabs
Lignocaine 1% for local anaesthetic with 2 ml syringe and 23 gauge needle
Syringe and heparinised 0.9% saline
Seldinger cannulation set:
    syringe
    needles
    Seldinger guide wire
    cannula
Suture material
Prepared infusion set
Tape

Procedure

Although initially described for use with arterial cannulation, this technique is very suitable for central venous cannulation and is associated with an increased success rate. It relies on the insertion of a guide wire into the vein over which a suitable catheter is passed. As a relatively small needle is used to introduce the wire, damage to adjacent structures is reduced.

Having decided which approach to use (see earlier), the skin must be prepared and towelled. Full aseptic precautions are necessary as a "no-touch" technique is impossible.

1. Check and prepare your equipment; in particular, identify the floppy end of the guide wire and ensure free passage of the guide wire through the needle.
2. Attach the needle to a syringe and puncture the vein.
3. After aspirating blood, remove the syringe taking care to avoid the entry of air (usually by placing a thumb over the end of the needle).

413

4. Insert the floppy end of the guide wire into the needle and advance 4–5 cm into the vein.
5. Remove the needle over the wire, taking care not to remove the wire with the needle.
6. Load the catheter on to the wire, ensuring that the proximal end of the wire protrudes from the catheter. Holding the proximal end of the wire, insert the catheter and wire together into the vein. It is important never to let go of the wire!
7. Remove the wire holding the catheter in position.
8. Reattach the syringe and aspirate blood to confirm placement of the catheter in the vein.

If it is difficult to insert the wire, the needle and wire must be removed together. Failure to do this may damage the tip of the wire as it is withdrawn past the needle point. After three minutes gentle pressure to reduce bleeding, the needle can be reintroduced.

Occasionally it may be necessary to make a small incision in the skin to facilitate the passage of the catheter.

29

Practical procedures: medical

PROCEDURES

- Joint aspiration
- Balloon tamponade of oesophageal varices
- Lumbar puncture
- Blood cultures
- Insertion of pulmonary arterial flotation (Swan–Ganz) catheter
- Pulmonary capillary wedge pressure

JOINT ASPIRATION

Diagnostic indications

- Suspected septic arthritis
- Crystal induced synovitis
- Haemarthrosis

Therapeutic indications

- Tense effusions
- Septic effusions
    recurrent aspiration
    lavage (rare)
- Haemarthrosis
- Steroid injection

Contraindications

- Overlying skin infection/cellulitis

Equipment

Antiseptic solution, e.g. ethanol, povidone iodine
Swabs

Sterile gloves
Syringes: 5, 10, 20 ml
Needles: large joint (21 gauge) green
         small joint (23 gauge) blue

Procedure

1. Explain to the patient what you are going to do.
2. Identify the bony margins of the joint space.
3. Ensure you have all the appropriate materials required.
4. Using a sterile technique prepare the skin.
5. Inject a small amount of local anaesthetic (1% lignocaine) into the skin over the joint to be aspirated.
6. Gently insert the needle into the joint space. Normally a green needle (21 gauge) will suffice for most joints, but for finger and toe joints a blue (23 gauge) needle is advised.
7. Aspirate fluid and send for microbiological assessment, crystals, cytology, protein, lactate dehydrogenase (LDH), and glucose estimation.

Specific procedures

Knee joint aspiration
1. Ensure the patient is as comfortable as possible.
2. Slightly flex the knee to ensure relaxation of the quadriceps muscles.
3. Palpate the posterior edge of the patella medially or laterally. Using the earlier general technique insert the needle horizontally or slightly downwards into the joint between the patella and femur (often a slight resistance is felt when the needle penetrates the synovial membrane).

Shoulder joint aspiration
This joint is easier to access through an anterior approach although a lateral and posterior approach is also possible. The anterior approach will be described.

1. Ensure that the patient is seated with their arm relaxed against the side of their chest.
2. Palpate the space between the head of the humerus and the glenoid cap, about 1 cm below the cricoid process.
3. Using the earlier general procedure insert the needle into the space with a slight medial angle (it should enter the joint easily and to almost the length of the green needle).

Complications

- Reaction to topical skin preparation.
- Inappropriate puncture of blood vessels or nerves.
- Introduction of infection into joint space.

BALLOON TAMPONADE OF OESOPHAGEAL VARICES

Equipment

Sengstaken–Blakemore tube
Two spigots

60 ml bladder syringe
Saline/contrast media
Tongue depressors
Tape
Anaeroid pressure gauge
Suction
Drainage bags

Procedure

Variceal bleeding can be controlled by balloon compression either at the cardia or within the oesophageal lumen. A large number of devices are available for this purpose, the commonest is a Sengstaken–Blakemore tube that has been modified to allow aspiration of gastric and oesophageal contents as well as inflation of gastric and oesophageal balloons.

Insertion of the tube usually occurs in conscious patients and, therefore, the nasal route is advocated. Unfortunately this can make insertion difficult but is subsequently better tolerated by the patient. If the airway is in jeopardy, ensure that it is cleared and secured before attempting to insert the tamponade tube. If the patient has an endotracheal tube *in situ*, the oral route is advocated. Although you may be faced with torrential bleeding from oesophageal varices, ensure that you have all the equipment available before you attempt insertion of this tube and, more importantly, that the associated oesophageal and gastric balloons will inflate and remain inflated.

It is important to realise that tamponade tubes are difficult to introduce and they require meticulous supervision whilst inflated.

1. Lubricate the tube with water soluble jelly.
2. Providing that there are no contraindications, insert the tube into the right nostril using a technique similar to that described for nasopharyngeal airway insertion in Chapter 30. Ensure you direct the tube backwards (not superior or inferior).
3. Advance the tube gently. It will follow the contour of the oropharynx into the oesophagus.
4. Advance the tube until you reach the 50 cm mark (note that the tube has 5 cm graduations). Advancing the tube to at least 50 cm will, in **most** patients, ensure that it is in the stomach. Aspiration of blood does not, however, verify this.
5. Inflate the gastric balloon with 200 ml of air or alternatively 200 ml of water soluble contrast material. Gentle traction of the nasal end of the tube will ensure that the inflated gastric balloon is adjacent to the cardia and gastro-oesophageal junction.
6. Tape the balloon to the side of the patient's face. Often inflation of the gastric balloon, with gentle traction, is all that is required to stem variceal bleeding as the feeding vessel to the varices, the left gastric vein, is tamponaded by this manoeuvre. If this fails to control the bleeding then inflate the oesophageal balloon with air to 4·5–5·4 kPa (30–40 mm Hg) using a pressure gauge. If a specific pressure gauge is not available then it is possible to adapt a sphygmomanometer for this purpose.
7. Ensure that both gastric and oesophageal aspiration ports are draining freely. Both the gastric and oesophageal balloons seal automatically once inflated by one-way valves. Continuous oesophageal suction reduces the risk of aspiration.
8. Deflate the balloon after 24 hours. This will reduce the risk of oesophageal mucosal ulceration and perforation.

It is important to realise that balloon tamponade is only a temporising procedure and once the bleeding has stopped the patient should undergo oesophageal sclerotherapy.

Complications

- Aspiration, especially without continuous aspiration of the oesophageal port
- Hypoxaemia, if the balloon is inadvertently inserted into the trachea
- Tracheal rupture, as above
- Oesophageal rupture. The procedure is performed blindly and with the presence of a hiatus hernia or an oesophageal stricture it is possible for the Sengstaken–Blakemore tube to coil in the oesophagus. Inflation produces catastrophic results
- Mucosal ulceration in the oesophagus and stomach
- Failure to stop variceal haemorrhage

LUMBAR PUNCTURE

Indications

- Suspected meningitis
- Subarachnoid haemorrhage
- Encephalitis
- Benign intracranial hypertension

Contraindications

- Raised intracranial pressure
- Spinal cord compression
- Local sepsis
- Bleeding disorders

Equipment

Antiseptic solution
Gauze swabs
Sterile drapes and gloves
1% lignocaine (max 5 ml)
5ml syringe
Needles: 25 gauge (orange)
          21 gauge (green)
Lumbar puncture needles
Manometer
Collection bottles
Tape

Procedure

1. Explain to the patient what you are going to do.
2. Place the patient in the left lateral position, ensuring that their back, in particular the lumbar spine, is parallel to the edge of the bed. The hips and knees should be flexed to greater than 90° and the knees separated by one pillow. Ensure that the head is supported on one pillow and that the patient's cervical and thoracic spine are gently flexed.
3. Check that you have all the necessary equipment.
4. Identify the fourth lumbar vertebra, i.e. a line drawn between the top of the iliac crests.
5. Thoroughly cleanse the skin using an aseptic technique.

6. Identify the interspace between the second and third or third and fourth lumbar vertebrae (hence the spinal cord will not be damaged). In the midline, inject a small amount of 1% lignocaine to raise a skin bleb.

7. Through the skin bleb, advance a green needle and ensuring that the blood vessel has not been punctured. Inject 1 ml local anaesthetic into the interspinous ligament in the respective interspace. Too much local anaesthetic will cause damage to these tissues and produce profound discomfort.

8. Using a sterile spinal needle advance through the anaesthetised tissues, directing the needle slightly cephalad and maintaining a midline position.

9. As you enter the subarachnoid space, a sudden change in resistance on advancing the needle is felt. Then gently remove the inner trochar and watch for a drop of cerebrospinal fluid appearing at the end of the needle. If this does not occur, replace the central trochar and advance the needle again, until a change in resistance is felt. Repeat the procedure until cerebrospinal fluid is seen.

10. Attach the manometer and measure the pressure of the cerebrospinal fluid.

11. Place five drops of cerebrospinal fluid sequentially in three tubes for red cell count, then five drops in a further two for microscopy culture and sensitivity. Similar samples should be taken for protein estimation, spectroscopy, virology, and glucose (the latter should be placed in a fluoride tube).

12. Note the colour of the cerebrospinal fluid, i.e. whether it is clear, opalescent or yellow (xanthochromia).

13. Remove the needle and ensure that the patient stays supine for four hours. Occasionally, postlumbar puncture headache may result which necessitates simple analgesia with paracetamol.

Complications

- Failure to obtain cerebrospinal fluid may be due to incorrect anatomical positioning, "a dry tap", degenerative or inflammatory changes in the lumbar spine
- Nerve root pain when inserting the needle – usually transient
- Introduction of sepsis
- Bleeding
- Headache
- Coning

BLOOD CULTURES

Indications

- Pyrexia of unknown origin
- Septicaemia
- Suspected infective endocarditis

Procedure

1. Thoroughly cleanse the skin, ideally with an alcohol based solution.
2. Whilst this is evaporating to dryness wash your hands thoroughly; under aseptic conditions don surgical gloves.
3. At the previously prepared site perform a venepuncture and aspirate 40 ml of blood.
4. Thoroughly cleanse the top of the blood culture bottle.
5. Insert 10 ml of blood into each blood culture bottle.

It is important to realise that if you suspect infective endocarditis, then two sets of blood cultures from three different sites should be taken.

Complications

- Bleeding
- Sepsis at venepuncture site

INSERTION OF PULMONARY ARTERIAL FLOTATION (SWAN–GANZ) CATHETER

Indications

- Measurement of pulmonary capillary wedge pressure (PCWP)
- Pulmonary artery end diastolic pressure (PAEDP)
- Cardiac output

Equipment

See central venous cannulation in Chapter 28.

The catheter

This is a balloon tipped device with a single distal hole. It can be inserted at the bedside without X-ray control or under fluoroscopy.

The balloon serves two purposes. Firstly as soon as the catheter is inserted into a central vein, inflation of the balloon with air will ensure that it acts as a "sail" navigating the catheter through the tricuspid and pulmonary valves. Changes in the pressure tracing, as described later, will enable these structures to be identified. Furthermore, once the catheter is inserted into a small pulmonary artery, the balloon may then be inflated, occluding the artery proximally. This will leave the catheter tip exposed to the pulmonary capillary wedge pressure.

Catheter insertion

1. Using the technique described for central venous access in Chapter 28, advance the catheter into a large vein. If an insertion sheath is used, ensure it is one size larger than the catheter, to ensure passage of the deflated balloon through the insertion sheath.
2. Connect to transducer.
3. Inflate the balloon.
4. Slowly advance the catheter tip, guided by the blood flow.
5. Advance the catheter through into the pulmonary artery bed, trying to find a position which gives a good pulmonary artery tracing with the balloon deflated and a good wedge pressure with the balloon inflated.
6. X-ray the chest.

Alternatively, the catheter can be inserted under fluoroscopic control. It is, however, still important to ensure that a good pulmonary artery tracing is obtained with the balloon deflated, and a good wedge pressure is obtained with the balloon inflated.

Measurement

Specific details of pulmonary capillary wedge pressure measurement will vary according to the equipment available. There are, however, certain common features.

1. Most equipment is designed for continuous monitoring; as such it is precalibrated. Therefore the only major adjustment is to zero the transducer to atmospheric pressure before recording. To do this ensure that the catheter is connected via a three-way tap to the manometer line; the other portholes of the three-way tap should be connected to a flushing system and to the air. It is also mandatory to ensure that, in setting up the equipment, you bleed all air bubbles from the system.
2. Move the three-way tap to ensure that blood cannot flow back from the catheter to the transducer but that the final port of the three-way tap is open to the air.
3. Adjust the tracing on the monitor to zero.
4. Close the transducer sidearm and open the transducer to the catheter. Ideally allow approximately 30 min for the transducer to "warm up".

Measurements are made with the patient flat and the transducer at the angle of Louis. You will note that during measurements the pressure swings related to respiration will impart a biphasic nature to the pulmonary wedge pressure. It is, therefore, important that the mean wedge pressure is used.

It is always important to check:

*   the transducer level
*   that the system is set at zero
*   that wedging does not occur.

Problems

*   Failure to wedge – reposition the catheter.
*   Flat/damp trace – unblock catheter. Ensure that there is no air in the system and that the transducer is not open to both the patient and air. Flush the system – usually a hand flush of 1 ml of saline is required, but ensure that no air is introduced.
*   Overwedging – occasionally the catheter is lodged in a pulmonary artery; unfortunately, the diameter of this vessel is less than that of the balloon and does not allow accurate pressure recording. This usually manifests by a fluctuating, steadily increasing pressure trace. Ideally deflate the balloon and reposition the catheter.

PULMONARY CAPILLARY WEDGE PRESSURE

This can be recorded as described earlier, along with pressures in the pulmonary artery, right ventricle, and right atrium (Table 29.1).

Table 29.1 Normal pressure ranges

Site	Pressure (mm Hg)
Right atrium (mean)	–1–6
Right ventricle	0–25
Pulmonary artery (mean)	10–20
Pulmonary capillary wedge pressure (mean)	8–15

The pulmonary capillary wedge pressure is an indirect reflection of left arterial pressure (LAP). This in turn is similar to left ventricular end diastolic pressure (LVEDP).

421

In certain acute medical conditions, the pulmonary capillary wedge pressure does not accurately reflect left ventricular end diastolic pressure. With pulmonary venous obstruction, for example, pulmonary emboli or raised intrathoracic pressure (for instance, intermittent positive pressure ventilation) the pulmonary capillary wedge pressure is less than the left ventricular end diastolic pressure – thus pulmonary capillary wedge pressure is a particularly useful measurement in patients with poor left ventricular function and it may be used to optimise fluid therapy.

CARDIAC OUTPUT

Cardiac output may be assessed using the Fick equation which relates cardiac output (CO) to oxygen uptake (VO_2). In this manner cardiac output equals oxygen uptake divided by the difference in arteriovenous oxygen content.

$$\text{Cardiac output} = \frac{\text{Oxygen uptake}}{\text{Arteriovenous oxygen content difference}}$$

$$\text{Therefore CO (l/min)} = \frac{VO_2 \text{ (ml/min)}}{CaO_2 - CvO_2 \text{ (ml/l)}}$$

To obtain these values a true mixed venous sample of blood must be taken from the tip of the pulmonary artery. This will allow the difference in the arteriovenous oxygen content to be assessed.

Complications

- As with central venous access
- Pulmonary parenchymal damage

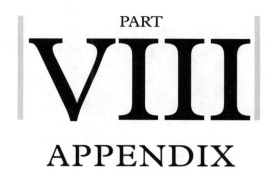

PART

VIII

APPENDIX

Drugs commonly used in the management of medical emergencies

Drug	Indications	Dose and route	Notes
N acetyl cysteine	Paracetamol poisoning Renal dysfunction in a patient with decompensated liver disease	IV infusion 150 mg/kg over 15 min then 50 mg/kg over 4 hours, then 100 mg/kg over 16 hours	Most effective if given less than 8 hours post overdose. Requirement for treatment based on blood paracetamol levels at least 4 hours post ingestion. Nomogram available on data sheet or British National Formulary. Treat at lower levels for at risk patients – alcoholics, anorexics and patients on liver enzyme inducing drugs Same dose for hepatorenal failure – continue 100 mg/kg every 16 hours until improvement
Aciclovir	Herpes simplex encephalitis, varicella zoster in immunocompromised	10 mg/kg IV 8 hourly	Most effective if started at onset of infection. Can be used orally, topically or intravenously at lower dose for immunocompetent adults with herpes infections or prophylaxis in immunocompromised patients
Adenosine	Cardioversion of paroxysmal supraventricular arrhythmias	3–12 mg by rapid IV injection (see notes)	Do not use in Wolff–Parkinson–White syndrome with atrial fibrillation as increased conduction via accessory pathways may result in circulatory collapse or ventricular fibrillation. Use lower initial dose (0·5–1 mg) if heart transplant patient or patient taking dipyridamole (avoid use unless essential). Antagonised by theophyllines
Adrenaline	Cardiac arrest	1 mg IV 2 mg ETT	Improves circulation achieved by chest compressions. Central line is the preferred route
	Anaphylaxis	0.5 ml; 1 in 1000 IM	Continue injection until clinical effect. ECG monitoring necessary. Will frequently require adrenaline infusion after (see inotropic support next)
	Inotropic support	0·1–0·5 µg/kg/min IV	Give by continuous infusion (through dedicated line to avoid boluses). Predominantly increases cardiac output at lower doses. Also causes vasoconstriction at higher doses
Aminophylline	Acute severe asthma	5 mg/kg IV over 20 minutes	Do not give this initial loading dose to patients on oral theophyllines
		0·5 mg/kg/hour IV	Vary infusion rate according to plasma theophylline levels (aim for 10–20 mg/l)

Drug	Indications	Dose and route	Notes
Amiodarone	Ventricular tachycardia, atrial fibrillation and flutter, supraventricular tachycardia	300 mg IV over 20–60 min, followed by 1200 mg/24 hours IV	Effective antiarrhythmic with many complications. When given intravenously must be via a central venous catheter. Hypotension or cardiovascular collapse possible with rapid administration
Atenolol	Myocardial infarction	5–10 mg IV, followed by 50 mg orally at 15 min and 12 hours, then 100 mg each day	Early use of atenolol post myocardial infarction reduces mortality. Should not be given to patients with a high degree of heart block, hypotension or overt left ventricular failure
Atropine	Asystole	3 mg IV 6 mg ETT	Used once only in the management of asystole
	Bradycardia	0·5 mg IV	Use incremental doses of 0·5 mg up to a maximum of 3 mg
Benzylpenicillin	Meningococcal septicaemia	2·4 g IV 4 hourly	Give immediately if meningococcal septicaemia suspected. If possible do blood cultures first. Do not delay for lumbar puncture
Ceftriaxone	Septicaemia, pneumonia, meningitis	1–4 g IV once daily	Third generation broad spectrum cephalosporin. Long half life; therefore given only once daily
Clarithromycin	Atypical pneumonia, other infections in penicillin allergic patients	500 mg IV 12 hourly	Similar spectrum of activity to erythromycin but slightly greater activity and higher tissue levels. Fewer gastrointestinal side effects than erythromycin
Diazepam	Fitting	5–10 mg IV, repeated if necessary 10–20 mg rectally	May cause respiratory depression and hypotension. Use of flumazenil to reverse this may precipitate further seizures. Use rectal route if IV access not easily attainable
Digoxin	Atrial fibrillation	500 µg IV over 30 min 62·5–500 µg/day orally or IV	Loading dose. Do not give if patient taking digoxin. Used to control ventricular response rate. Does not cause chemical cardioversion. Maintenance dose. Be wary that arrythmias may be caused by digoxin toxicity
Dobutamine	Cardiogenic shock	2·5–20 µg/kg/min	Inodilator. Give by continuous infusion. May cause paradoxical hypotension with increasing doses as a result of tachycardia and vasodilatation
Dopamine	Shock with inadequate urine output	1–3 µg/kg/min	Used as an adjunct to inotropic support. Increases renal blood flow and urine output
Frusemide	Pulmonary oedema secondary to left ventricular dysfunction	50–100 mg IV	Works initially by vasodilator effect, and later as diuretic. Use with extreme caution in hypotensive patients as severe hypotension may develop; consider use in conjunction with inotropic support. In the acutely anuric patient, bumetanide may be a better alternative as excretion of the drug into the tubule is not required. Higher doses required in patients on large oral doses of a loop diuretic or with known renal impairment
Glucagon	Hypoglycaemia	1 mg SC/IV/IM	Mobilises glycogen from the liver. If not recovered within 10 min give IV glucose
	β blocker overdose	50–150 µg/kg IV	Useful in shock refractory to atropine therapy in patients with β blocker overdose. Is only available as 1 mg vials. Total dose required is up to approximately 10 mg

Drug	Indications	Dose and route	Notes
Glyceryl trinitrate	Pulmonary oedema secondary to left ventricular dysfunction	1–10 mg/hour IV	In hypotensive patients, use only in conjunction with inotropic support
	Ischaemic chest pain	500 µg sublingual 1–5 mg buccal 1–10 mg/hour IV	If chest pain not rapidly relieved by nitrates, myocardial infarction should be excluded and alternative diagnoses considered
Hydrocortisone	Anaphylaxis and angiooedema	100–300 mg IV	Of secondary benefit as onset of action delayed for several hours. Use in more severely affected patients
	Acute adrenocortical insufficiency	100 mg IV 6–8 hourly	
Ipratropium bromide	Acute asthma	500 µg nebulised 4 hourly	Indicated in life threatening asthma in conjunction with a β_2 agonist. In severe acute asthma use as a second line treatment. Beneficial in a small group of patients with chronic obstructive pulmonary disease
Lignocaine	Ventricular tachycardia	100 mg IV 1–4 mg/min	Commonly used to treat ventricular tachycardia. Myocardial depressant. Use cautiously if impaired left ventricular function. Treat underlying cause of arrhythmia – usually myocardial ischaemia
	Local anaesthetic	3 mg/kg maximum	Infiltrate locally or perineurally. Facilitates procedures – large IV line, intercostal tube insertion, lumbar puncture. Increased dose (7 mg/kg) may be used if infiltrated with adrenaline (not fingers, nose, ears, or penis)
Lorazepam	Status epilepticus	4 mg IV	May cause respiratory depression or apnoea. Longer duration of action compared to diazepam
Morphine	Myocardial infarction	2·5–20 mg IV (titrate against response)	Anxiolysis and analgesia reduce catecholamine levels, decreasing heart rate, afterload and hence myocardial oxygen consumption
	Pulmonary oedema	2·5–10 mg IV	Acts as above. Also effects on pulmonary vasculature reduce left ventricular preload
	Pain	2·5–20 mg IV (titrate against response)	Diamorphine is an alternative as may cause less hypotension and nausea. Powerful analgesic. May cause respiratory depression
Naloxone	Opiate poisoning	0·4–2 mg IV 4 µg/min IV (increase dose as required to maintain required response)	Deliberate self harm, iatrogenic or recreational use of opiates may result in respiratory arrest. Beware opiates with long half lives, especially methadone. IV infusion should be used if long acting opiate involved or recurrent coma or respiratory depression
Phenytoin	Status epilepticus	15 mg/kg loading dose IV at <50 mg/min Maintenance 100 mg IV 6–8 hourly	Second line drug in status epilepticus. Phenytoin offers theoretical advantages as can be infused rapidly. May cause central nervous system or cardiovascular depression, more marked with rapid infusion rates
Salbutamol	Acute asthma	2·5–5 mg nebulised as required 250 µg IV	β_2 agonist. Nebulise with high flow oxygen. In severe or life threatening acute asthma not responding to nebulised β_2 agonist, IV therapy is indicated. Consider need for anaesthetic help
		3–20 µg/min IV	Infusions of salbutamol are used following IV bolus
Streptokinase	Myocardial infarction	1·5 million units IV over 1 hour	Reduces mortality post myocardial infarction. Indicated when potential benefits outweigh risks. Risks mainly relate to haemorrhage (see Chapter 10)

Drug	Indications	Dose and route	Notes
tPA	Myocardial infarction	15 mg bolus followed by 50 mg over 30 min, then 35 mg over 60 min IV	See streptokinase. May have mortality benefits in some subgroups compared to streptokinase. Use dictated by local protocols, commonly including patients with anterior myocardial infarction or hypotension related to myocardial infarction
	Pulmonary embolism	10 mg bolus followed by 90 mg over 2 hours	Use in haemodynamically significant pulmonary embolus or pulmonary embolus causing severe hypoxaemia despite high FiO_2

IM, intramuscular; IV, intravenous; ETT, endotracheal tube; SC, subcutaneous.

Answers to Time Out Questions

CHAPTER 2: RECOGNITION OF THE MEDICAL EMERGENCY

2.1, a. Clinical features to diagnose potential respiratory failure are respiratory rate, symmetry of respiration, effort of respiration and effectiveness of breathing.

b. The signs of potential circulatory failure are heart rate, blood pressure and capillary refill.

The presence of peripheral and/or central pulses, i.e. radial pulse, will disappear if the systolic blood pressure falls below 80 mmHg, the femoral pulse will disappear if the systolic blood pressure falls below 60 mmHg and the carotid pulse will disappear if the systolic blood pressure is below 60 mmHg.

c. The signs of potential central neurological failure are conscious level, posture and pupillary response.

Remember also that hypoxemia will produce a tachycardia or peripheral vasoconstriction and affect mental function. Similarly shock will cause tachypnea, peripheral vasoconstriction and reduce both cerebral and renal perfusion. Furthermore central neurological failure can influence both the effort and pattern of respiration as well as the pulse rate and blood pressure.

These features can be summarised as:

- Breathing – check rate, effort and symmetry
- Circulation – assess pulse for rate rhythm and character, measure blood pressure and assess peripheral perfusion
- Disability – assess pupil size and reactions along with evaluation of the conscious level (either the AVPU system or the Glasgow Coma Score is appropriate).

CHAPTER 3: A STRUCTURED APPROACH TO MEDICAL EMERGENCIES

3.1 The primary assessment would comprise:

- Airway – assess patency. As the patient is talking no intervention at this stage is required except for high flow oxygen (FiO$_2$ 0·85)
- Breathing – assess rate, effort and symmetry of respiration. Look for an elevated JVP whilst palpating the trachea for tug or deviation. Percuss the anterior chest wall in upper, middle and lower zones, and in the axillae. Listen to establish whether breath sounds are absent, present or masked by added sounds. As no abnormality has been detected arterial saturation can be measured using the pulse oximeter.
- Circulation – assess pulse – rate rhythm and character; blood pressure and capillary refill time. If there is no evidence of shock, a single cannula is inserted and blood taken for baseline haematological and biochemical values including a serum glucose. A bedside measurement of glucose is also important. Continuous monitoring of pulse blood pressure and ECG will provide valuable baseline information as will a 12-lead ECG. The BM stix shows the glucose to be 1·2 mmol/l. The patient is therefore immediately treated with 10% dextrose 250 mls while the assessment continues.
- Disability – assessment of pupils – mildly dilated, symmetrical and slowly reacting to light. GCS 13/15: E4, V4, M5, no obvious lateralising signs.
- Exposure – no evidence of acute skin rash. Core temperature 36·8°C. This assessment would be repeated and the patient would be monitored until the blood glucose had returned to normal. If the patient's conscious level did not change, however, treatment would continue to prevent secondary brain injury while reassessment and further investigations were requested. In contrast, if the patient's condition did improve then it would be appropriate to start the secondary assessment.

3.2 Primary Assessment:

a. Reassess the patient
b. Shock – likely hypovolaemic
c. Continue with high flow oxygen and give a fluid challenge, then reassess the patient.

CHAPTER 4: AIRWAY ASSESSMENT

4.1
- Look – paradoxical (see-saw movement of the chest and abdomen in complete obstruction due to increased respiratory effort), accessory muscle use.

- Listen – stridor indicates upper airway obstruction, wheezes usually signify obstruction of the lower airways. Crowing accompanies laryngeal spasm while snoring indicates that the pharynx is partially occluded by the tongue. Gurgling usually signifies presence of semi-solid material.

- Feel – for expired air against the side of your cheek, chest movement, the position of trachea, any tracheal tug and the presence of first subcutaneous emphysema.

CHAPTER 5: BREATHING ASSESSMENT

5.1 This is the amount of air inspired per breath and is equivalent to 7–8 mls per kilogram bodyweight or 500 mls for the 70 kg patient.

(ii) This is the amount of air inspired each minute and is calculated by multiplying the respiratory rate by the tidal volume.

15 breaths per minute × 500 mls = 7·5 litres per minute.

b(i) Alveolar ventilation can be calculated from the respiratory rate x (tidal volume – anatomical dead space). The anatomical dead space is constant. However as the respiratory rate increases, the amount of inspired air per breath or tidal volume is reduced. Therefore as the respiratory rate increases in particular over 20 breaths per minute, the tidal volume is reduced dramatically as is the alveolar ventilation. For further details the reader is referred to Chapter 5.

b(ii) This is shown in Chapter 5. The important feature however is that the relationship between the PaO_2 and O_2 saturation of haemoglobin is not linear. This means that haemoglobin O_2 saturation is initially well maintained over a very wide arterial oxygen concentration from 50 to 100 mmHg.

c
- Airway obstruction
- Breathing – bronchospasm, pulmonary oedema, tension pneumothorax

CHAPTER 6: CIRCULATION ASSESSMENT

6.1 Please see Figure 6.2.

6.2
- History of asystole;
- When there is any pause ≥3 seconds in the presence of Mobitz Type II or complete heart block with wide QRS complexes. Clinical features that indicate treatment with atropine include low cardiac output, cardiac failure, hypotension (systolic blood pressure ≤90 mmHg). Heart rate <40 beats per minute; presence of ventricular arrhythmias that require suppression.

6.3 There are many ways to remember the causes of shock and one system in use is the preload, pump, afterload, (peripheral classification often referred to as the three Ps). Preload causes of shock are due to hypovolaemia that may be real, for example following haemorrhage, profuse diarrhoea or vomiting; and apparent, due to venodilation following treatment with intravenous nitrates. In addition venous return can also be obstructed by the gravid uterus, severe asthma or tension pneumothorax. Pump problems include severe left or right ventricular failure, cardiac tamponade. Peripheral or afterload causes are associated with widespread vasodilation (reduced systemic vascular resistance seen with anaphylaxis, systemic inflammatory response syndrome including septicaemia and toxaemia) and neurogenic shock.

CHAPTER 7: DISABILITY ASSESSMENT

7.1 See Figure 7.5 showing dermatomes

CHAPTER 8: THE PATIENT WITH BREATHING DIFFICULTIES

8.1 Key components of the assessment so far:

- Look
- Listen
- Feel
- Look – colour, sweating, posture, respiratory effort, rate and symmetry
- Feel – tracheal position, tracheal tug, chest expansion
- Percuss
- Listen

8.2, a. Rapid primary assessment and treatment with:

A   High flow oxygen
B   Assessment indicates pulmonary oedema
C   Supports the diagnosis of left ventricular failure with hypertension therefore cardiogenic shock, so the patient requires intravenous access and, after appropriate bloods have been taken including markers of myocardial damage, inotropes should be started.

b. Investigations should include a full blood count to ensure that there is no instance of anaemia, baseline renal function and blood glucose, chest X-ray and 12 lead ECG. The patient will also require appropriate monitoring including pulse oximetry and continuous ECG.

8.3, a. This is a chronic inflammatory condition resulting in reversible narrowing of the airways.

b. A susceptible airway in which bronchospasm may occur precipitated by IgE mass cell degranulation or exposure to environmental factors which will induce chronic inflammation. Bronchial contraction, mucosal oedema, increased mucous production and epithelial cell damage will drive the inflammatory response and exacerbate the airway narrowing. Persisting inflammation will induce collagen deposition under the basement membrane.

c. Airway narrowing.

d. It reduces the forced expiratory volume and peak expiratory flow rate. There is also increased functional residual capacity due to air trapping but no change in total lung capacity. Thus because of increased airways resistance, the work of breathing is increased and hence the patient feels breathless. In addition, in an acute attack some of the airways may be blocked by mucous plugs resulting in hypoxemia due to ventilation perfusion mismatch. This will increase the work of breathing.

e. By giving high flow oxygen.

Nebulised – a) salbutamol 5 mg or terbutaline 10 mg; b) iprotroprium bromide 0·5 mg or given via an oxygen driven nebuliser.

Intravenous – a) hydrocortisone 200 mg; b) salbutamol 250 µg over 10 minutes. Alternatively terbutaline or aminophylinne can be used.

Chest X-ray to exclude a pneumothorax.

f. i.   Hypoxemia (PaO_2 <8 kPa despite FiO_2 >0·6)
    ii. Hypercapnia ($PaCO_2$ >6 kPa)
    iii. Exhaustion
    iv. Altered conscious level
    v.   Respiratory arrest

8.4 The immediate management comprises a rapid primary assessment to ensure airway patency. Her FiO_2 should be increased to 0·85. Breathing must be reassessed to exclude life threatening bronchospasm, tension pneumothorax and pulmonary oedema. She should be treated with nebulised bronchodilators including salbutamol and iprotroprium, along with intravenous hydrocortisone and a bronchodilator. An urgent chest

X-ray is required. The result is a right sided pneumothorax. Whilst there are no clinical features to indicate underlying tension, even a small pneumothorax in a person with pre-existing chest disease can cause rapid decompensation. Therefore a chest drain is also required.

8.5, a. *Streptococcus pneumoniae*

b. The patient may experience prodromal features of malaise anorexia, myalgia, arthralgia and headache, there may also be a history of pyrexia and sweating. In addition the patient will have had a cough productive of sputum and experience breathlessness, possible pleuritic pain and even haemoptysis. One third of patients may develop herpes simplex labialis. It is important to remember however that elderly patients may remain afebrile.

c. High flow oxygen, titrated to the arterial blood gas results, intravenous fluids and a combination of cephtriaxone 2 g and clarithromycin 1 g daily.

d. High risk factors in patients with pneumonia are: clinical confusion, respiratory rate >30 per minute, diastolic blood pressure <60 mmHg, recent onset atrial fibrillation.

Investigations: a) Blood urea >7 mmol/l; b) White cell count $<4 \times 10^9$ or $>20 \times 10^9/l$, PaO$_2$ <8 kPa (60 mmHg); serum albumin <25 g/l, multilobe involvement on chest X-ray.

8.6, a. This is pneumonia developing more than 48 hours after admission to hospital.

b. Those patients who are ill, bed-bound and who have impaired consciousness. This may be exacerbated by an inability to clear bronchial secretions for example after a general anaesthetic or thoracic and abdominial surgery where coughing is impaired. The risk of a post operative pneumonia is also exacerbated in the elderly and those patients who have a history of smoking, obesity and underlying chronic illness.

c. Make sure that they are on supplemental oxygen and intravenous fluids along with an appropriate antibiotic regime. As there is a wide range of potential organisms, an early liaison with a microbiologist is advocated. Approprite antibiotic regimes include cephtriaone, metronidazole or cephtriaxone plus gentamicin. If pseudomonas is suspected then ticarcillin may be required.

8.8 Larger emboli that block larger branches of the pulmonary artery provoke a rise in pulmonary artery pressure and rapid shallow respiration. Tachypnea is also a reflex response to activation of vagal innovated luminal stretch receptors and interstitial J receptors within the alveolar and capillary network.

CHAPTER 9: THE PATIENT WITH SHOCK

9.1, a.   i.   Concentration of oxygen reaching the alveoli
      ii.   Pulmonary perfusion
      iii. Adequacy of pulmonary gas exchange
      iv. Capacity of blood to carry oxygen
      v.   Blood flow to the tissues

9.1, b. The sympathetic nervous system can help in several ways – increasing venous return by reducing the diameter of the veins and the capacity of the venous system; positively inotropic and the positively chromotropic effect.

9.2 Sepsis is term reserved for the systemic inflammatory response syndrome and is driven by an infection. Circulating inflammatory mediators have a negative inotropic effect, cause vasodilatation and impair energy utilisation at a cellular level. Furthermore prime inflammatory cytokines increase capillary permeability and indirectly paralyse precapillary spincters further exacerbating capillary leakage and hypovolaemia. The end result is both a fall in preload, myocardial depression and a full and systemic vascular resistance.

9.3 The clinical features are in keeping with a diagnosis of hypovolaemic shock. The patient should therefore receive high flow oxygen. Venous access is required and from the insertion of the first cannula, a litre of warmed balanced salt solution can be given. Bloods can be taken from the second cannula before a further litre of fluid is given. Appropriate investigations include a full blood count, baseline clotting, renal function and blood glucose. A rapid reassessment of the patient is required to provide further details in particular about breathing and also the response to a fluid challenge. The patient is in grade 3 shock – at least 4 units of type specific and 6 units of cross matched blood should be requested. He will require continuous monitoring of saturations, pulse, blood pressure and ECG. Surgical colleagues should be informed. Clues to the underlying cause of his haematemesis may be noted during the primary assessment such as stigmata of chronic liver disease and this would raise the possibility of oesophageal varices. Thus octreotide 25 µg should be given initially followed by an infusion at 25 µg per hour. Any abnormalities in blood clotting should be corrected, guided by further results. The presence of a soft systolic murmur is likely to represent a hyperdynamic circulation but further reassessment and investigations may be warranted.

If the patient becomes haemodynamically normal then an appropriate secondary assessment can be done. If however this is not possible then the patient should be transferred to high dependency for further treatment and according to liaisons with the consultant may require endoscopy in theatre enroute.

CHAPTER 11: THE PATIENT WITH ALTERED CONSCIOUS LEVEL

11.1, a. Consciousness is a function of the integrated action of the brain. The two interlinked key areas are the reticular formation and the cerebral cortex.

b. This assessment comprises:

- Pupillary response
- Eye movement
- Corneal response
- Respiratory pattern

11.2, a. These develop on medium sized arteries at the base of the brain and the commonest sites are the distal internal carotid/posterior communicating artery and the anterior communicating artery complex.

b. 1. Intracranial saccular aneurysm
   2. Arterio venous malformation

c. >12 hours

d. 25%

e. *Streptococcal pneumoniae* and *neisseria meningitidis.*

f. The immuno-compromised patients including those with the human immuno deficiency virus; immigrants from Pakistan, India, Africa and the West Indies; alcoholics and intravenous drug users; patients with previous pulmonary tuberculosis.

g. Gustatory and olfactory hallucinations, amnesia, expressive dysphasia, temporal lobe seizures, anosmia and behavioural abnormalities. This specific symptom complex occurs because herpes simplex encephalitis involves primarily the temporal and frontal cortex.

h. Cerebral malaria should be considered a differential diagnosis of any acute febrile illness until it can be excluded by – definite lack of exposure; repeat examination of blood smears; following a therapeutic trial of antimalarial chemotherapy.

i. Non-neurological features of *Plasmodium falciparum* infection include – anaemia, spontaneous bleeding from the GI tract, jaundice, hypoglycaemia, shock, oliguria, acute renal failure and pulmonary oedema.

j. Although intracranial abscesses can be caused by infection from sinuses or penetrating trauma, intracerebral abscesses can also follow septicaemia due to infective endocarditis, pulmonary abscess and bronchiectasis. Extradural abscesses are difficult to diagnose and may present with a localised headache in association with mastoiditis and sinusitis. In contrast subdural and intracerebral abscesses present with headache, vomiting, impaired consciousness and neurological signs.

k. Extradural haematoma classically follows a tear to the meningeal artery. It is a classic sequence of events after the head injury when the patient becomes unconscious, develops a lucid interval and then becomes comatosed. In contrast subdural haematoma usually occurs in patients who are over anticoagulated or following falls in the elderly or alcoholic patients. Intracerebral haematoma occurs spontaneously and the clinical features and signs will be dictated by the area of the brain that has been affected.

CHAPTER 12: THE COLLAPSED PATIENT

12.1, a. Stroke is a syndrome characterised by an acute onset of focal, but occasionally global, loss of function lasting more than 24 hours. This can be brought about by a number of causes including reduction in cerebral blood flow along a known vascular pathway affecting neurological tissue; generalised cerebral hypoperfusion from whatever cause; localised vascular disease; epilepsy; metabolic disturbances leading to neurological dysfunction e.g. hyperglycaemia.

b. The patient should have a rapid primary assessment with reference to a serum glucose estimation.

CHAPTER 14: THE PATIENT WITH A HEADACHE

14.1, a. These can be classified as intracranial e.g. meningitis, encephalitis and subarachnoid haemorrhage or extracranial – acute sinusitis, acute viral illness, malaria or typhoid.

b. Weakness usually affects the proximal and distal limb muscles equally, wasting occurs but is not prominent, reflexes are diminished or absent. Sensation may be unaffected although there may be variable loss.

14.2, a. Initial diagnosis includes acute sinusitis, cervical spondylosis, giant cell arteritis and acute glaucoma.

b. Acute sinusitis – orbital cellulitis/abscess, meningitis, cerebral abscess, osteomyelitis and cavernous sinus thrombosis.

Cervical spondylosis – spinal cord compression.

Giant Cell arteritis – visual problems including blindness ischaemia/infarction of the heart, intestine and brain, acute glaucoma. Ischaemia of the optic nerve and retina.

14.3, a. Tension headache – diffuse, commonly at the vertex frequently bilateral and described as a pressure tight band or squeezing.

Migrainous headaches can be paroxysmal, unilateral, bilateral and are often described as throbbing. In the minority of patients 20% will develop visual aura or some sensory disturbance.

Cluster headaches – unilateral with ipsilateral corneal injection, nasal congestion, and possibly a Transient Horner's syndrome. The headache is usually centred around the orbit and lasts for between 30 minutes and 2 hours each day for between 4 and 16 weeks.

In a tension type headache it usually starts in the morning and increases throughout the day. There is no vomiting and no visual disturbance.

b. A lumbar puncture must be considered in any patient who has an acute onset of a headache that is new, progressive and awakes them from a sleep, especially those people who have a history suggestive of coital migraine.

CHAPTER 15: THE PATIENT WITH ABDOMINAL PAIN

15.1, a. i) Consider:
- Leaking abdominal aortic aneurysm
- Gastrointestinal bleeding (e.g. bleeding peptic ulcer)
- Acute pancreatitis
- Severe gastroenteritis
- Cardiogenic shock (acute myocardial infarction)
- Small bowel infarction (mesenteric artery occlusion)
- Sepsis (e.g. colonic perforation, pneumonia)

ii) Consider:
- Ectopic pregnancy
- Gastrointestinal bleeding (e.g. bleeding peptic ulcer)
- Acute pancreatitis
- Severe gastroenteritis/ulcerative colitis
- Diabetic ketoacidosis
- Ruptured spleen (spontaneous rupture occurs rarely in infectious mononucleosis)
- Sepsis (e.g. lower lobe pneumonia, meningococcal septicaemia)
- Acute adrenal insufficiency

b.
- Is the airway unprotected and is there a risk of aspiration (particularly in the patient with vomiting and/or a depressed level of consciousness)? If so, secure the airway. Start high flow oxygen by facemask with a non rebreathing reservoir bag.
- Examine the chest. Is ventilation and gas exchange adequate? If not, consider the need for intubation and ventilation (e.g. in patients with severe acute pancreatitis or septic shock).
- Assess degree of circulatory failure. Obtain vascular access with two large bore (peripheral) cannulae; take samples for blood cross match, baseline haematology and biochemistry (including amylase and glucose stick test), blood gas analysis, and – when appropriate – coagulation screen, β-hCG pregnancy test and sickle cell screen. For hypovolaemia initiate fluid resuscitation with 0·9% saline, followed by blood for haemorrhagic shock.
- 12 lead ECG if myocardial infarction/arrhythmia/pulmonary embolism suspected; urgent CXR for pneumonia or other chest pathology; establish monitoring of SaO_2, ECG and BP.
- Perform abdominal, rectal and – if indicated – vaginal examination.
- Urgent surgical or gynaecological referral and/or other emergency treatment (analgesia, antibiotics), as appropriate.
- Consider the need for nasogastric tube and/or urinary catheter.
- Perform/arrange a portable ultrasound scan where this may confirm the diagnosis (e.g. suspected abdominal aortic aneurysm).
- Reassess and go on to complete the secondary assessment.

15.2 Adverse prognostic factors in acute pancreatitis (within 48 hours)

- Age >55 years
- White blood cell count $>15 \times 10^9/l$
- Blood glucose >10 mmol/l (no diabetic history)
- Serum urea >16 mmol/l (no response to IV fluids)
- PaO_2 <8 kPa
- Serum calcium <2·0 mmol/l
- Serum albumin <32 g/l
- Lactate dehydrogenase >600 U/l

CHAPTER 16: THE PATIENT WITH HOT RED LEGS OR COLD WHITE LEGS

16.1 Post-operative, immobile, pregnant patients, women on the oral contraceptive pill, family history of coagulopathy.

16.2
- Arterial emboli tend to occur at the bifurcation of arteries. These will depend on the extent of the occlusion of the circulation and the degree of co-lateral circulation.

- Medical features include pain, pallor, pulselessness, parathesia, paralysis and perishing cold.

- In contrast a closed compartment syndrome is caused by a swollen or a contused muscle or bleeding into the muscle from inside a rigid fascial envelope. Pain and parasthesia are early symptoms but the affected limb may also be pale and cool with slow capillary refill. However the presence of a distal pulse does not help diagnosis.

CHAPTER 17: THE PATIENT WITH HOT AND/OR SWOLLEN JOINTS

17.1   There are many algorithms but the key important step is the first step. The first step is to exclude a septic arthritis.

CHAPTER 18: THE PATIENT WITH A RASH

18.1, a.   i.   Urticaria
ii.   Erythema
iii.   Purpura and vasculitis
iv.   Blistering disorders

b.   The reader is referred to chapter 18 for the algorithms for each of these conditions.

CHAPTER 19: ORGAN FAILURE

19.1, a. (i) Acute asthma; pulmonary embolus; cardiac e.g. dysrhythmia; neurological e.g. status epilepticus; neuromuscular e.g. myasthenia gravis.

(ii)   The commonest cause is ischaemic heart disease. Others include valvular pathology, acute hypertension, cardiomyopathy.

(iii)   Any chronic neurological disorder can have the final common pathway of brain failure. Dementia is another cause. These are not acute medical emergencies, however, the important point is to be able to differentiate these conditions from potentially treatable problems such as a patient with an acute confusional state or underlying depression.

(iv)   These may be classified as prerenal, intrinsic renal or post renal conditions. The commonest group is the prerenal which usually arises as secondary to hypovolaemia. The second most common cause is post renal or obstructive uropathy for example in association with prostatic pathology. Intrinsic renal disease in comparison is rare.

(v)   Acute liver failure is usually caused by drugs such as an overdose of paracetamol and with increasing frequency Ecstacy. It can also occur in pregnancy.

Acute on chronic liver failure is commonly caused by alcoholic liver disease.

(vi)   Will depend upon the particular gland that is affected and also the hormone or hormones that are not being produced. Irrespective of these conditions considered there are common features that influence all aspects of the primary assessment.

CHAPTER 20: THE ELDERLY PATIENT

20.1 10%

CHAPTER 21: TRANSPORTATION OF THE SERIOUSLY ILL PATIENT

21.1 A 27 year old mechanic with a subarachnoid haemorrhage is stable with a respiration rate of 14 per minute, sinus tachycardia 110 per minute, BP 120/70, BM 7 mmol/l, GCS 15/15 PERLA. The decision has been made to transfer this patient to the local neurological centre for assessment before surgery.

ASSESSMENT

Male, 27, clinical details as described above

- *What is the problem?*
  Diagnosis – subarachnoid haemorrhage.

- *What has been done?*
  Prevention of secondary brain injury, CT scan and lumbar puncture.

- *What was the effect?*
  Maintaining the status quo and preventing secondary brain injury.

- *What is needed now?*
  Transfer for further assessment.

There are potential problems that may arise during transfer:

Airway – obstruction, hypoxaemia

Breathing – hypocarbia respiratory arrest

Circulation – cardiac arrest, dysrhythmia, hypoglycaemia, hypoatremia

Disability – deterioration in Glasgow Coma Score, fit, extension of subarachnoid haemorrhage, development of raised intracranial pressure

CONTROL

A comprehensive assessment by the clinician in charge and the decision has been made to transfer the patient to hospital for further investigation.

COMMUNICATION
With:
The consultant
Intensive care consultant
Patient's relatives
Accepting consultant
Ambulance control

Communication also includes determining the lines of responsibility and using the assessment questions to provide a structure to tell the receiving team the salient points before transfer. In addition the reason for transfer and what is needed for the receiving centre should be explained.

EVALUATION

The specialist care has already been determined as part of the initial assessment.

PACKAGE AND PREPARATION

The patient has been stabilised before transfer and all baseline blood tests including arterial gases have been requested, reviewed and appropriate action taken. All relevant equipment monitoring and treatment has been prepacked and checked. Furthermore this also includes contingency equipment that should be required in case the patient deteriorates and incurs one of the problems that was listed earlier. The neurosurgical centre is 30 miles away by motorway with no predicted problems and a stable patient, so the decision has been made to transport by ambulance.

PERSONNEL

The ambulance crew
One doctor
One nurse
Part of the regular transfer team has been briefed and has the appropriate personal equipment. Lastly a transportationally equipped ambulance is available with appropriate monitoring equipment and back up systems including oxygen should any problems arise. Shortly before transfer all the patient's documentations have been photocopied and appropriate forms are available to record the patient's condition during transfer.

INDEX

Page numbers in **bold** type refer to figures; those in *italic* refer to tables or boxed material

441